theclinics.com

EMERGENCY MEDICINE CLINICS OF NORTH AMERICA

Infectious Diseases in Emergency Medicine

GUEST EDITOR
Daniel R. Martin, MD

CONSULTING EDITOR
Amal Mattu, MD

May 2008 • Volume 26 • Number 2

SAUNDERS

An Imprint of Elsevier, Inc.
PHILADELPHIA   LONDON   TORONTO   MONTREAL   SYDNEY   TOKYO

W.B. SAUNDERS COMPANY
A Division of Elsevier Inc.

1600 John F. Kennedy Boulevard, Suite 1800 • Philadelphia, Pennsylvania 19103-2899

http://www.theclinics.com

EMERGENCY MEDICINE CLINICS	Volume 26, Number 2
OF NORTH AMERICA	ISSN 0733-8627
May 2008	ISBN-13: 978-1-4160-5855-7
Editor: Patrick Manley	ISBN-10: 1-4160-5855-9

Emergency Medicine Clinics of North America (ISSN 0733-8627) is published quarterly by Elsevier Inc., 360 Park Avenue South, New York, NY, 10010-1710. Months of issue are February, May, August, and November. Business and Editorial Offices: 1600 John F. Kennedy Boulevard, Suite 1800, Philadelphia, PA 19103-2899. Customer Service Office: 6277 Sea Harbor Drive, Orlando, FL 32887-4800. Periodicals postage paid at New York, NY, and additional mailing offices. Subscription prices are $109.00 per year (US students), $212.00 per year (US individuals), $339.00 per year (US institutions), $145.00 per year (international students), $285.00 per year (international individuals), $400.00 per year (international institutions), $145.00 per year (Canadian students), $261.00 per year (Canadian individuals), and $400.00 per year (Canadian institutions). International air speed delivery is included in all *Clinics'* subscription prices. All prices are subject to change without notice. POSTMASTER: Send address changes to *Emergency Medicine Clinics of North America*, Elsevier Periodicals Customer Service, 6277 Sea Harbor Drive, Orlando, FL 32887-4800. Customer Service: 1-800-654-2452 (US). From outside the United States, call 1-407-563-6020. Fax: 1-407-363-9661. E-mail: JournalsCustomerService-usa@elsevier.com.

Emergency Medicine Clinics of North America is covered in *Index Medicus, Current Contents/Clinical Medicine, EMBASE/Excerpta Medica, BIOSIS, SciSearch, CINAHL, ISI/BIOMED,* and *Research Alert.*

Printed in the United States of America.

CONSULTING EDITOR

AMAL MATTU, MD, Program Director, Emergency Medicine Residency; and Associate Professor, Department of Emergency Medicine, University of Maryland School of Medicine, Baltimore, Maryland

GUEST EDITOR

DANIEL R. MARTIN, MD, Professor and Emergency Medicine Residency Director, Department of Emergency Medicine, The Ohio University Medical Center, Columbus, Ohio

CONTRIBUTORS

MARK E. BRAUNER, DO, Resident Physician, Department of Emergency Medicine, The Ohio State University Medical Center, Columbus, Ohio

JEFFREY M. CATERINO, MD, Assistant Professor, Department of Emergency Medicine; and Assistant Professor, Department of Internal Medicine, The Ohio State University, Columbus, Ohio

JESMIN P. EHLERS, MD, Medical Student, University of Iowa Carver College of Medicine, Iowa City, Iowa

BRADLEY W. FRAZEE, MD, Associate Clinical Professor of Medicine, Department of Emergency Medicine, Alameda County Medical Center-Highland Campus, University of California at San Francisco, Oakland, California

DIANE L. GORGAS, MD, Associate Professor and Co-Residency Director, Department of Emergency Medicine, The Ohio State University Medical Center, Columbus, Ohio

DIANA HANS, DO, Department of Emergency Medicine, Maricopa Medical Center, Phoenix, Arizona

H. GENE HERN, MD, Associate Clinical Professor of Medicine, Department of Emergency Medicine, Alameda County Medical Center-Highland Campus, University of California at San Francisco, Oakland, California

HANS R. HOUSE, MD, FACEP, Associate Professor, Clinical, Department of Emergency Medicine; and Director, Emergency Medicine Residency Program, University of Iowa Hospitals and Clinics, Iowa City, Iowa

COLIN G. KAIDE, MD, FACEP, FAAEM, Clinical Associate Professor of Emergency Medicine, Department of Emergency Medicine; and Associate Director of Hyperbaric Medicine, The Ohio State University Medical Center, Columbus, Ohio

ERIC D. KATZ, MD, Program Director, Emergency Medicine Residency, Department of Emergency Medicine, Maricopa Medical Center, Phoenix, Arizona

ERIN KELLY, MD, Department of Emergency Medicine, Maricopa Medical Center, Phoenix, Arizona

SORABH KHANDELWAL, MD, Clinical Associate Professor of Emergency Medicine, Department of Emergency Medicine; and Director of Hyperbaric Medicine, The Ohio State University Medical Center, Columbus, Ohio

NICHOLAS E. KMAN, MD, Assistant Professor, Department of Emergency Medicine, The Ohio State University Medical Center, Columbus, Ohio

SHARON E. MACE, MD, FACEP, FAAP, Professor, Cleveland Clinic Lerner College of Medicine of Case Western Reserve University; and Faculty, Cleveland Clinic/ MetroHealth Medical Center Emergency Medicine Residency; and Director, Pediatric Education/Quality Improvement; and Director, Observation Unit, Emergency Services Institute, Cleveland Clinic, Cleveland, Ohio

CATHERINE A. MARCO, MD, FACEP, Professor, Department of Surgery, Division of Emergency Medicine, University of Toledo College of Medicine, Toledo, Ohio

DANIEL R. MARTIN, MD, Professor and Emergency Medicine Residency Director, Department of Emergency Medicine, The Ohio University Medical Center, Columbus, Ohio

HOWARD K. MELL, MD, MPH, Assistant Professor, Department of Emergency Medicine, College of Medicine, The Ohio State University; Medical Director for Education, The Ohio State University Medical Centers, Center for Emergency Medical Services, Columbus, Ohio

RICHARD N. NELSON, MD, Professor and Vice Chair, Department of Emergency Medicine, The Ohio State University Medical Center, Columbus, Ohio

DONALD L. NORRIS II, MD, Assistant Professor, Department of Emergency Medicine, The Ohio State University Medical Center, Columbus, Ohio

DAVID C. PIGOTT, MD, Associate Professor of Emergency Medicine and Vice Chair for Academic Development, Department of Emergency Medicine, The University of Alabama at Birmingham, Birmingham, Alabama

JESSE M. PINES, MD, MBA, MSCE, Assistant Professor of Emergency Medicine and Epidemiology, Department of Emergency Medicine, Hospital of the University of Pennsylvania; Senior Scholar, Center for Clinical Epidemiology and Biostatistics, University of Pennsylvania School of Medicine; Senior Fellow, Leonard Davis Institute of Health Economics, University of Pennsylvania, Philadelphia, Pennsylvania

JOSEPH F. PLOUFFE, MD, Sarasota, Florida; Formerly Professor Emeritus, Division of Infectious Diseases, Department of Internal Medicine, The Ohio State University Medical Center, Columbus, Ohio

RICHARD E. ROTHMAN, MD, PhD, FACEP, Associate Professor, Department of Emergency Medicine, Johns Hopkins University School of Medicine, Baltimore, Maryland

THOMAS R. WALLIN, MD, Emergency Medicine Resident, Department of Emergency Medicine, Alameda County Medical Center-Highland Campus, Oakland, California

KRISTA WILHELMSON, MD, Department of Emergency Medicine, Maricopa Medical Center, Phoenix, Arizona

JEREMY D. YOUNG, MD, MPH, Assistant Professor, Division of Infectious Diseases, Department of Internal Medicine, The Ohio State University Medical Center, Columbus, Ohio

CONTENTS

The importance of antibiotic timing is a common clinical question encountered in emergency medicine practice for patients who have severe infections. Various studies in the medical literature have reported associations between early antibiotic timing and improved survival for meningitis, pneumonia, and septic shock. Understanding the evidence behind antibiotic timing and survival is vital to emergency physicians, because they must balance the potential benefits of early antibiotic administration and the potential for antibiotic overuse and misuse. The measurement of antibiotic timing in pneumonia has been shown to be associated with antibiotic misuse in emergency departments. Quality organizations should study carefully the intended and unintended consequences of measuring and reporting antibiotic timing to make policy decisions on current and future performance measures in this area.

Emergency physicians are trained to separate "sick" from "not sick" patients during their training. Nevertheless, every emergency physician will face situations in which early intervention is critical to their patient's outcome. Infectious diseases are responsible for many of these potentially poor outcomes. This article discusses early identification and treatment for several rapidly fatal infections, including two newly identified travel-related illnesses.

clinical presentations, differential diagnosis, early treatment strategies, and disposition options is crucial to the effective emergency department management of HIV infections and AIDS.

Pneumonia in the Emergency Department
Joseph F. Plouffe and Daniel R. Martin

Pneumonia remains one of the most common reasons for admission of emergency department (ED) patients to the hospital. Pneumonia also remains one of the most common causes of death in our patients. As with many emergent conditions, the ED management of these patients initiated by ED physicians contributes greatly to the survival and successful management of these patients. Specifically, the recognition of severe pneumonias, precise choice of diagnostic tests, and appropriate antibiotics can have an impact on the outcome.

Urinary Tract Infections: Diagnosis and Management in the Emergency Department
Donald L. Norris II and Jeremy D. Young

With the emergence of increasing resistance to common antibiotics used to treat urinary tract infections (UTIs), including ciprofloxacin and trimethoprim-sulfamethoxazole (TMP-SMX), the choice of antibiotics for these infections has become more challenging. In this article, the authors review the evidence-based guidelines for the evaluation and treatment of cystitis and pyelonephritis in the emergency department. They review the pathophysiology and describe the initial diagnostic workup, spending some time discussing the urine dipstick. The authors discuss whether hospital antibiograms are useful in making the initial antibiotic choice. The treatment section reviews the current recommendations and also highlights the use of nitrofurantoin in the treatment of uncomplicated UTIs. The authors also discuss the appropriate use of ciprofloxacin and TMP-SMX in the treatment of UTIs.

Community-Associated Methicillin-Resistant *Staphylococcus aureus*
Thomas R. Wallin, H. Gene Hern, and Bradley W. Frazee

Community-associated methicillin-resistant *Staphylococcus aureus* (CA-MRSA) has emerged over the last decade across the United States and the world, becoming a major pathogen in many types of community-acquired infections. Although most commonly associated with minor skin and soft tissue infections, such as furuncles, CA-MRSA also can cause necrotizing fasciitis, pyomyositis, osteoarticular infections, and community-acquired pneumonia. This article discusses the epidemiology, diagnosis, and management of these infections from the perspective of the emergency physician.

in the medical community. Bioterrorism is the use of a biologic weapon to create terror and panic. Biologic weapons, or bioweapons, can be bacteria, fungi, viruses, or biologic toxins. Because the emergency department represents the front line of defense for the recognition of agents of bioterrorism, it is essential that emergency physicians have the ability to quickly diagnose victims of bioterrorism. This review examines the most deadly and virulent category A agents of bioterrorism, that is, anthrax, smallpox, plague, botulism, hemorrhagic fever viruses, and tularemia. The focus is on epidemiology, transmission, clinical manifestations, diagnosis, and treatment.

Influenza and pneumococcal pneumonia remain among the most significant causes of morbidity and mortality of any of the infectious disease emergencies presenting to emergency departments (EDs). Because the ED has become a recommended location at which immunizations have been administered to prevent several infections, pneumococcal and influenza vaccinations can have an impact on the care of ED patients. ED personnel are uniquely positioned to vaccinate a substantial number of patients who would not otherwise be vaccinated, including many high-risk populations. In addition to decreasing vaccine-preventable mortality and morbidity from influenza and pneumococcal diseases, EDs that implement and monitor a systematic approach to these vaccinations can attenuate ED overcrowding and facilitate patient flow. ED vaccination strategies have been proved to be successful and reimbursable and are advocated by several major clinical practice advisory groups.

This article reviews the applications of hyperbaric oxygen (HBO) as an adjunctive treatment of certain infectious processes. Infections for which HBO has been studied and is recommended by the Undersea and Hyperbaric Medicine Society include necrotizing fasciitis, gas gangrene, chronic refractory osteomyelitis (including malignant otitis externa), mucormycosis, intracranial abscesses, and diabetic foot ulcers that have concomitant infections. In all of these processes, HBO is used adjunctively along with antimicrobial agents and aggressive surgical debridement. This article describes the details of each infection and the research that supports the use of HBO.

FORTHCOMING ISSUES

RECENT ISSUES

The Clinics are now available online!

Access your subscription at
www.theclinics.com

GOAL STATEMENT

The goal of *Emergency Medicine Clinics of North America* is to keep practicing physicians up to date with current clinical practice in emergency medicine by providing timely articles reviewing the state of the art in patient care.

ACCREDITATION

The *Emergency Medical Clinics of North America* is planned and implemented in accordance with the Essential Areas and Policies of the Accreditation Council for Continuing Medical Education (ACCME) through the joint sponsorship of the University of Virginia School of Medicine and Elsevier. The University of Virginia School of Medicine is accredited by the ACCME to provide continuing medical education for physicians.

The University of Virginia School of Medicine designates this educational activity for a maximum of *15 AMA PRA Category 1 Credits*™. Physicians should only claim credit commensurate with the extent of their participation in the activity.

The Emergency Medicine Clinics of North America CME program is approved by the American College of Emergency Physicians for 60 hours of ACEP Category I Credit per year.

The American Medical Association has determined that physicians not licensed in the US who participate in this CME activity are eligible for *15 AMA PRA Category 1 Credits*™.

Credit can be earned by reading the text material, taking the CME examination online at http://www.theclinics.com/home/cme, and completing the evaluation. After taking the test, you will be required to review any and all incorrect answers. Following completion of the test and evaluation, your credit will be awarded and you may print your certificate.

FACULTY DISCLOSURE/CONFLICT OF INTEREST

The University of Virginia School of Medicine, as an ACCME accredited provider, endorses and strives to comply with the Accreditation Council for Continuing Medical Education (ACCME) Standards of Commercial Support, Commonwealth of Virginia statutes, University of Virginia policies and procedures, and associated federal and private regulations and guidelines on the need for disclosure and monitoring of proprietary and financial interests that may affect the scientific integrity and balance of content delivered in continuing medical education activities under our auspices.

The University of Virginia School of Medicine requires that all CME activities accredited through this institution be developed independently and be scientifically rigorous, balanced and objective in the presentation/discussion of its content, theories and practices.

All authors/editors participating in an accredited CME activity are expected to disclose to the readers relevant financial relationships with commercial entities occurring within the past 12 months (such as grants or research support, employee, consultant, stock holder, member of speakers bureau, etc.). The University of Virginia School of Medicine will employ appropriate mechanisms to resolve potential conflicts of interest to maintain the standards of fair and balanced education to the reader. Questions about specific strategies can be directed to the Office of Continuing Medical Education, University of Virginia School of Medicine, Charlottesville, Virginia.

The authors/editors listed below have identified no professional or financial affiliations for themselves or their spouse/partner:
Mark E. Brauner, DO; Jeffrey M. Caterino, MD; Jesmin P. Ehlers, MD; Bradley W. Frazee, MD; Diane L. Gorgas, MD; Diana Hans, DO; H. Gene Hern, MD; Hans R. House, MD, FACEP; Colin G. Kaide, MD, FACEP, FAAEM; Eric D. Katz, MD; Erin Kelly, MD; Sorabh Khandelwal, MD; Nicholas E. Kman, MD; Sharon E. Mace, MD, FACEP, FAAP; Patrick Manley (Acquisitions Editor); Catherine A. Marco, MD, FACEP; Daniel R. Martin, MD (Guest Editor); Amal Mattu, MD (Consulting Editor); Howard K. Mell, MD, MPH; Richard N. Nelson, MD; Donald L. Norris, II, MD; David C. Pigott, MD; Jesse M. Pines, MD, MBA, MSCE; Joseph F. Plouffe, MD; Richard E. Rothman, MD, PhD, FACEP; Thomas R. Wallin, MD; Krista Wilhelmson, MD; and Jeremy D. Young, MD, MPH.

The authors/editors listed below have identified the following professional or financial affiliations for themselves of their spouse/partner:

Disclosure of Discussion of non-FDA approved uses for pharmaceutical products and/or medical devices:
The University of Virginia School of Medicine, as an ACCME provider, requires that all faculty presenters identify and disclose any "off label" uses for pharmaceutical and medical device products. The University of Virginia School of Medicine recommends that each physician fully review all the available data on new products or procedures prior to instituting them with patients.

TO ENROLL

To enroll in the Emergency Medicine Clinics of North America Continuing Medical Education program, call customer service at 1-800-654-2452 or visit us online at www.theclinics.com/home/cme. The CME program is available to subscribers for an additional fee of $195.00.

ELSEVIER
SAUNDERS

Emerg Med Clin N Am
26 (2008) xv–xvi

EMERGENCY
MEDICINE
CLINICS OF
NORTH AMERICA

Foreword

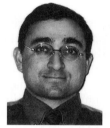

Amal Mattu, MD
Consulting Editor

Thousands of years before physicians began focusing their attention on advanced resuscitation, cardiology, critical care, and surgery, "healers" primarily concerned themselves with ridding the body of "tiny creatures" that could cause illness: "certain minute animals, invisible to the eye...[that] reach the inside of the body...and cause disease" (Varro, 1st century B.C.) [1]. For thousands of years, plagues and epidemics caused by "simple" infections have affected national leaders, armies, cultures, societies, and even world history. Infections small enough to be transmitted by the bite of a mosquito are responsible for more loss of human life than all the wars in human history combined. Some of the greatest physicians in recent centuries, including Lister, Jenner, Pasteur, Koch, Reed, and Ehrlich, made their mark by way of their discoveries that helped fight infections. It is argued easily that the very profession of medicine was born from the fight against infectious disease.

Despite the advances in medical therapies and biomedical technology, the modern medical profession is, still in many ways, at the mercy of infections. Although we appear to have conquered or limited some infectious diseases, the re-emergence of "old" infections and the emergence of newer ones continue to challenge us. Tuberculosis, once thought to be well-controlled, has re-emerged with a vengeance, resistant to many standard therapies. The constant threat of terrorism threatens to return diseases that were once thought to be "conquered," such as smallpox and the plague. Viruses, such as HIV and influenza, are a constantly changing international threat. Bacteria that once were considered "simple," such as *Staphylococcus aureus*, have evolved

0733-8627/08/$ - see front matter © 2008 Elsevier Inc. All rights reserved.
doi:10.1016/j.emc.2008.02.006

emed.theclinics.com

to develop resistance against usual antibiotics. Also, pneumonia continues to be a leading killer among the elderly. The medical profession's war against infections rages on, and physicians continue the struggle to minimize the toll in human lives.

In this issue of *Emergency Medicine Clinics of North America*, Dr. Daniel R. Martin (Guest Editor) has assembled an outstanding group of authors who provide updates on the "current state of war" against infectious disease in emergency medicine. They discuss the common diseases that are encountered in everyday clinical practice, such as urinary infections, community acquired pneumonia, and food borne infections. They also discuss less common but high-risk diseases, such as central nervous system and other rapidly fatal infections. Separate articles are devoted to special populations, including elderly patients, pregnant patients, and patients who have HIV. Controversies related to the timing of antibiotics, treatment of methicillin-resistant *Staphylococcus aureus*, and the use of vaccine programs in the emergency department are addressed. Finally, the recent increased use of hyperbaric oxygen for treatment of certain infections is discussed as well.

If knowledge is to be considered a weapon in the war against infectious disease, this issue of the *Emergency Medicine Clinics of North America* represents an important addition to our arsenal. Dr. Martin and his colleagues have summarized, in a single source, the most up-to-date knowledge of large portions of an ever-changing and ever-threatening field. It is critically important that emergency physicians stay apprised of these newest concepts to continue the battle against infections. My thanks go to Dr. Martin and his colleagues for their valuable work.

Amal Mattu, MD
Program Director
Emergency Medicine Residency
Associate Professor
Department of Emergency Medicine
University of Maryland School of Medicine
110 S. Paca Street, 6th Floor, Suite 100
Baltimore, MD 21201, USA

E-mail address: amattu@smail.umaryland.edu

Reference

[1] Lyons AS. Infection. In: Lyons AS, Petrucelli RJ, editors. Medicine: An illustrated history. New York: Harry N. Abrams, Inc.; 1987. p. 549–64.

ELSEVIER
SAUNDERS

Emerg Med Clin N Am
26 (2008) xvii–xviii

EMERGENCY
MEDICINE
CLINICS OF
NORTH AMERICA

Preface

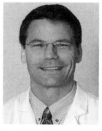

Daniel R. Martin, MD
Guest Editor

The interest in infectious diseases in emergency medicine stems from the fact that most acute infections present to our emergency departments (EDs). Even mild bothersome symptoms (such as those caused by infections originating from the skin, respiratory, or urinary tract) usually cannot wait for a distant appointment in a primary care provider's office. Emergency medicine physicians rapidly must recognize and distinguish minor infections from the most severe and acutely life threatening infections. Several of the articles in this issue deal with a wide spectrum of infectious disease severity, how to rapidly and appropriately diagnose these conditions, and which empiric therapies should be administered.

In a changing infectious environment, knowledge of local and national resistance patterns plays a major role in the management of infections in the ED, because most of our therapeutic options are empiric. External pressures in most EDs—such as increasing ED volumes, ED overcrowding, and additional institutional pressures designed to emphasize rapid treatment of infectious emergencies—further complicates the management of these patients. Even more difficult is that many "rules" and "requirements" for treating infections in the ED are based on very little evidence. The first three articles discuss the controversies of using rapid antibiotic therapy for a variety of potentially life threatening infections, and they address whether the severity of the infections at presentation may be more important than the rapidity of antibiotic administration.

The next several articles describe infectious presentations that are varied and greatly depend upon an unusual host condition that complicates the diagnosis and management of infections in populations, such as the elderly, obstetric patients, and immunocompromised patients (ie, patients who have HIV). Although there are overlapping areas, the description of how these host conditions affect infectious presentations and the diagnosis and management of these illnesses often presents a challenge for the ED physician.

Common traditional infections, such as pneumonia, urinary tract infections, skin infections, travel related illnesses, and food-borne illnesses, continue to present to emergency departments and account for many patients admitted for inpatient treatment. However, increasing resistance patterns, new diagnostic approaches, and an increasing number of antibiotic possibilities create the need for a state of the art review of these entities. Furthermore, examples of unusual infections, such as methicillin-resistant *Staphylococcus aureus* (MRSA), are described, because this infectious agent has become ubiquitous in our environment after initially being found predominately as an etiology of skin and soft tissue infections. MRSA now accounts for more serious infections such as MRSA sepsis and pneumonia.

Infectious agents used for the purpose of bioterrorism represent a critical area with which emergency medicine physicians must be familiar. These types of infections have tied our knowledge of infectious diseases to disaster preparedness. Newer therapies in the armamentarium of emergency physicians for these infections and unusual therapies, such as hyperbaric oxygen and ED immunizations, have become therapies often administered in our emergency departments and soon will become more standard.

Having an attitude of gratitude, I recognize and thank the talented authors who have helped to make this issue possible. These gifted individuals made my role as editor and author extremely easy, and, as great team players, made us all better for their involvement with this project. I anxiously awaited each article's arrival, because each manuscript was extremely enlightening and informative. I also thank some of the most important people in my life, whose support in this endeavor was key to the success of the project: my emergency medicine residents; Ellen, our residency coordinator; and Janine and Mary Jane from our department. Finally, I thank those closest to me: my three daughters, Jennifer, Jacquelyn and Jessica, and my wife, Eileen, who always put up with my academic distractions and continue to root for me.

Daniel R. Martin, MD
Department of Emergency Medicine
The Ohio University Medical Center
410 West 10th Avenue
Columbus, OH 43210, USA

E-mail address: martin.23@osu.edu

ELSEVIER
SAUNDERS

Emerg Med Clin N Am
26 (2008) 245–257

EMERGENCY
MEDICINE
CLINICS OF
NORTH AMERICA

Timing of Antibiotics for Acute, Severe Infections

Jesse M. Pines, MD, MBA, MSCE[a,b,c,*]

[a]Department of Emergency Medicine, Hospital of the University of Pennsylvania,
3400 Spruce Street, Ground Ravdin, Philadelphia, PA 19104, USA
[b]Center for Clinical Epidemiology and Biostatistics, University of Pennsylvania
School of Medicine, 423 Guardian Drive, Philadelphia, PA 19104, USA
[c]Leonard Davis Institute of Health Economics, University of Pennsylvania,
Colonial Penn Center, 3641 Locust Walk, Philadelphia, PA 19104, USA

Patients who have a range of infections initially are diagnosed and treated in emergency departments (ED). According to the National Hospital Ambulatory Medical Care Survey, 15 million of the 114 million ED visits in United States in 2005 involved the administration of one or more antimicrobial agents [1]. The importance of antibiotic timing in the ED is a common clinical question, because some infections may be time-sensitive, where earlier antibiotics are associated with improved outcomes. There are also risks in providing early empiric antibiotic therapy in infections without definitive source, however, because of the potential for worsening antibiotic resistance. There is a tradeoff between the expected benefits of early antibiotic therapy compared with waiting for complete test results. Although waiting for test results may prevent antibiotic overuse and allow for more tailored antibiotic regimens, the concern is that waiting in itself may result in progressive infection/sepsis and lead to poorer outcomes.

When patients present to the ED, they may not have a definitive diagnosis or clear source for infection. Some infections require considerable care coordination and time to definitively identify a source, including those that are diagnosed using radiography and/or cerebrospinal fluid testing. Diagnostic testing in the ED creates time lags between patient arrival, physician evaluation, identification of a definitive infectious source, and antibiotic administration. These time lags sometimes can be on the order of hours

Dr. Pines is supported by the Emergency Medicine Foundation, the Institute on Aging at Penn, and the Thomas McCabe Fund.

* Department of Emergency Medicine, Hospital of the University of Pennsylvania, 3400 Spruce Street, Ground Ravdin, Philadelphia, PA 19104.

E-mail address: pinesj@hotmail.com

spent in the ED waiting for test results. If culture results or molecular testing are required, identification of a definitive source may take days.

Understanding disease entities where antibiotic timing is associated with outcomes is vital to the practice of emergency medicine. For patients who have minor infections, delays in antibiotics on the order of hours spent in the ED likely are not associated with substantial differences in outcomes. Studies, however, have investigated the impact of antibiotic timing on outcomes in patients who have more severe infections such as meningitis and septic shock, and those admitted for pneumonia. Studies regarding the importance of early antibiotics are conflicting. Although some studies report that use of early antibiotics on the order of hours is associated with improved outcomes, others who have studied the same outcomes in the same diseases have reported no association. The inconsistent nature of the literature makes evidence-based decisions on early antibiotics a challenge.

Studies that have reported associations between antibiotic timing and survival have prompted quality organizations and specialty groups to release guidelines regarding the appropriateness of specific time intervals from patient presentation to administration of antibiotics for severe sepsis/septic shock and pneumonia [2,3]. These guidelines have sparked controversy because of inherent methodological limitations of the data supporting these associations, where it is impossible to draw a causal relationship between antibiotic timing and outcomes [4–6]. In addition, there have been concerns raised that measurement of antibiotic timing may promote antibiotic overuse and may worsen antibiotic resistance [7].

The objectives of this article are to:

Discuss antibiotic timing in acute, severe infections in the ED through an assessment of the data and the limitations in the conclusions that can be drawn from observational studies
Provide an overview of the controversy behind the measurement of time to antibiotics in guidelines and performance measures
Provide practical recommendations to emergency physicians on the use of empiric antibiotics in suspected and documented severe infections

The article focuses on studies that report the time-sensitive nature of care on the order of hours instead of days, because this issue is more central to bedside emergency care.

Theoretic basis for early antibiotics in severe infections

Empiric antibiotics aimed at the likely source of infection are the cornerstone in therapy for patients who have acute life-threatening infections [8]. Mortality in acute infections frequently is caused not by the infection itself, but the physiologic response to the infection and the multisystem organ failure (MSOF) that ensues. In patients who have severe infections, administration of early antibiotics makes good clinical sense. The administration of antibiotics, by killing the offending agent, may halt or reduce the likelihood of physiologic progression to MSOF. In addition, as infection progresses and bacterial load increases, the cytokine release that occurs when antibiotics are given may be more dramatic and increase the likelihood of progression to MSOF. There is also variability in a host's ability to mount an immune response to specific infections. In the preantibiotic era, some diseases like community-acquired pneumonia were not uniformly fatal, while other more severe infections such as those involving the central nervous system and those involving sepsis carried a much higher mortality rate.

Animal data on early antibiotics

There are a few animal studies that demonstrate the impact of antibiotic timing on survival on the order of hours. Two studies have reported a direct association between antibiotic timing on bacterial propagation rates in mice after an intraperitoneal inoculation of *Streptococcus pneumoniae* [9,10]. In the latter study, although there was no difference in effectiveness when mice were treated with high-dose penicillin at 1 hour and 16 hours after inoculation and at 24-hours after inoculation, antibiotics were considerably less effective in their ability to reduce intraperitoneal bacterial counts, indicating a time-dependent effect on the antibiotic pharmacokinetics. Another study in mice reported that after intraperitoneal or intravenous inoculation with a 90% to 100% lethal dose of *Escherichia coli*, *Proteus mirabilis*, or *Klebsiella pneumoniae*, delays in antibiotics were associated with proportionally higher mortality [11].

More recently, a study by Kumar and colleagues demonstrated an association between antibiotic timing and survival in a mouse model [12]. This study illustrated numerous important points in the pathophysiology of septic shock and timing of antibiotic therapy. The study found that antibiotic timing had little effect on survival in the early stages of infection. There was a critical inflection point, however, where antibiotic timing became important to survival outcomes. This inflection point was the onset of septic shock (ie, sepsis with hypotension). During this high-risk period, antibiotic timing was related directly to survival. In later phases of infection when sustained hypotension was present, there was a point beyond which the injury was irreversible, and the progression to MSOF and death was inevitable regardless of intervention. Beyond this point, the use of or timing of antibiotics was not associated with survival. This confirmed an animal model for hemorrhagic shock that found that resuscitation invariably will fail if resuscitation with antibiotics is initiated beyond a critical point of irreversible injury [13].

Methodological limitations of data in people

Because of ethical implications, no controlled trials have investigated the impact of withholding antibiotics on patients who have severe infections.

Because studies reporting data on antibiotic timing and outcomes are observational, inherent limitations make it nearly impossible to conclude causality in the association between antibiotic timing and outcomes. In observational studies, the risk is that there are unmeasured confounding factors that may explain associations. That is, something that is not measured may be responsible for the observed differences in survival. A confounder in the association between antibiotic timing and survival is the clinical presentation of disease. When the clinical presentation is atypical, and/or classic symptoms are absent, this may reflect information about both the disease host, severity of disease, and the host response to infection [14]. Host responses to infection may be associated with survival. In addition, host response and clinical manifestation of disease also may be associated with the time of treatment initiation. For example, patients who do not manifest a dramatic physiologic response to infection with vital sign abnormalities may not prompt clinicians to perceive a need for early antibiotic initiation. These same patients also may experience poorer outcomes, because their immune system is not mounting an appropriate response to infection.

Teasing out the interaction among clinical presentation of disease, antibiotic timing, and survival is central to the question on whether the clinical decision to give early antibiotics makes a difference. One hypothesis is that the association between antibiotic timing and survival is merely a statistical artifact, because there is something clinically different about patients who get recognized and treated later. That is, some other factor that augments either the host response to the disease or a clinician's decision to worry about them and expedite tests or treat them empirically is what is associated with better survival outcomes. By that logic, time to antibiotics itself may be the confounder, and something else associated with the disease host may be the causal factor that permits earlier recognition and more timely treatment. The alternative hypothesis is that it is the antibiotic timing in itself that affects survival. Therefore, those patients with time-sensitive infections who are recognized earlier and treated earlier will have better outcomes. Currently, there are no definitive data that prove or disprove either hypothesis. Fig. 1 shows a schematic of these two hypotheses.

Another methodological issue in research on antibiotic timing is that theoretically the time course of the illness itself should be an important determinant of outcome. Time course of illness may not correlate directly with what is being measured (ie, time course of presentation to the hospital). Therefore, using door-to-treatment time has substantial face validity issues. Patients may be ill for days or weeks before presenting to the ED or doctor's office for their care. This makes it difficult to believe that associations between door to antibiotics and survival are real when antibiotic timing is measured on the order of hours, particularly in populations who are not critically ill and where the disease course is not rapidly progressive such as pneumonia.

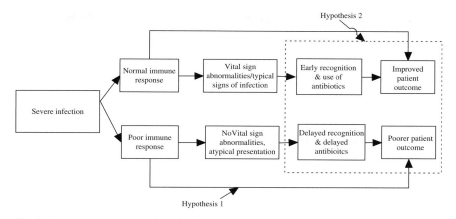

Fig. 1. Two hypotheses regarding the importance of early antibiotics. In the face of a severe infection, hosts will mount a normal immune response or a poor immune response, which will manifest as vital sign abnormalities and typical symptoms of infection or the lack of these findings. The presence of these findings may prompt early recognition and use of antibiotics. Hypothesis 1 is that outcomes are improved, because antibiotics were given earlier. Hypothesis 2 is that early antibiotic use is associated with typical symptoms and early recognition/antibiotic use and that those who have a poor immune response would have experienced the same outcome regardless of antibiotic timing.

In addition, studying antibiotic timing across multiple hospitals presents a challenge in data analysis. Because most multicenter studies on antibiotic timing do not account for hospital-level effects, this additional factor may confound the association. It makes sense that hospitals that are more likely to rapidly diagnose and treat infections also may be more likely to provide better overall care. Therefore, the impact of antibiotic timing may be confounded at the hospital level.

Disease-specific data in humans

The three disease states in people where antibiotic timing on the order of hours has been associated with survival are meningitis, pneumonia, and septic shock. Along with supportive care, the use of antibiotics is a vital to the treatment of all these conditions.

Bacterial meningitis

Bacterial meningitis carries a high risk for significant morbidity and mortality. Prompt recognition and antibiotic therapy for patients who have bacterial meningitis are the standard of care, because meningitis can be a rapid progressive illness [15]. Certainly, when a diagnosis of bacterial meningitis is established, antibiotics should be given immediately. The clinical question arises in cases of suspected bacterial meningitis without definitive diagnosis whether antibiotic therapy should be given empirically. Clinically, patients who have suspected bacterial meningitis fall into two broad, sometimes overlapping categories. The first is the group at high risk for bacterial meningitis based on the clinical presentation. This would include patients who have clear signs of bacterial meningitis (ie, fever, altered mental status, neck stiffness). There are substantial data and face validity that support the assertion that antibiotics should be given before a definitive diagnosis in high-risk patients. The second group is patients who are at lower-risk for bacterial meningitis but need definitive testing to rule out the disease (ie, diagnostic lumbar puncture). This would include patients who have more nonspecific symptoms. In this group, the data regarding the importance of antibiotics on the order of hours are less clear-cut.

Multiple observational studies have demonstrated a strong association between antibiotic timing and survival in meningitis [16–21]. One study investigated reported that patients who received antibiotics in the ED had a mortality rate of 7.9% compared with a mortality rate of 29% for those who received antibiotics after hospital admission [19]. Another found that antibiotic timing was important in patients who deteriorated clinically in the ED [18].

Others studies, however, have not demonstrated an association between antibiotic timing and survival [22,23]. A 1997 *New England Journal of Medicine* review of meningitis reported that of the papers that had been published on the association between antibiotic timing and survival in meningitis up to that point, only half reported a significant association [24]. A 1992 evidence-based review concluded that the association between treatment delays and outcomes is highly dependent on clinical presentation [25]. For presentations of meningitis that are associated with nonspecific illness, treatment delays are not associated with the risk of morbidity and mortality. Additionally, when meningitis is fulminant, delays in initiating antibiotics are also not associated with outcomes. For patients who have clinically overt meningitis (ie, fever, neck stiffness and altered mental status), however, antibiotic delays are associated with both morbidity and mortality outcomes. These data seem to correlate well with animal data, where outcomes of less severe infections are not time-sensitive with regard to antibiotics. More severe infections that may be more clinically overt are time-sensitive, and there is point beyond which antibiotic timing or any intervention will not impact outcome [12,13].

More recent data have aimed to control for clinical presentation and time to antibiotics from a clinically important starting point (time of altered consciousness) [26]. This study reported that a delay in antibiotics of greater than 6 hours from presentation was associated with an adjusted odds of death of 8.4 (95% CI 1.7 to 40.9). In addition, the association was incremental, and longer delays were associated with a higher risk of death.

Septic shock

Early antibiotic therapy in patients who have severe sepsis and septic shock is the standard of care and recommended by guidelines [2]. Studies reporting survival improvements in patients who have severe sepsis and septic shock have included early antibiotics as part of their treatment strategies [27–30]. These protocols, however, involve other therapies such as aggressive fluid resuscitation, transfusions, vasopressors, vasodilators, inotropes, invasive monitoring techniques, and adjunctive therapy such as activated protein C. No peer-reviewed studies have reported data on antibiotic timing and survival in ED patients.

Antibiotic timing has been isolated in a large study of ICU patients who had septic shock [31]. In this multicenter, retrospective cohort study, the authors reported a strong association between delays in antibiotic therapy and in-hospital mortality in patients who had recurrent or persistent hypotension. The authors reported a 7.6% higher risk of death per hour of delay in antibiotic therapy. These results were impressive and important because of the incremental relationship, where there was poorer survival per hour of delay. This study, however, was limited in that it did not account for hospital-level effects. Another study of 88 ICU patients who had cancer found that a delay in antibiotic therapy of more than 2 hours was associated with a higher risk of death, odds ratio 7.1 (95% CI 1.2 to 42.2) in adjusted analysis [32]. This study was limited, however, because it was confined to one hospital and did not control for patient presentation.

Pneumonia

Antibiotic timing in pneumonia has been associated with improved survival in two large, retrospective studies and before–after studies of pneumonia protocols that include early antibiotics as one element of care [33–39]. There also have been studies that have reported no association between antibiotic timing and survival in patients who had pneumonia [40,41]. The first study to report an association between antibiotic timing and survival investigated processes of care at multiple hospitals and reported a survival difference using a 4-hour time-to-antibiotic cutoff (14.8% versus 20.2%) [34]. Another before–after study investigated the impact of a pneumonia protocol at three hospitals and reported a significant survival improvement (10.2% to 6.8%) and a reduction in hospital length of stay after implementation of the protocol [35]. In this study, improving antibiotic timing was only one element of the protocol and was not studied in isolation. Other studies have reported shortened lengths of stay after implementation of pneumonia pathways; however, these studies also did not isolate antibiotic timing [36,37].

The two large studies that investigated large, retrospective cohorts of Medicare (at least 65 years of age) patients reported adjusted mortality differences at various cutoffs (4 hours and 8 hours after arrival) for antibiotic timing [38,39]. The absolute, adjusted survival differences in these studies was about 1% between early and delayed antibiotics. These studies were limited in that they were retrospective in nature and did not account for hospital characteristics. In addition, these studies included both ED and direct admissions. Smaller studies have reported no difference in survival by antibiotic timing [40,41].

Several studies have investigated the impact of antibiotic delays on survival in inpatients who had nosocomial pneumonia. One study found that the likelihood of death in patients who had ventilator-associated pneumonia was eight times higher in patients where appropriate antibiotic coverage was delayed by 24 hours or more [42]. Other studies have reported poorer survival in patients who had ventilator-associated or ICU-associated pneumonia when the initial antibiotic was inappropriate, indicating a delay in definitive therapy [43–45].

Antibiotic delays

There is much literature on reasons for antibiotic delays in the ED. Studies have focused on presentation-level factors, patient-level factors, and system-level factors such as ED crowding and delays in diagnostic testing. Presentation-level factors that are associated with delays include the presence of atypical symptoms of the disease, and patient-level factors include demographics such as age and comorbid conditions that predispose patients to having atypical presentations.

Factors that have been associated with shortened antibiotic times include a history of vomiting, no history of headache, hypotension, a bulging fontanelle, and a sick presentation [17]. Treatment delays also have been associated with a failure to consider the diagnosis [46]. In meningitis, systematic delays are associated with sequential care, where patients first receive a head CT, then a diagnostic lumbar puncture before initiation of antibiotic therapy [16,19]. In addition, failure to administer therapy before transfer to another hospital has been associated with significant antibiotic delays in patients who have meningitis [19]. In meningitis, patient factors that have been associated with treatment delays include the absence of fever and severely impaired mental status [20].

In pneumonia, atypical presentations have been associated with both delayed antibiotics and also survival. In one study of 451 patients who had pneumonia, the authors identified a difference in survival outcomes with delayed antibiotics [47]. When the presence of an atypical presentation was controlled for, in multivariable analysis, the survival difference disappeared, however. This supports the contention that the association between antibiotic timing and survival and pneumonia may be a function of the presentation (ie, host response to infection) and not the antibiotic timing in itself. Systematic factors that have been associated delays in pneumonia include extended waiting times for evaluation, diagnosis, and treatment

[48]. In addition, recent literature has suggested that a patient-level exposure to ED crowding is associated with longer waits for antibiotics in pneumonia [49–51].

Measurement of antibiotic timing and potential misuse

Currently, the Surviving Sepsis guidelines recommend the first dose of antibiotic be given within 1 hour of patient arrival for patients admitted to intensive care settings and that the first dose of antibiotics be given to patients within 3 hours for those admitted to floor beds [2]. The guidelines recognize that there is little direct evidence for these recommendations. Guideline authors, however, support these recommendations by arguing that in critically ill patients who have sepsis, the risk of antibiotic overuse outweighs the risks of withholding antibiotics. This is primarily because patients who have severe sepsis/septic shock are at high risk for rapid progression of disease. In addition, more recent laboratory and human data support both the theoretic and actual importance of antibiotic timing by demonstrating an incremental relationship between where progressive antibiotic delays and poorer survival on the order of almost 8% per hour [12,31].

There has been considerable debate over the use of antibiotic timing as a performance measure in pneumonia [4–6,52,53]. Central to the argument over the use of antibiotic timing in performance measurement is the quality of the studies that support the association [4]. What differentiates pneumonia from septic shock and meningitis is the natural history of disease. Most cases of pneumonia are not rapidly progressive on the order of hours, while meningitis and septic shock are. Proponents of using antibiotic timing in pneumonia as a performance measure support the validity of the association by arguing that there is a preponderance of evidence and that the association is maintained in stratified analysis [50]. Based on strong beliefs that the provision of early antibiotics will lead to improved outcomes, they support the use of antibiotic timing as a performance measure. The group that supports these recommendations also advises The Joint Commission (TJC) and Center for Medicare & Medicaid Services (CMS) on performance measurement and have persisted in supporting antibiotic timing despite considerable controversy and specialty group guidelines that do not continue to support its use [54]. Under the current version of TJC/CMS Core Measures, administration of antibiotics within 4 hours of hospital arrival is measured and reported publicly as a quality measure [3]. This time interval will be changed to 6 hours in future versions of the Core Measures [55].

Groups that have argued against the use of antibiotic timing in performance measurement have disputed the quality of the data supporting the association between antibiotic timing and survival and argued that measurement in itself is associated with misuse [4–6,56]. A recent study of academic EDs found that one third have policies where patients who have suspected pneumonia receive empiric antibiotics before chest radiograph results [7].

There are also data to suggest that a higher proportion of patients have been admitted with a diagnosis of pneumonia without radiographic abnormalities after the implementation of pneumonia guidelines [57]. A large multicenter study demonstrated that increased success in meeting antibiotic timing measures in pneumonia is associated with increases in overuse of antibiotics for conditions such as chronic obstructive pulmonary disease, asthma, and heart failure [58].

Recommendations for good, evidence-based clinical practice

Reviewing data on antibiotic timing in aggregate, numerous important observations can be made. The first observation is that because of methodological limitations of studies, no definitive statements can be made about a causal relationship between antibiotic timing and survival. Presentation of disease appears to confound the association, because host response to disease is associated with survival, rapidity of diagnosis, and decisions behind antibiotic timing. Both animal and clinical data in people suggest however, that patients who are critically ill may benefit from early antibiotic administration. The most convincing data on the association have been reported in septic shock and meningitis, supporting the use of early, empiric antibiotics in cases where patients are at high risk for bacterial meningitis based on clinical presentation or demonstrate physiology consistent with septic shock. This is supported by observational data that show strong associations between early antibiotics and survival outcomes, even in studies that adjust for severity of illness and patient presentation.

The importance of antibiotic timing in pneumonia is more controversial. Because patients admitted with pneumonia are a broader cohort that includes both critically ill and noncritically ill patients, the risk associated with delayed antibiotics is smaller than in meningitis and septic shock. Studies that report this association are at high risk for confounding at the level of both the clinical presentation and the hospital. Although there are no data that have reported increases in antibiotic resistance that have resulted from performance measures for antibiotic timing in pneumonia, data suggest that the use of these measures is associated with overuse of antibiotics for antibiotic nonresponsive conditions. There are little data to suggest that emergency physicians should empirically treat patients with suspected pneumonia who are not critically ill before definitive diagnosis. Based on the data supporting the use of early antibiotics in septic shock, however, emergency physicians should consider empiric antibiotics in patients who have severe pneumonia and/or those who have septic shock. As studies continue to be published documenting misuse surround the measurement of antibiotic timing, it is the hope of this author that TJC/CMS will follow the American Thoracic Society/Infectious Disease Society of America guidelines and remove any timing-specific recommendation for antibiotics in pneumonia [53].

Summary

The importance of antibiotic timing is controversial, and a causal relationship has not been well-established. For patients who are critically ill with septic shock and meningitis, however, data suggest that early antibiotics are associated with higher survival rates. Emergency physicians need to weigh carefully decisions to treat patients with potentially severe infections empirically or wait for further testing based on both the best available evidence and bedside estimate of risk. There is a growing literature that demonstrates that measurement of antibiotic timing is associated with antibiotic overuse and misuse. Quality measurement organizations need to study carefully both the intended and unintended consequences of measuring antibiotic timing before making broad recommendations that may promote overuse and misuse.

References

[1] Middleton K, Hing E, Xu J. National hospital ambulatory medical care survey: 2005 outpatient department summary. Adv Data 2007;389:1–34.

[2] Dellinger RP, Carlet JM, Masur H, et al. Surviving sepsis campaign guidelines for management of severe sepsis and septic shock. Crit Care Med 2004;32:858–73.

[3] The Joint Commission for the Accreditation of Hospitals and Organization Specification Manual. Available at: http://www.jointcommission.org/PerformanceMeasurement/PerformanceMeasurement/Current+NHQM+Manual.htm. Accessed October 22, 2007.

[4] Pines JM. Measuring antibiotic timing for pneumonia in the emergency department: another nail in the coffin. Ann Emerg Med 2007;49:561–3.

[5] Pines JM. Profiles in patient safety: antibiotic timing in pneumonia and pay for performance. Acad Emerg Med 2006;13:787–90.

[6] Seymann GB. Community-acquired pneumonia: defining quality care. J Hosp Med 2006;1: 344–53.

[7] Pines JM, Hollander JE, Lee H, et al. Emergency department operational changes in response to pay for performance and antibiotic timing in pneumonia. Acad Emerg Med 2007;14:545–8.

[8] Deresinski S. Principles of antibiotic therapy in severe infections: optimizing the therapeutic approach by use of laboratory and clinical data. Clin Infect Dis 2007;45(Suppl 3):S177–83.

[9] Frimodt-Moller N, Thomsen VF. The pneumococcus and the mouse protection test: inoculum, dosage and timing. Acta Pathol Microbiol Immunol Scand [B] 1986;94:33–7.

[10] Knudsen JD, Frimodt-Moller N, Espersen F. Pharmacodynamics of penicillin are unaffected by bacterial growth phases of *Streptococcus pneumoniae* in the mouse peritonitis model. J Antimicrob Chemother 1998;41:451–9.

[11] Greisman SE, DuBuy JB, Woodward CL. Experimental gram-negative bacterial sepsis: prevention of mortality not preventable by antibiotics alone. Infect Immun 1979;25:538–57.

[12] Kumar A, Haery C, Paladuga B, et al. The duration of hypotension before the initiation of antibiotic treatment is a critical determinant of survival in a murine model of Escherichia coli septic shock: association with serum lactate and inflammatory cytokine levels. J Infect Dis 2006;193:251–8.

[13] Wiggers CJ. The present status of the shock problem. Physiol Rev 1942;22:74–123.

[14] Metlay JP, Schulz R, Li YH, et al. Influence of age on symptoms at presentation in patients with community-acquired pneumonia. Arch Intern Med 1997;157:1453–9.

[15] van de Beek D, de Gans J, Tunkel AR. Community-acquired bacterial meningitis in adults. N Engl J Med 2006;354:44–53.

[16] Talan DA, Zibulewsky J. Relationship of clinical presentation to time to antibiotics for the emergency department management of suspected bacterial meningitis. Ann Emerg Med 1993;22:1733–8.

[17] Lebel MH. Adverse outcome of bacterial meningitis due to delayed sterilization of cerebro-spinal fluid. Antibiot Chemother 1992;45:226–38.

[18] Miner JR, Heegaard W, Mapes A, et al. Presentation, time to antibiotics, and mortality of patients with bacterial meningitis at an urban county medical center. J Emerg Med 2001; 21:387–92.

[19] Proulx N, Frechette D, Toye B, et al. Delays in the administration of antibiotics are associated with mortality from adult acute bacterial meningitis. QJM 2005;98:291–8.

[20] Strang JR, Pugh EJ. Meningococcal infections: reducing case fatality by giving penicillin before admission to hospital. Br Med J 1992;305:141–3.

[21] Cartwright K, Reilly S, White D, et al. Early treatment with parenteral penicillin in menin-gococcal disease. BMJ 1992;305:143–7.

[22] Meadow WL, Lantos J, Tanz RR, et al. Ought standard care be the standard of care? A study of the time to administration of antibiotics in children with meningitis. Am J Dis Child 1993; 147:40–4.

[23] Hussein AS, Shafran SD. Acute bacterial meningitis in adults. A 12-year review. Medicine 2000;79:360–8.

[24] Quagliarello VJ, Scheld MJ. Treatment of bacterial meningitis. N Engl J Med 1997;336: 708–16.

[25] Radetsky M. Duration of symptoms and outcome in bacterial meningitis: an analysis of causation and the implications of a delay in diagnosis. Pediatr Infect Dis J 1992;11:694–8.

[26] Lepur D, Barsic B. Community-acquired bacterial meningitis in adults: antibiotic timing in disease course and outcome. Infection 2007;35:225–31.

[27] Rivers E, Nguyen B, Havstad S, et al. Early goal-directed therapy in the treatment of severe sepsis and septic shock. N Engl J Med 2001;345:1368–77.

[28] Trzeciak S, Dellinger RP, Abate NL, et al. Translating research to clinical practice: a 1-year experience with implementing early goal-directed therapy for septic shock in the emergency department. Chest 2006;129:225–32.

[29] Shapiro NI, Howell MD, Talmor D, et al. Implementation and outcomes of the Multiple Urgent Sepsis Therapies (MUST) protocol. Crit Care Med 2006;34:1025–32.

[30] Nguyen HB, Corbett SW, Menes K, et al. Early goal-directed therapy, corticosteroid, and recombinant human activated protein c for the treatment of severe sepsis and septic shock in the emergency department. Acad Emerg Med 2006;13:109–13.

[31] Kumar A, Roberts D, Wood KE, et al. Duration of hypotension before initiation of effective antimicrobial therapy is the critical determinant of survival in human septic shock. Crit Care Med 2006;34:1589–96.

[32] Larche J, Azoulay E, Fieux F, et al. Improved survival of critically ill cancer patients with septic shock. Intensive Care Med 2003;29:1688–95.

[33] Dean NC, Silver MP, Bateman KA, et al. Decreased mortality after implementation of a treatment guideline for community-acquired pneumonia. Am J Med 2001;110:451–7.

[34] Kahn KL, Rogers WH, Rubenstein LV, et al. Measuring quality of care with explicit process criteria before and after implementation of the DRG-based prospective payment system. JAMA 1990;264:1969–73.

[35] McGarvey RN, Harper JJ. Pneumonia mortality reduction and quality improvement in a community hospital. QRB Qual Rev Bull 1993;19:124–30.

[36] Rosenstein AH, Brooks Hanel J, Martin C. Timing is everything: impact of emergency department care on hospital length of stay. J Clin Outcomes Manag 2000;7:31–6.

[37] Battleman DS, Callahan M, Thaler HT. Rapid antibiotic delivery and appropriate antibiotic selection reduce length of hospital stay of patients with community-acquired pneumonia: link between quality of care and resource utilization. Arch Intern Med 2002;162:682–8.

[38] Meehan TP, Fine MJ, Krumholz HM, et al. Quality of care, process, and outcomes in elderly patients with pneumonia. JAMA 1997;278:2080–4.

[39] Houck PM, Bratzler DW, Nsa W, et al. Timing of antibiotic administration and outcomes for Medicare patients hospitalized with community-acquired pneumonia. Arch Intern Med 2004;164:637–44.

[40] Dedier J, Singer DE, Chang Y, et al. Processes of care, illness severity, and outcomes in the management of community-acquired pneumonia at academic hospitals. Arch Intern Med 2001;161:2099–104.

[41] Silber SH, Garrett C, Singh R, et al. Early administration of antibiotics does not shorten time to clinical stability in patients with moderate-to-severe community-acquired pneumonia. Chest 2003;124:1798–804.

[42] Iregui M, Ward S, Sherman G, et al. Clinical importance of delays in the initiation of appropriate antibiotic treatment for ventilator-associated pneumonia. Chest 2002;122:262–8.

[43] Rello J, Gallego M, Mariscal D, et al. The value of routine microbial investigation in ventilator-associated pneumonia. Am J Respir Crit Care Med 1997;156:196–200.

[44] Luna CM, Vujacich P, Niederman MS, et al. Impact of BAL data on the therapy and outcome of ventilator-associated pneumonia. Chest 1997;111:676–85.

[45] Alvarez-Lerma F. Modification of empiric antibiotic treatment in patients with pneumonia acquired in the intensive care unit. ICU-acquired pneumonia study group. Intensive Care Med 1996;22:387–94.

[46] Wilks D, Lever AML. Reasons for delay in administration of antibiotics to patients with meningitis and meningococcaemia. J Infect 1996;32:49–51.

[47] Waterer GW, Kessler LA, Wunderink RG. Delayed administration of antibiotics and atypical presentation in community-acquired pneumonia. Chest 2006;130:11–5.

[48] Pines JM, Morton MJ, Datner EM, et al. Systematic delays in antibiotic administration in the emergency department for adult patients admitted with pneumonia. Acad Emerg Med 2006;13:939–45.

[49] Pines JM, Hollander JE, Localio AR, et al. The association between emergency department crowding and hospital performance on antibiotic timing for pneumonia and percutaneous intervention for myocardial infarction. Acad Emerg Med 2006;13:873–8.

[50] Pines JM, Localio AR, Hollander JE, et al. The impact of emergency department crowding measures on time to antibiotics for patients with community-acquired pneumonia. Ann Emerg Med 2007;50:510–6.

[51] Fee C, Weber EJ, Maak CA, et al. Effect of emergency department crowding on time to antibiotics in patients admitted with community-acquired pneumonia. Ann Emerg Med 2007; 50:501–9.

[52] Houck PM, Bratzler DW. Administration of first hospital antibiotics for community-acquired pneumonia: does timeliness affect outcomes? Curr Opin Infect Dis 2005;18:151–6.

[53] Thompson D. The pneumonia controversy: hospitals grapple with 4-hour benchmark. Ann Emerg Med 2006;47:259–61.

[54] Mandell LA, Wunderink RG, Anzueto A, et al. Infectious Diseases Society of America/ American Thoracic Society consensus guidelines on the management of community-acquired pneumonia in adults. Clin Infect Dis 2007;44(Suppl 2):S27–72.

[55] Mitka M. JCAHO tweaks emergency departments' pneumonia treatment standards. JAMA 2007;298:1397–8.

[56] Kelen GD, Rothman RE. Community pneumonia practice standard mandates: can't see the forest for the trees. Acad Emerg Med 2006;13:986–8.

[57] Kanwar M, Brar N, Khatib R, et al. Misdiagnosis of community-acquired pneumonia and inappropriate utilization of antibiotics: side effects of the 4-h antibiotic administration rule. Chest 2007;131(6):1865–9.

[58] Drake DE, Cohen A, Cohn J. National antibiotic hospital timing measures and antibiotic overuse. Qual Manag Health Care 2007;16:113–22.

ELSEVIER
SAUNDERS

Emerg Med Clin N Am
26 (2008) 259–279

EMERGENCY
MEDICINE
CLINICS OF
NORTH AMERICA

Rapidly Fatal Infections

Diana Hans, DO[a], Erin Kelly, MD[a],
Krista Wilhelmson, MD[a], Eric D. Katz, MD[b],*

[a]Department of Emergency Medicine, Maricopa Medical Center, 2601 E. Roosevelt,
Phoenix, AZ 85008, USA
[b]Emergency Medicine Residency, Department of Emergency Medicine,
Maricopa Medical Center, 2601 E. Roosevelt, Phoenix, AZ 85008, USA

Every emergency physician will encounter a patient with a rapidly fatal infection. More importantly, every emergency physician will see many stable patients whose differential diagnoses include one or more potentially rapidly fatal infections. The challenge is to identify and initiate care as rapidly as possible. This article explores several of these diagnoses and provides the information needed to diagnose and begin therapy.

Rapidly fatal infections of the central nervous system

A nearly infinite list of organisms can cause a wide variety of central nervous system (CNS) infections. These organisms include bacteria, viruses, fungi, and parasites. This section focuses on the etiology, presentation, diagnosis, and treatment modalities of a few organisms that can lead to a rather speedy death. More indolent and nonfulminant disease progressions are not discussed.

Bacterial meningitis

Meningitis is an inflammation of the thin membranes (dura, arachnoid, and pia mater) that surround the brain and spinal cord. Bacterial meningitis was first described by Viesseux [1] in 1805. The fatality rate approached 100%. In 1913, Flexner [2] first reported some treatment success with the use of an intrathecal equine meningococcal antiserum. Since then much has changed; the use of antibiotics and the introduction of the *Haemophilus influenzae* type b conjugate vaccine have decreased mortality rates as well as shifted the relative frequency of the various bacteria that are responsible for

* Corresponding author. Emergency Medicine Residency, Department of Emergency Medicine, Maricopa Medical Center, 2601 E. Roosevelt, Phoenix, AZ 85008.
E-mail address: eric_katz@medprodoctors.com (E.D. Katz).

community-acquired bacterial meningitis [3,4]. In addition, a dramatic increase in the median age of patients with bacterial meningitis has been observed. In less than a decade, the median age of presenting patients has soared from 15-month-old toddlers to 25-year-old adults [5].

Etiology

Today the leading cause of bacterial meningitis after the neonate stage is *Streptococcus pneumoniae*, followed by *Neisseria meningitidis* and *Listeria monocytogenes* [3]. In addition, nosocomial meningitis appears to be an increasingly relevant contributor among reported adult cases [4]. In general, bacterial meningitis can occur at any age in otherwise healthy individuals; however, the patient's age and certain predisposing factors can give important clues as to which organism might be involved in the disease process. Table 1 exhibits characteristics and common associations of organisms that can cause bacterial meningitis [4–7].

Signs and symptoms

Classic textbook signs and symptoms include fever, nuchal rigidity, altered mental status (such as lethargy), and headache. Patients who are

Table 1
Characteristics and common associations of organisms that can cause bacterial meningitis

Organism	Age	Other associations
Streptococcus pneumoniae (gram-positive diplococci)	Any age	Sickle cell disease and asplenia
Neisseria meningitidis (gram-negative diplococci)	Any age, but often associated with young adults (college freshmen and military recruits)	Crowded living conditions, classic petechial rash, purulent pericarditis, Waterhouse-Friderichsen syndrome
Listeria monocytogenes (gram-positive rods)	Any age, but often associated with neonates and immunocompromised adults aged more than 50 years	May form small brain abscesses
Haemophilus influenzae type b (gram-negative bacilli)	Children and adults	Children who are not vaccinated, otorhinorrhea
Streptococcus agalactiae group B streptococcus (gram-positive cocci)	Infants less then 1 month of age and adults aged more than 50 years	Most common cause of meningitis in newborns
Gram-negative bacilli (other than *Haemophilus influenzae*) and gram-positive staphylococci	Any age	Nosocomial meningitis, history of neurosurgery, recent head trauma, ventricular shunts, and cerebrospinal fluid leaks

very young, elderly, or immunocompromised may present atypically and can have a paucity of these symptoms; however, studies consistently report that the vast majority will have at least one traditional finding [4,8]. Other classic associations include Brudzinski's and Kernig's signs. The former is seen when the clinician flexes the patient's neck and this, in turn, causes the patient to flex his or her hips. The latter can be observed with the patient lying supine in hip flexion at 90 degrees. The patient will resist the clinician's attempt to fully extend the knee secondary to pain [9]. Patients can also present with photophobia, sore throat, and a rash [10]. A classic petechial rash is most commonly associated with *Neisseria meningitidis* but can also occur with *Streptococcus pneumoniae* and other bacteria. The same is true for an often associated complication of meningococcal meningitis, the Waterhouse-Friderichsen syndrome. It manifests as meningococcemia (or pneumococcal meningitis [6]) with hypotension and bilateral adrenal hemorrhage. In general, an adverse outcome and increased mortality have been observed in persons aged more than 60 years and in patients who initially present with seizure activity or severely altered mental status [4,5].

Diagnosis

Bacterial meningitis is a clinical diagnosis, and antibiotic treatment must not be delayed for lumbar puncture or CT scan. If a high index of suspicion exists, the patient must be treated empirically; the definitive diagnosis is often not revealed until lumbar puncture results are available. A definitive diagnosis is important not to satisfy one's own curiosity but to keep statistics current and to better allow the Centers for Disease Control (CDC) to analyze trends and make recommendations. Furthermore, empiric antibiotic regimens can and should be modified when a particular organism has been identified [11,12]. There is ongoing debate over whether a CT scan should be performed before lumbar puncture [4]. In general, it may be advisable if the patient has focal neurologic signs, papilledema, or is in a state of coma. The yield of a CT scan is low in the absence of such findings [11,13]. Antibiotics should be given first even if the clinician decides to obtain a head CT before lumbar puncture.

Lumbar puncture and cerebrospinal fluid analysis. A conventional emergency department lumbar puncture tray includes four vials. A 1- to 1.5-mL sample of cerebrospinal fluid (CSF) is collected per vial. A cell count with differential, protein and glucose concentrations, as well as culture and Gram stain are routinely requested. Typical CSF findings are depicted in Table 2. As is true for any analysis, absolute numbers should be treated with caution. Bacterial meningitis cannot necessarily be ruled out in a patient who has a negative Gram stain and an absolute CSF white blood cell (WBC) count of less than 100 cells/mm^3 [5]; rather, a wider range of less than 100 WBC/mm^3 to greater than 10,000 WBC/mm^3 may sometimes be encountered [12] in bacterial meningitis.

Table 2
Cerebrospinal fluid analysis in bacterial meningitis

Cerebrospinal fluid	Values that denote a normal range[a]	Bacterial meningitis
White blood cell count (cells/mm^3)	≤5	>5 Abnormal, a commonly expected range (1000–5000)
Differential	≤1 Polymorphonuclear leukocytes	Polymorphonuclear leukocyte predominance
Protein (mg/dL)	15–45	>45, Often elevated > 150
Glucose (mg/dL)	50–80	<50

[a] Exact reference values often depend on the laboratory where the fluid is analyzed.

Treatment

Even though we have a much better understanding of the disease today and newer antibiotics have been introduced, during the past 35 years, overall case fatality rates have remained high at 20% to 25% [4,5,8]. Bacterial meningitis is a rapidly fatal infection; therefore, empiric intravenous antibiotic treatment is appropriate and necessary. The drawback is the increasing antimicrobial resistance, especially among pneumococci [11]. A better understanding of the pathophysiology and the involvement of inflammatory cytokines in the disease process has led to the use of corticosteroids as an adjunct treatment. Although early reports stated that steroids did not affect overall mortality, it was soon recognized that they decrease the rate of complications associated with bacterial meningitis, especially sensorineural hearing loss [3]. Other sequelae include brain damage, learning disabilities, and mental retardation [5,14]. In 2007 the Cochrane Database of Systematic Reviews stated that the use of corticosteroids in community-acquired bacterial meningitis reduced mortality, hearing loss, and other neurologic complications in children and adults [15]. As a result, dexamethasone is the drug of choice to be given before or with the first antibiotic dose [12,15]. Table 3 shows the current recommendations for antibiotic treatment in suspected bacterial meningitis cases [11,12].

Table 3
Empiric intravenous antibiotic therapy

Patient age	Treatment
<1 mo	Cefotaxime and ampicillin (vancomycin and ceftazidime if the infant is preterm, has a low birth weight, and there is an increased risk for nosocomial infections with gram-negative and staphylococcal organisms)
>1 mo	Ceftriaxone and vancomycin
>50 y	Ceftriaxone and vancomycin and ampicillin

Rationale: Ampicillin is added for suspected *Listeria monocytogenes* or *Streptococcus agalactiae*. Vancomycin helps with cephalosporin-resistant *Streptococcus pneumoniae*. In addition, ceftazidime and aminoglycosides can provide good coverage for gram-negative organisms.

Antibiotic prophylaxis for close contacts of patients with meningococcal meningitis is currently recommended. Close contacts include members of the same household or day care center, and those with direct contact with oral secretions (may include emergency medical service or emergency department personnel). Current regimens for prophylaxis include single-dose ciprofloxacin, 400 mg orally, or rifampin, 600 mg orally q12 hrs for four doses. Respiratory isolation is recommended for all suspected meningitis patients [14].

Viral encephalitis

Viral encephalitis is caused by an inflammation of the brain parenchyma itself. The multitude of viruses that can cause such an inflammation is vast. Described herein are two arboviruses, the St. Louis encephalitis virus and the Eastern equine virus. Both viruses are associated with high mortality rates as well as a high incidence of neurologic sequelae among survivors [16]. The CDC has reported a 5% to 15% mortality rate for St. Louis encephalitis [17]. Eastern equine encephalitis has a somewhat higher mortality rate of 33%; therefore, it is one of the most fatal arthropod-borne diseases in the United States [18].

Etiology

Arboviruses cause disease in humans via the bite of an infected mosquito. The St. Louis encephalitis virus is a small RNA virus that belongs to the Flaviviridae family. Cases have been reported in most US states, but the central and eastern regions are primarily affected [17]. Eastern equine encephalitis virus is also a small RNA virus and a member of the Togaviridae family; transmission occurs mostly along the East and Gulf Coast regions [18].

Signs and symptoms

Both viruses have similar incubation periods and clinical presentations. After the mosquito bite, 2 to 15 days may pass before a viral illness develops. There is great variability of signs and symptoms, ranging from mild headache, fever, and neck stiffness to altered mental status and coma [17–21]. Especially with Eastern equine encephalitis, gastrointestinal manifestations such as nausea, vomiting, and abdominal pain are common [19]. Once neurologic symptoms start, deterioration is rapid. Seizures may also be seen and have been associated with a poor outcome in St. Louis encephalitis [21]. Even mild forms of twitching around the mouth and eyebrows are poor prognostic indicators [22]. One study found no such correlation with Eastern equine encephalitis; however, bad outcomes were related to a high initial WBC count in the CSF and the degree of hyponatremia in the serum [19].

Forms of parkinsonian movement disorders have also been described with St. Louis encephalitis, which are most likely associated with the viral inflammation of the basal ganglia [20]. Focal radiographic signs and early basal ganglia involvement are also characteristic of Eastern equine encephalitis; these disease entities can be distinguished from herpes simplex encephalitis which shows temporal lobe involvement [19,23,24]. Typical radiographic signs in herpes simplex encephalitis include inflammatory changes on MRI consistent with increased water content. CT may show nonspecific edema but may be normal in up to 30% of cases [23,24].

In St. Louis encephalitis, adults are more often affected than are children, but both groups can have severe disease manifestations. Adults and elderly patients usually have a worse outcome [20]. Eastern equine encephalitis used to be more commonly seen in younger patients, but some reported series have not found this to be true. Furthermore, neither age nor the length of the prodrome can be correlated with outcome [19]. According to the CDC, patients aged more than 50 years and those younger 15 years are at greater risk for severe disease [18].

Diagnosis

Serology testing is currently the best diagnostic modality. ELISA is used for antibody detection of IgM in serum and CSF; however, this test can often be negative when the patient initially presents, because antibodies may not be detectable at the time of presentation. Lumbar punctures may have to be repeated [19–21]. These viruses often demonstrate basal ganglia involvement, and repeat radiographic imaging can be of value. The CSF analysis usually shows an elevated WBC count that is predominately lymphocytic in St. Louis encephalitis, whereas in Eastern equine encephalitis a polymorphonuclear leukocyte (PMN) pleocytosis is seen [19]. Glucose levels are often normal with normal or mildly elevated protein levels [19,22]. Especially in St. Louis encephalitis, viremia is infrequent; therefore, the virus cannot be isolated from the CSF. It comes as no surprise that in cases in which virus isolation has been possible, the patients have died rather quickly [20].

Treatment

Currently, there is no antiviral treatment, and all efforts should be directed toward supportive care such as correcting electrolyte imbalances and preventing secondary bacterial infections. Early treatment of St. Louis encephalitis with interferon-alfa may decrease the severity of neurologic sequelae [25]. Corticosteroids and antiepileptic medications as adjunct therapy have been tested for Eastern equine encephalitis, but the outcomes were disappointing. In one case report, improvement was observed secondary to immunotherapy [26]; however, the majority of patients in another study actually did worse when compared with patients who were not treated with any steroids or anticonvulsants [19]. Although there is no treatment, fast diagnosis is essential, especially if it involves index cases. Early involvement of public health authorities may lessen the endemic case burden via public awareness. Preventing mosquito bites in the first place is the only effective way to avoid these diseases [17,18].

Meningoencephalitis

Meningoencephalitis describes a more diffuse inflammatory process of the meninges as well as the brain parenchyma. It is commonly seen with fungi and parasites. A well-established disease entity is primary amoebic meningoencephalitis. Caused by the parasitic amoeba *Naegleria fowleri*, it is a rare but rapidly fatal disease that leads to fulminant inflammation and necrosis of the brain [27]. According to the CDC, the mortality rate is greater than 95%, and few survivors have been reported. In the United States, 23 cases secondary to primary amoebic meningoencephalitis have been documented between 1995 and 2004 [28]. *Naegleria fowleri* infections have been on the rise, and stories have appeared on national news casts. The total number of fatal cases for 2007 was six [29].

Etiology

Naegleria fowleri is a free living amoeba that flourishes in fresh water at temperatures of around 28°C or above [30]. It gains entry into the CNS via the nasal mucosa and the cribiform plate when swimming in rivers, fresh water lakes, hot springs, or insufficiently chlorinated swimming pool. Person-to-person transmission is not possible [28,31]. More recently, microbiologists have identified *Naegleria fowleri* as a reservoir for pathogenic bacteria [32], although the clinical significance of this is unclear.

Signs and symptoms

Usually, 1 to 12 days pass before a viral like illness develops. Presenting signs and symptoms are similar to those seen in meningitis. Patients may complain of fever, headache, nausea, vomiting, and neck stiffness [27–29]. Altered mental status and seizures can occur [33]. Altered taste and smell sensations have also been reported [27]. Coma and death usually occur within a few days after the onset of symptoms [28].

Diagnosis

Diagnosis is challenging, and most cases can only be confirmed at autopsy [33]. Although it is a rare disease, the fact that it is so rapidly fatal makes it an important entity. It should be on the differential diagnosis list when a patient with fever, headache, and a history of recent swimming or water sport activity presents to the emergency department. CSF analysis resembles the clinical presentation of bacterial meningitis, with an increased PMN pleocytosis, elevated protein, and decreased glucose concentrations, with potentially visible motile organisms seen on microscopy [27,33,34].

Treatment

Fast diagnosis is essential, but only limited treatment options exist at this time. Survival has been documented on rare occasions. Based on the limited information available, intravenous or intrathecal amphotericin B in combination with intravenous or oral rifampin as an adjunct should be given as quickly as possible [32,34].

Toxic shock syndrome

Epidemiology

Toxic shock syndrome (TSS) is a disease entity characterized by sudden onset fever, chills, vomiting, diarrhea, and rash which can quickly progress to hypotension, multiorgan system failure, and even death. Reports have suggested a mortality rate of 30% to 70% despite aggressive treatment [35] TSS is most commonly caused by *Staphylococcus aureus* and group A streptococcus. *S aureus* TSS has a strong association with tampon use, intravaginal contraceptive devices, nasal packing, and postoperative wound infections, whereas group A streptococcus TSS has been linked to minor trauma, surgical procedures, and viral infections, particularly varicella [36]. Of the total cases of *S aureus* TSS, 93% percent involve women [37]. Group A streptococcus TSS affects all ages and genders equally. The last active surveillance performed in the United States in 1987 by the CDC showed an annual incidence of 1 to 2 cases per 100,000 population in women aged 15 to 44 years; however, the current incidence is likely much lower after the withdrawal of highly absorbent brands of tampons from the market in the late 1980s. Cases of menstrual-related *S aureus* TSS accounted for over 90% of total TSS cases in 1980 and have significantly decreased to 59% in 1996, with a predicted annual incidence of 1 case per100,000 women [38]. The incidence of group A streptococcus TSS has maintained a consistent level of approximately 3.5 cases per 100,000 people since the 1980s [39]. Menstrual-related cases are more likely to occur in women who use higher absorbency tampons, who keep a single tampon in place for a longer period of time, and who use tampons continuously for more days in their cycle [40]. Nonmenstrual TSS is quickly gaining ground on menstrual-related cases. Women account for 76% of nonmenstrual cases, perhaps because many cases are related to postpartum wound infections and mastitis. Other causes include surgical wounds, sinusitis, burns, respiratory infections, and skin infections. The number of postsurgical-related cases increased nearly twofold from 1986 to 1996, now accounting for 27% of all cases of nonmenstrual-related TSS [37,41].

Pathophysiology

Both *S aureus* and group A streptococcus cause TSS by releasing exotoxins that act as superantigens. Superantigens activate large numbers of T cells to produce cytokines, including interleukin-1, tumor necrosis factor, and interferon, which results in capillary leakage and tissue damage and development of the signs and symptoms of TSS. In contrast to typical antigens, superantigens do not need to be processed by an antigen-presenting cell to produce the T-cell activation cascade, allowing them to activate many T cells at once and in a very short period of time [42]. *S aureus* produces TSS toxin-1 (TSST-1) and various enterotoxins, whereas group A streptococcus produces an assortment of pyrogenic exotoxins [43–46]. The M protein of group A streptococcus is an important virulence factor and gives the organism antiphagocytic properties. Serotypes of group A streptococcus are based on their M type. Those most commonly associated with TSS are M types 1, 3, 12, and 28.

Clinical presentation

The CDC developed a case definition for the diagnosis of TSS in 1981 which is still used today [47]. The definition includes fever ($> 38.9°C$), hypotension, rash, desquamation within 1 to 2 weeks after onset of illness, involvement of three or more organ systems, and negative results for any other pathogen.

A multitude of skin manifestations have been reported in TSS [48,49]. The typical initial presentation is a diffuse, erythematous, macular rash involving all skin and mucosal surfaces including the palms and soles resembling sunburn. Infections of surgical wounds can have more intense erythema around the surgical sites. One to 3 weeks into the disease process, desquamation begins on the palms and soles and can progress diffusely. Some patients even have hair and nail loss months after the onset of illness.

There is little difference in the presentation of menstrual and nonmenstrual TSS. One small study showed an earlier onset of rash and fever, less musculoskeletal involvement, and more severe renal and CNS complications in nonmenstrual TSS [50].

Treatment

Clinicians must remember that the working definition for TSS was created for epidemiologic surveillance. If one has a strong suspicion of TSS, treatment should not be delayed if all criteria are not met, and antibiotics should not be withheld if there is concern for non-staphylococcal TSS. Supportive care should be initiated immediately and remains the mainstay of treatment. Hypotension is often severe and unresponsive to large volumes of intravenous fluid resuscitation. Patients may require 10 to 20 L of fluid per day to maintain perfusion in addition to vasopressors. Surgical intervention is commonly needed for group A streptococcus infections, and it is best to consult surgeons early on in patients who have this TSS diagnosis. Deep-seated infections often require debridement, fasciotomy, amputation, or aspiration [51].

Staphylococcus aureus *toxic shock syndrome*

The addition of antibiotics has not been proven to alter the course of acute *S aureus* TSS [52,53]. Despite the fact that studies suggest a decrease in the recurrence rate with antibiotics, episodes are shown to resolve without antibiotics [54]. Clindamycin has been used for the treatment of *S aureus* TSS since the syndrome was initially defined. Its use is hypothetically supported by its suppression of protein synthesis and, hence, toxin synthesis, and it has been shown to suppress TSST-1 synthesis in vitro by 90% even at levels below inhibitory concentrations [55]. The same study showed that beta-lactam antibiotics actually increased levels of TSST-1, most likely because of their mechanism of action on the cell wall leading to cell lysis or increased membrane permeability resulting in increased release of toxin. A more recent 2006 in vitro study showed that clindamycin and linezolid completely suppressed TSST-1, whereas maximum toxin production occurred with nafcillin and vancomycin [56]. The most appropriate treatment regimen can be selected based on culture and sensitivity results. Patients with suspected *S aureus* TSS should be treated empirically with clindamycin plus vancomycin or linezolid. If sensitivity results show methicillin-sensitive *S aureus*, vancomycin can be changed to oxacillin or nafcillin.

Group A streptococcus toxic shock syndrome

Antibiotic regimens for simple group A streptococcus infections are relatively simple because group A streptococcus remains nearly universally sensitive to penicillins. Unfortunately, complicated group A streptococcus infections are shown to have a high mortality rate despite aggressive antibiotic therapy, and penicillin has been shown to have limited effects if not initiated early in the disease. Studies suggest that penicillin loses its effectiveness once large numbers of group A streptococcus are present. This loss is attributed to the fact that penicillins and beta-lactams work best against rapidly growing bacteria. Once concentrations of group A streptococcus build up, replication slows down, reducing the effectiveness of the antibiotic [57]. Clindamycin is now used as an alternative to penicillin for several key reasons. First, clindamycin is not affected by the number of group A streptococcus or the stage of growth. Second, as mentioned previously, clindamycin suppresses protein synthesis, including toxins. Third, it allows phagocytosis of group A streptococcus by inhibiting M-protein synthesis [58–60]. In addition, clindamycin has a longer postantibiotic effect than penicillin and suppresses the production of tumor necrosis factor. Current guidelines for antibiotic regimens for group A streptococcus TSS are based on limited retrospective trials, which suggest use of a protein synthesis–inhibiting antibiotic (eg, clindamycin) with a cell wall–inhibiting antibiotic (eg, beta-lactams) [61].

The use of intravenous immune globulin and corticosteroids are less conventional treatments that have been suggested for TSS, but neither has been extensively studied. Multiple small studies of the use of intravenous immune globulin suggest little effect on outcome in *S aureus* TSS and mild improvement for group A streptococcus TSS [62–64]; however, more studies are needed before recommendations can be made regarding its routine use. Corticosteroid use has been shown to decrease the duration and severity of symptoms but has no measurable effect on mortality rates and is not recommended for routine treatment of TSS [65].

Methicillin-resistant *Staphylococcus aureus* necrotizing pneumonia

Epidemiology

Methicillin was introduced to the public in 1959 as a narrow spectrum beta-lactam antibiotic. Shortly after its introduction, outbreaks of methicillin-resistant *Staphylococcus aureus* (MRSA) infections began to appear [66]. MRSA began primarily as a hospital-acquired infection; however, it is quickly becoming a common community-acquired pathogen. In fact, the rate of community-acquired MRSA (CA-MRSA) is increasing so rapidly that it now accounts for the majority of community-acquired skin and soft tissue infections and approximately 5% of all community-acquired pneumonias. Necrotizing pneumonia is caused almost exclusively by the CA-MRSA strains. The exact prevalence of necrotizing pneumonia caused by MRSA is unknown; however, the mortality rate of documented cases is significant (30% to 75%) [42,50,63,64]. The prevalence of CA-MRSA colonization and soft tissue infections which include pneumonia is more extensively studied.

In 2004, a prospective study followed adults with skin and soft tissue infections at 11 emergency departments in the United States. MRSA was present in 59% of cases, and 97% were consistent with CA-MRSA strains [67]. In 2005, a case-control study was conducted to determine the rate of MRSA carriage by performing surveillance cultures on more than 700 patients at hospital admission. Fifty-three percent of the patients were positive for MRSA, and the risk factors associated with colonization included recent antibiotic use (within 3 months), hospitalization within the past year, skin or soft tissue infection on admission, and HIV infection [68]. A 2003 meta-analysis study found that the CA-MRSA prevalence among total hospital-diagnosed MRSA cases was 30.2% in 27 retrospective studies and 37.3% in five prospective studies [69]; however, study samples obtained from community members outside of the health care setting showed a colonization rate of only 1.3%. In addition, studies that excluded people with any health care contacts had an MRSA prevalence of only 0.2%, suggesting that the distinction between hospital-acquired and CA-MRSA is becoming blurred. The term *CA-MRSA* is now defined by the genetic traits of the strain rather than the means by which colonization or infection occurred.

Pathophysiology

Panton-Valentine leukocidin (PVL) is a pore-forming cytotoxin that causes leukocyte destruction and tissue necrosis. PVL is produced by fewer than 5% of *S aureus* strains but is found in the majority of CA-MRSA strains that cause soft tissue infections and necrotizing pneumonia [67,70–72]. It is rarely found in hospital-acquired MRSA. One study found PVL genes in 93% of MRSA strains associated with furunculosis and in 85% of those associated with severe necrotic hemorrhagic pneumonia [70]. PVL genes were not found in strains that caused endocarditis, mediastinitis, hospital-acquired pneumonia, TSS, and urinary tract infections [70]. Studies on a mouse model of acute pneumonia showed that PVL alone was sufficient to cause necrotizing pneumonia [73].

In addition to PVL, a strong link between the influenza virus and MRSA necrotizing pneumonia has been reported in multiple instances [74–77]. During the 2003 to 2004 influenza season, the CDC received reports of severe pneumonia caused by *S aureus* and MRSA among previously healthy children and adults after influenza virus infection [75]. Of the 17 case patients identified, 5 died (median age, 28 years), and only 1 had underlying illness. Most died within 1 week of symptom onset. Most infections were caused by MRSA (76%), 85% had the PVL genes, and all were uniformly resistant to macrolides [75]. Another study of 10 cases of CA-MRSA pneumonia occurred in association with the influenza season in 2006 to 2007 [76]. Sixty percent of the patients who were co-infected died of their illness. Various mechanisms by which influenza interacts with *S aureus* to increase the risk of co-infection have been suggested. They include an influenza-induced increase in *S aureus* adhesion to the respiratory tract and an increase in *S aureus* proteases which leads to a synergistic increase in severity of both the influenza and *S aureus* infection [78–80].

Clinical presentation

MRSA necrotizing pneumonia can be difficult to differentiate from other causes of community-acquired pneumonia based on symptoms alone. The key distinguishing features are the severity of symptoms, the rapid progression of disease, the age of patients, the association of disease onset and recent viral illness, the lack of comorbidities, and the significantly increased mortality [70]. Similar to patients who have community-acquired pneumonia, patients with MRSA pneumonia present with cough, fever, respiratory distress, and malaise. Patients with PVL-positive MRSA pneumonia are more likely to present with shock, hemoptysis, leukopenia, and even death [70,72,81].

Between 1986 and 1999, eight cases of necrotizing pneumonia caused by *S aureus* in France were reported [82]. All of the strains were found to produce PVL, which prompted a prospective surveillance study of staphylococcal pneumonia [77,83]. A total of 52 cases were studied, 16 of which were positive for PVL. PVL-positive *S aureus* pneumonia typically occurred in younger patients (median age, 14.8 years) who were previously healthy, and 75% were found to have had a viral infection in the preceding days. Other remarkable features of PVL pneumonia versus non-PVL pneumonia were the frequency of shock (81% versus 53%), respiratory distress (75% versus 53%), hemoptysis (38% versus 3%), and mortality (75% versus 47%) [77,83]. A retrospective study of 50 cases reported in France from 1986 to 2005 showed a mortality rate of 56%. The factors most closely linked to death were leukopenia, airway bleeding, and erythroderma [82].

Treatment

In recent years, vancomycin has remained the cornerstone of pharmacologic therapy for severe MRSA infections; however, failure rates of up to 40% have been reported [84]. Most antimicrobial studies are performed on hospital-acquired MRSA infections, making antibiotic decision making difficult for CA-MRSA pneumonia. Linezolid is a bacteriostatic choice with activity against MRSA that is relatively new to the market. Some studies suggest that linezolid and clindamycin are superior to vancomycin due to their ability to inhibit exotoxin production, specifically PVL [81]; however, an open-label trial of linezolid versus vancomycin for MRSA pneumonia showed equivalent rates of clinical cure (75% versus 75%) [85]. A retrospective analysis of two prospective double-blind clinical trails of hospital-acquired pneumonia suggested that cure rates of linezolid were superior to that of vancomycin (59% versus 36%); however, no differences in outcomes for patients with concomitant bacteremia were appreciated [81,86–88]. To date, no study has demonstrated superiority of linezolid over vancomycin for MRSA pneumonia; therefore, the choice remains one of physician preference. Other antibiotics, including trimethoprim-sulfamethoxazole, clindamycin, quinupristin-dalfopristin, and daptomycin, have undergone limited trials with poor demonstrable efficacy.

Other options for treatment have been suggested but not extensively studied, including percutaneous drainage, thoracoscopic decortication, and surgical debridement. Surgical management of acute necrotizing pneumonia is rarely performed due to unclear indications and high risks of complications. A retrospective review of 35 patients undergoing resection for lung necrosis showed an 8.5% postoperative death rate, and 11% of patients remained ventilator dependent [89].

With the increasing prevalence of CA-MRSA colonization and newly emerging drug-resistance strains of S aureus, necrotizing pneumonia is likely to become an increasing problem. Rapid disease progression and significant mortality demand aggressive diagnosis and treatment. Particular attention and consideration need to be given to younger patients who present with a history of recent viral illness, sudden onset cough and hemoptysis, leukopenia, and chest radiographs consistent with pneumonia.

Severe acute respiratory syndrome and avian influenza

Viral infections have the potential of being rapidly fatal infections. Fatal viral infections, although rare, are particularly ominous because of the lack

of effective treatments. Two deadly viral infections that have emerged in recent years include severe acute respiratory syndrome (SARS) and influenza A
(H5N1), also known as avian influenza or bird flu. Although there have been
no recent cases of SARS and although avian influenza is still rare, both infections have the potential to be rapidly fatal and to reach pandemic status.

Severe acute respiratory syndrome

From its emergence in Guangdong Province in China in November 2002
until July 31, 2003, there were 8096 probable SARS coronavirus (SARS-
CoV) cases, with a case fatality ratio of 9.6% [90]. According to the CDC
definition, key clinical features of SARS-CoV are an incubation period of
2 to 10 days, early systemic symptoms followed within 2 to 7 days by dry
cough or shortness of breath, the development of radiographically confirmed pneumonia by day 7 to 10, and lymphocytopenia in many cases [91].

One of the more disturbing aspects of SARS is its ability to start with one
index case and to spread rapidly to many contacts of that individual. One
such case was studied in March of 2003 at the Prince of Wales Hospital
in Hong Kong. A 26-year-old man was admitted with fever and productive
cough. He was not placed in respiratory precautions, and, subsequently,
SARS infection developed within the next 2 weeks in 138 people, mainly
hospital personnel [92]. A similar case occurred in Singapore and began
when a 23-year-old woman resided at a hotel in Hong Kong on the same
floor as other individuals infected with SARS. This patient returned to Singapore and infected 20 close contacts, including hospital workers [93].

At the Prince of Wales Hospital from March 11, 2003 to March 25, 2003,
156 patients were treated for SARS. Many of them were hospital personnel
exposed to the index case discussed previously. Complaints on initial presentation included fever in 100% of patients, cough, muscle aches, and
headache. Common laboratory findings included leukopenia, lymphocytopenia, and thrombocytopenia, and elevated activated partial thromboplastin time, aspartate transaminase (AST), creatinine kinase, and lactate
dehydrogenase (LDH). Abnormal chest radiographs were found in 78%
of patients, often with one-sided consolidation. Twenty-three percent of patients required ICU care, and nearly 14% of patients needed ventilatory support. In total, five patients died by day 21 [94].

Staying at the same hotel as the index case for Singapore discussed previously was the index case for a Toronto outbreak. An elderly woman traveling from Hong Kong to Toronto brought the infection with her. A cohort
of 144 patients was studied in Toronto, with 14 physicians and 29 nurses infected. Signs and symptoms of the illness were similar to those seen in Hong
Kong. Twenty-one patients needed ICU admission, and the 21-day mortality rate was 6.5% [95]. Poor prognostic indicators for SARS have included
male sex, hyponatremia, left shift, elevated LDH, and age greater than 60
years [93–95].

Unfortunately, there is no rapid test for SARS. Reverse transcription–polymerase chain reaction (RT-PCR) can be used to evaluate for SARS, but the yield depends on the duration of symptoms and the type of sample [96]. There is also no known effective treatment. Anecdotally, some Hong Kong patients seemed to respond to corticosteroid and ribavirin therapy, but no randomized control trials have been done [94].

Due to its high fatality, lack of treatment options, and the frightening ability to spread among contacts, it is important to have a plan to control any new infections and prevent spread. According to World Health Organization (WHO) guidelines, patients with suspected SARS should have a separate triage area. These patients need to wear a mask, and triage staff should wear mask and eye protection. Probable cases should be isolated in a single negative pressure room if available and be placed on droplet, airborne, and contact precautions. Disposable devices such as stethoscopes should be used for each patient. If single rooms are not available, patients should be placed in cohort rooms [97]. There have been no cases of SARS in the past few years; however, there is always the potential for this deadly virus to re-emerge.

Avian influenza

Another emerging deadly virus is avian influenza, otherwise known as influenza A (H5N1). Although there have been relatively few cases, this virus is especially disturbing owing to its pathogenic nature. The reservoir for avian influenza is wild poultry. It is present in wild birds in Asia, Europe, the Near East, and Africa. Most infections in humans are related to exposure to ill birds. Human-to-human transmission is currently rare [98].

According to WHO statistics, there have been 332 total reported cases from 2003 to October 2007 and 204 reported deaths in that period [99]. The majority of cases have been in Indonesia and Viet Nam. Up to this point, there have been no reported cases in North or South America [99].

In January 2004, 10 cases of avian influenza were diagnosed by RT-PCR or viral culture in Viet Nam. The ages of these patients ranged from 5 to 24 years. Eight of the ten patients had a known contact with poultry. Every patient was found to have abnormalities on chest radiography that significantly progressed during the course of their illness (although there is no report on a characteristic radiographic finding). Signs and symptoms of infection included fever, cough, diarrhea, shortness of breath, lymphocytopenia, and thrombocytopenia. Disturbingly, eight patients required mechanical ventilation within 48 hours of admission, and all of these patients died between day 6 and 14 [100].

Similarly in Turkey in 2006, there were eight WHO-confirmed cases of patients infected with avian influenza [101]. These patients were between 5 and 15 years of age. All of the patients had been exposed to live poultry in their homes. Fever was present in each patient. Cough, sore throat, myalgia, and diarrhea were also common complaints. Lymphocytopenia, thrombocytopenia, and elevated AST, LDH, and creatinine kinase were common laboratory findings, similar to the cases studied in Viet Nam. Four of the patients needed mechanical ventilatory support within 48 to 72 hours. All of the eight patients died within 7 days of hospitalization [101].

The worrisome factors in both of these case series include not only the obviously high mortality but also the young age of the patients involved and the rapidity at which their disease progressed. Indeed, according to the CDC, the overall mortality rate of avian influenza is currently 60%. Strikingly, mortality is highest in patients aged 10 to 19 years, similar to the influenza outbreak of 1918 [98].

Health care providers should entertain the diagnosis of avian influenza when addressing a patient with fever and respiratory illness who is from or has traveled to areas where avian influenza infection has been found in poultry [102]. These areas include Azerbaijan, Cambodia, China, Djibouti, Egypt, Indonesia, Iraq, Nigeria, Thailand, Turkey, and Viet Nam [99]. Rapid influenza detection kits should not be used for identifying avian influenza. Specimens should be sent to a WHO-recognized laboratory for identification [102].

As is true for many illnesses that are rare and rapidly fatal, only anecdotal information is available regarding the treatment of avian influenza. No randomized control trials are available at this time that address antiviral therapy. According to WHO guidelines, oseltamivir should be used for antiviral therapy. Anecdotal data suggest that it can reduce mortality. In patients with severe disease, amantadine or rimantadine can be added to the oseltamivir regimen. These drugs should not be used alone. Corticosteroids should only be considered in patients with septic shock and possible adrenal insufficiency. If adult respiratory distress syndrome develops, lung protective mechanical ventilation should be used [102].

As is true for SARS, there is no clinically proven treatment for avian influenza, making prevention of the spread of disease very important. Currently, person-to-person spread is rare, but influenza viruses in general are known for their ability to change. Because the virus has its reservoir in poultry, there is an embargo on birds from affected countries to the United States in an attempt to prevent the spread of infection [103].

It is important to maintain contact and airborne precautions when dealing with patients with suspected avian influenza. Whenever possible, patients should be in a negative pressure isolation room. The expiratory ports of ventilators and oxygen masks should contain a high-efficiency particulate air filter to decrease aerosol production and spread of the disease [102,104].

Although avian influenza and SARS infections are rare, they clearly have the potential to be rapidly fatal. Travel by air can easily cause spread of infection to previously infection-free sites. Health care providers need to be aware of these infections and keep them in mind when evaluating patients with febrile respiratory illnesses, especially those who have traveled from affected areas.

References

[1] Glikman D, Matushek S, Kahana M, et al. Pneumonia and empyema caused by penicillin-resistant Neisseria meningitidis: a case report and literature review. Pediatrics 2006;117(5): e1061–6.
[2] Flexner S. The results of the serum treatment in thirteen hundred cases of epidemic meningitis. J Exp Med 1913;17:553–76.
[3] Swartz M. Bacterial meningitis: a view of the past 90 years. N Engl J Med 2004;351:1826–8.
[4] Durand M, Calderwood S, Weber D, et al. Acute bacterial meningitis in adults: a review of 493 episodes. N Engl J Med 1993;328:21–8.
[5] Schuchat A, Robinson K, Wenger J, et al. Bacterial meningitis in the United States in 1995. N Engl J Med 1997;337:970–6.
[6] Rosenstein N, Perkins B, Stephens D. Meningococcal disease. N Engl J Med 2001;344: 1378–88.
[7] Dee RR, Lorber B. Brain abscess due to *Listeria monocytogenes*: case report and literature review. Rev Infect Dis 1986;8:968.
[8] Pizon A, Bonner M, Wang H, et al. Ten years of clinical experience with adult meningitis at an urban academic medical center. J Emerg Med 2006;31(4):367–70.
[9] Lavoie F, Saucier J. Central nervous system infections. In: Marx J, Hockberger R, Walls R, et al. Rosen's emergency medicine: concepts and clinical practice. 6th edition, vol. 2. Philadelphia: Mosby Elsevier; 2006. p. 1710–23.
[10] Drumheller B, D'Amore J, Nelson M. A simple clinical decision rule to predict bacterial meningitis in patients presenting to the emergency department. Annals Emergency Medicine 2007;50(3):S10.
[11] Quagliarello V, Scheld W. Treatment of bacterial meningitis. N Engl J Med 1997;336: 708–16.
[12] Menaker J, Martin IB, Hirshorn JM, et al. Marked elevation of CSF white blood cell count: an unusual case of S pneumoniae meningitis, differential diagnosis, and a brief review of current epidemiology and treatment recommendations. J Emerg Med 2005;29(1):37–41.
[13] Cabral D, Flodmark O, Farrell K, et al. Prospective study of computed tomography in acute bacterial meningitis. J Pediatr 1987;111:201–5.
[14] Centers for Disease Control and Prevention. Division of bacterial and mycotic diseases. Available at: http://www.cdc.gov/ncidod/dbmd/diseaseinfo/meningococcal-g.html. Accessed October15, 2007.
[15] van de Beek D, de Gans J, McIntyre P, et al. Corticosteroids for acute bacterial meningitis. Cochrane Database Syst Rev 2007;(1):CD004405 DOI:10.1002/14651858.
[16] Anderson J. Viral encephalitis and its pathology. Curr Top Pathol 1988;76:23–60.
[17] Centers for Disease Control and Prevention. Division of vector borne infectious diseases: St. Louis encephalitis. Available at: http://www.cdc.gov/ncidod/dvbid/sle/index.html. Accessed October15, 2007.
[18] Centers for Disease Control and Prevention. Division of vector borne infectious diseases: Eastern equine encephalitis. Available at: http://www.cdc.gov/ncidod/dvbid/eee/index.html. Accessed October 15, 2007.
[19] Deresiewicz R, Thaler S, Hsu L, et al. Clinical and neuroradiographic manifestations of Eastern equine encephalitis. N Engl J Med 1997;336:1867–74.
[20] Solomon T. Flavivirus encephalitis. N Engl J Med 2004;351:370–8.
[21] Sothern PM, Smith JW, Luby JP, et al. Clinical and laboratory features of epidemic St. Louis encephalitis. Ann Intern Med 1969;71:681–9.
[22] Wasay M, Diaz-Arrastia R, Suss R, et al. St. Louis encephalitis: a review of 11 cases in a 1995 Dallas, Texas epidemic. Arch Neurol 2000;57:114–8.

[23] Demaerel P, Wilms G, Robberecht W, et al. MRI of herpes simplex encephalitis. Neurora-diology 1992;34:490–3.

[24] Farber S, Hill A, Connerly ML, et al. Encephalitis in infants and children caused by the virus of the eastern variety of equine encephalitis. JAMA 1940;114:1725–31.

[25] Rahal JJ, Anderson J, Rosenberg C, et al. Effect of interferon alpha 2b therapy on St. Louis viral meningoencephalitis: clinical and laboratory results of a pilot study. J Infect Dis 2004; 190:1084–7.

[26] Golomb MR, Durand ML, Schaefer PW, et al. A case of immunotherapy-responsive eastern equine encephalitis with diffusion-weighted imaging. Neurology 2001;56:420–1.

[27] Bennett N. Naegleria. Available at: http://www/emdicine.com/ped/topic2807.htm. Accessed October 18, 2007.

[28] Centers for Disease Control and Prevention. Division of parasitic diseases. Available at: http://www.cdc.gov/ncidod/dpd/parasites/naegleria.htm. Accessed October 18, 2007.

[29] Kahn C. Arizona teen becomes sixth victim this year of brain eating amoeba. Available at: http://www.foxnews.com/story/0,2933,298338,00.html. Accessed October 26, 2007.

[30] Pernin P, Pélandakis M, Rouby Y, et al. Comparative recoveries of Naegleria fowleri amoebae from seeded river water by filtration and centrifugation. Appl Environ Microbiol 1998; 64(3):955–9.

[31] US Food and Drug Administration, Department of Health and Human Services. Acanthamoeba spp., Naegleria fowleri and other Amoebae. Available at: http://www/cfsan.fda.gov/~mow/chap29.html. Accessed September 22, 2007.

[32] Marciano-Cabral F, Cabral GA. The immune response to Naegleria fowleri amebae and pathogenesis of infection. FEMS Immunol Med Microbiol 2007;51(2):243–59.

[33] Centers for Disease Control and Prevention. Primary amebic meningoencephalitis, Georgia, 2002. MMWR Morb Mortal Wkly Rep 2003;52(40):962–4.

[34] Seidel JS, Harmatz P, Visvesvara GS, et al. Successful treatment of primary amebic meningoencephalitis. N Engl J Med 1982;306:346–8.

[35] Stevens DL. Invasive group A streptococcus infections. Clin Infect Dis 1992;14:2–13.

[36] Laupland KB, Davies HD, Low DE, et al. Invasive group A streptococcal disease in children and association with varicella-zoster virus infection: Ontario Group A Streptococcal Study Group. Pediatrics 2000;105:E60.

[37] Hajjeh RA, Reingold A, Weil A, et al. Toxic shock syndrome in the United States: surveillance update, 1979–1996. Emerg Infect Dis 1999;5:807.

[38] Reduced incidence of menstrual toxic-shock syndrome: United States 1980–1990. MMWR Morb Mortal Wkly Rep 1990;39:421.

[39] O'Brien KL, Beall B, Barrett NL, et al. Epidemiology of invasive group A streptococcus disease in the United States, 1995–1999. Clin Infect Dis 2002;35:268.

[40] Reingold AL, Broome CV, Gaventa S, et al. Active surveillance for toxic shock syndrome in the United States, 1986. Rev Infect Dis 1989;11(Suppl 1):S28.

[41] Bartlett P, Reingold AL, Graham DR, et al. Toxic shock syndrome associated with surgical wound infections. JAMA 1982;247:1448.

[42] Schlievert PM. Role of superantigens in human disease. J Infect Dis 1993;167:997.

[43] Schlievert PM. Staphylococcal enterotoxin B and toxic-shock syndrome toxin-1 are significantly associated with non-menstrual TSS. Lancet 1986;1:1149.

[44] Bohach GA, Fast DJ, Nelson RD, et al. Staphylococcal and streptococcal pyrogenic toxins involved in toxic shock syndrome and related illnesses. Crit Rev Microbiol 1990; 17:251.

[45] Hauser AR, Stvens DL, Kaplan EL, et al. Molecular analysis of pyrogenic exotoxins from Streptococcus pyogenes isolates associated with toxic shock-like syndrome. J Clin Microbiol 1991;29:1562.

[46] Norrby-Teglund A, Newton D, Kotb M, et al. Superantigenic properties of the group A streptococcal exotoxin SpeF. Infect Immun 1994;62:5227.

[47] Case definitions for infectious conditions under public health surveillance. Centers for Disease Control and Prevention. MMWR Recomm Rep 1997;46(RR-10):1.

[48] Vuzevski VD, van Joost T, Wagenvoort JH, et al. Cutaneous pathology in toxic shock syndrome. Int J Dermatol 1989;28:94.

[49] Chesney PJ, Davis JP, Purdy WK, et al. Clinical manifestations of toxic shock syndrome. JAMA 1981;246:741.

[50] Kain KC, Schulzer M, Chow AW. Clinical spectrum of nonmenstrual toxic shock syndrome (TSS): comparison with menstrual TSS by multivariate discriminant analyses. Clin Infect Dis 1993;16:100.

[51] Bisno AL, Stevens DL. Streptococcal infections in skin and soft tissues. N Engl J Med 1996; 334:240.

[52] Davis JP, Chesney PJ, Want PJ, et al. Toxic shock syndrome. N Engl J Med 1980;303:1429.

[53] Reingold AL, Hargrett NT, Shands KN, et al. Toxic shock syndrome surveillance in the United States, 1980 to 1981. Ann Intern Med 1982;96:875.

[54] Davis JP, Osterholm MT, Helms CM, et al. Tri-state toxic-shock syndrome study. II. Clinical and laboratory findings. J Infect Dis 1982;145:441.

[55] Schlievert PM, Kelly JA. Clindamycin-induced suppression of toxic-shock syndrome: associated exotoxin production. J Infect Dis 1984;149:471.

[56] Stevens DL, Wallace RJ, Hamilton SM, et al. Successful treatment of staphylococcal toxic shock syndrome with linezolid: a case report and in vitro evaluation of the production of toxic shock syndrome toxin type 1 in the presence of antibiotics. Clin Infect Dis 2006;42:729.

[57] Eagle H. Experimental approach to the problem of treatment failure with penicillin. I. Group A streptococcal infection in mice. Am J Med 1952;13:389.

[58] Stevens DL, Bryant AE, Yan S. Invasive group A streptococcal infection: new concepts in antibiotic treatment. Int J Antimicrob Agents 1994;4:297.

[59] Mascini EM, Jansze M, Schouls LM, et al. Penicillin and clindamycin differentially inhibit the production of pyrogenic exotoxins A and B by group A streptococci. Int J Antimicrob Agents 2001;18:395.

[60] Gemmell CG, Peterson PK, Schmeling D, et al. Potentiation of opsonization and phagocytosis of *Streptococcus pyogenes* following growth in the presence of clindamycin. J Clin Invest 1981;67:1249.

[61] Zimbelman J, Palmer A, Todd J. Improved outcome of clindamycin compared with beta-lactam antibiotic treatment for invasive *Streptococcus pyogenes* infection. Pediatr Infect Dis J 1999;18:1096.

[62] Barry W, Hudgins L, Donta S, et al. Intravenous immunoglobulin therapy for toxic shock syndrome. JAMA 1992;267:3315.

[63] Darenberg J, Ihendyane N, Sjolin J, et al. Intravenous immunoglobulin G therapy in streptococcal toxic shock syndrome: a European randomized, double-blind, placebo-controlled trial. Clin Infect Dis 2003;37:333.

[64] Darenberg J, Soderquist B, Normark BH, et al. Differences in potency of intravenous polyspecific immunoglobulin G against streptococcal and staphylococcal superantigens: implications for therapy of toxic shock syndrome. Clin Infect Dis 2004;38:836.

[65] Todd JK, Ressman M, Caston SA, et al. Corticosteroid therapy for patients with toxic shock syndrome. JAMA 1984;252:3399.

[66] Benner EJ, Kayser FH. Growing clinical significance of methicillin-resistant *Staphylococcus aureus*. Lancet 1968;2:741.

[67] Moran GJ, Krishnadasan A, Gorwitz RJ, et al. Methicillin-resistant *S aureus* infections among patients in the emergency department. N Engl J Med 2006;355:666.

[68] Hidron AI, Kourbatova EV, Halvosa JS, et al. Risk factors for colonization with methicillin-resistant *Staphylococcus aureus* (MRSA) in patients admitted to an urban hospital: emergence of community-associated MRSA nasal carriage. Clin Infect Dis 2005;41:159.

[69] Salgado CD, Farr BM, Calfee DP. Community-acquired methicillin-resistant *Staphylococcus aureus*: a meta-analysis of prevalence and risk factors. Clin Infect Dis 2003;36:131.

[70] Lina G, Piedmont Y, Godail-Gamot F, et al. Involvement of Panton-Valentine leukocidin-producing *Staphylococcus aureus* in primary skin infections and pneumonia. Clin Infect Dis 1999;29(5):1128–32.

[71] Naimi TS, LeDell KH, Como-Sabetti K, et al. Comparison of community- and health care-associated methicillin-resistant *Staphylococcus aureus* infection. JAMA 2003;290: 2976.

[72] Boyle-Vavra S, Daum RS. Community-acquired methicillin-resistant *Staphylococcus aureus*: the role of Panton-Valentine leukocidin. Lab Invest 2007;87:3.

[73] Labandeira-Rey M, Couzon F, Boisset S, et al. *Staphylococcus aureus* Panton-Valentine leukocidin causes necrotizing pneumonia. Science 2007;315:1130.

[74] Francis JS, Doherty MC, Lopatin U, et al. Severe community-onset pneumonia in healthy adults caused by methicillin-resistant *Staphylococcus aureus* carrying the Panton-Valentine leukocidin genes. Clin Infect Dis 2005;40:100.

[75] Hageman JC. Severe community-acquired pneumonia due to *Staphylococcus aureus*, 2003–04 influenza season. Emerg Infect Dis 2006;12:894.

[76] Severe methicillin-resistant *Staphylococcus aureus* community-acquired pneumonia associated with influenza: Louisiana and Georgia, December 2006–January 2007. MMWR Morb Mortal Wkly Rep 2007;56:325.

[77] Dufour P, Gillet Y, Bes M, et al. Community-acquired methicillin-resistant *Staphylococcus aureus* infections in France: emergence of a single clone that produces Panton-Valentine leukocidin. Clin Infect Dis 2002;35:819.

[78] Sanford BA, Ramsay MA. Bacterial adherence to the upper respiratory tract of ferrets infected with influenza A virus. Proc Soc Exp Biol Med 1987;185:120–8.

[79] Tashiro M, Ciborowski P, Reinacher M, et al. Synergistic role of staphylococcal proteases in the induction of influenza virus pathogenicity. Virology 1987;157:421–30.

[80] Wunderink RG, Rello J, Cammarata SK, et al. Linezolid versus vancomycin: analysis of two double-blind studies of patients with methicillin-resistant *Staphylococcus aureus* nosocomial pneumonia. Chest 2003;124:1789–97.

[81] Micek ST, Dunne M, Kollef MH. Pleuropulmonary complications of Panton-Valentine leukocidin-positive community-acquired methicillin-resistant *Staphylococcus aureus*: importance of treatment with antimicrobials inhibiting exotoxin production. Chest 2005; 128(4):2732–8.

[82] Gillet Y, Vanhems P, Lina G, et al. Factors predicting mortality in necrotizing community-acquired pneumonia caused by *Staphylococcus aureus* containing Panton-Valentine leukocidin. Clin Infect Dis 2007;45(3):315–21.

[83] Gillet Y, Issartel B, Vanhems P, et al. Association between *Staphylococcus aureus* strains carrying gene for Panton-Valentine leukocidin and highly lethal necrotizing pneumonia in young immunocompetent persons. Lancet 2002;359:753.

[84] Moise PA, Schentag JJ. Vancomycin treatment failures in *Staphylococcus aureus* lower respiratory tract infection. Int J Antimicrob Agents 2000;16:S31–4.

[85] Stevens DL, Herr D, Lampiris H, et al. Linezolid versus vancomycin for the treatment of methicillin-resistant *Staphylococcus aureus* infections. Clin Infect Dis 2002;34: 1481–90.

[86] Kollef MH, Rello J, Cammarata SK, et al. Clinical cure and survival in gram-positive ventilator-associated pneumonia: retrospective analysis of two double-blind studies comparing linezolid with vancomycin. Intensive Care Med 2004;30:388–94.

[87] Rubinstein E, Cammarata SK, Oliphant TH, et al. Linezolid versus vancomycin in the treatment of hospitalized patients with nosocomial pneumonia: a randomized, double-blind, multicenter study. Clin Infect Dis 2001;32:402–12.

[88] Powers JH, Ross DB, Lin D, et al. Linezolid and vancomycin for methicillin-resistant *Staphylococcus aureus* nosocomial pneumonia. Chest 2004;126:314–6.

[89] Reimel BA, Krishnadasen B, Cuschieri J, et al. Surgical management of acute necrotizing lung infections. Can Respir J 2006;13(7):369–73.

[90] WHO Summary of probable SARS cases with onset of illness from 1 November 2002 to 31 July 2003. Geneva (Switzerland): World Health Organization; 2003. Available at: http://www.who.int/csr/sars/country/table2004_04_21/en/print.html. Accessed October 26, 2007.

[91] In the absence of SARS-CoV transmission worldwide: guidance for surveillance, clinical, and laboratory evaluation, and reporting version 2. Atlanta (GA): Centers for Disease Control; 2005. Available at: http://www.cdc.gov/ncidod/sars/absenceofsars.htm. Accessed October 26, 2007.

[92] Wong RS, David SH. Index patient and SARS outbreak in Hong Kong. Emerg Infect Dis 2004;10:339–41.

[93] Hsu LY, Lee CC, Green JA, et al. Severe Acute Respiratory syndrome (SARS) in Singapore: clinical features of index patient and initial contacts. Emerg Infect Dis 2003;9:713–7.

[94] Lee N, Hui D, Wu A, et al. A major outbreak of severe acute respiratory syndrome in Hong Kong. N Engl J Med 2003;348:1986–94.

[95] Booth CM, Matukas LM, Tomlinson GA, et al. Clinical features and short-term outcomes of 144 patients with SARS in the greater Toronto area. JAMA 2003;289:2801–9.

[96] Chan PK, To WK, Ng KC, et al. Laboratory diagnosis of SARS. Emerg Infect Dis 2004;10: 825–31.

[97] WHO hospital infection control guidance for severe acute respiratory syndrome. Geneva (Switzerland): World Health Organization; 2003. Available at: http://www.who.int/csr/sars/infectioncontrol/en/. Accessed October 26, 2007.

[98] Avian influenza: current situation. Atlanta (GA): Centers for Disease Control; 2007. Available at: http://www.cdc.gov/flu/avian/outbreaks/current.htm. Accessed October 26, 2007.

[99] WHO cumulative number of confirmed human cases of avian influenza A/(H5N1) reported to WHO. Geneva (Switzerland): World Health Organization; 2007. Available at: http://www.who.int/xsr/disease/avian_influenza/country/cases_table_2007_10_25/en/print/. Accessed October 26, 2007.

[100] Hien TT, Liem NT, Dung NT, et al. Avian influenza A (H5N1) in 10 patients in Vietnam. N Engl J Med 2004;350:1179–88.

[101] Oner AF, Bay A, Arslan S, et al. Avian influenza A (H5N1) in Eastern Turkey in 2006. N Engl J Med 2006;355:2179–85.

[102] WHO clinical management of human infection with avian influenza A (H5N1) virus. Geneva (Switzerland): World Health Organization; 2007. Available at: http://www.who.int/csr/disease/avian_influenza/guidelines/clinicalmanage07/en/index.html. Accessed October 26, 2007.

[103] Centers for Disease Control. Embargo of birds from specified countries. Atlanta (GA): Centers for Disease Control; 2007. Available at: http://www.cdc.gov/flu/avian/outbreaks/embargo.htm. Accessed October 26, 2007.

[104] Interim recommendations for infection control in health care facilities caring for patients with known or suspected avian influenza. Atlanta (GA): Centers for Disease Control; 2004. Available at: http://www.cdc.gov/flu/avian/professional/infect-control.htm. Accessed October 26, 2007.

ELSEVIER
SAUNDERS

Emerg Med Clin N Am
38 (2008) 281–317

EMERGENCY
MEDICINE
CLINICS OF
NORTH AMERICA

Acute Bacterial Meningitis

Sharon E. Mace, MD, FACEP, FAAP[a,b,c,d],*

[a]*Cleveland Clinic Lerner College of Medicine of Case Western Reserve University, E19, Cleveland Clinic, 9500 Euclid Avenue, Cleveland, OH 44195, USA*
[b]*Cleveland Clinic/MetroHealth Medical Center Emergency Medicine Residency, E19, Cleveland Clinic, 9500 Euclid Avenue, Cleveland, OH 44195, USA*
[c]*Pediatric Education/Quality Improvement, Cleveland Clinic, Cleveland, OH, USA*
[d]*Observation Unit, Emergency Services Institute, E19, Cleveland Clinic, 9500 Euclid Avenue, Cleveland, OH 44195, USA*

In spite of the availability of antibiotics and the introduction of vaccines for immunoprophylaxis, bacterial meningitis remains a common disease worldwide, with high morbidity and mortality. Meningitis can occur at any age and in previously healthy individuals, although some patients have an increased risk of meningitis including: the immunosuppressed patient and patients at the extremes of age; young children, especially infants; and geriatric patients. The clinical triad of meningitis—fever, neck stiffness, and altered mental status—is, unfortunately, present in less than half of adult patients who have bacterial meningitis. Furthermore, certain patient populations, such as infants (especially neonates) and the elderly, often have a subtle presentation with nonspecific signs and symptoms. Analysis of cerebrospinal fluid (CSF) remains the key to diagnosis. The goal of therapy remains the early administration of appropriate antibiotics, although in selected patients, adjuvant therapy with dexamethasone also may be administered.

Etiology

Meningitis, also termed arachnoiditis or leptomeningitis, is an inflammation of the membranes that surround the brain and spinal cord, thereby involving the arachnoid, the pia mater, and the interposed CSF. The inflammatory process extends throughout the subarachnoid space around the brain, the spinal cord, and the ventricles (Fig. 1).

---

* Corresponding author. Department of Emergency Medicine, E19, Cleveland Clinic, 9500 Euclid Avenue, Cleveland, OH 44195.
E-mail address: maces@ccf.org

0733-8627/08/$ - see front matter © 2008 Elsevier Inc. All rights reserved.
doi:10.1016/j.emc.2008.02.002
emed.theclinics.com

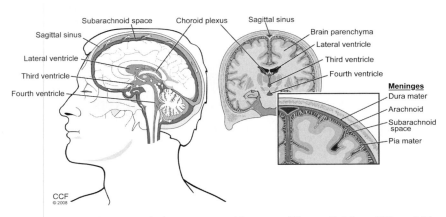

Fig. 1. Anatomy of the central nervous system. (*Courtesy of* Sharon E. Mace, MD, and Mr. Dave Schumick, of the Cleveland Clinic Center for Art and Photography; with permission.)

Meningitis has been divided into bacterial meningitis and aseptic meningitis. Bacterial or pyogenic meningitis is an acute meningeal inflammation secondary to a bacterial infection that generally evokes a polymorphonuclear response in the CSF. Aseptic meningitis refers to a meningeal inflammation without evidence of pyogenic bacterial infection on Gram's stain or culture, usually accompanied by a mononuclear pleocytosis (Fig. 2). Aseptic meningitis is subdivided into two categories: nonbacterial meningeal infections (typically viral or fungal meningitis), and noninfectious meningeal inflammation from systemic diseases (such as sarcoidosis), neoplastic disease (leptomeningeal carcinomatosis or neoplastic meningitis), or drugs.

Epidemiology

Bacterial meningitis is a common disease worldwide. Meningitis still has high morbidity and mortality in spite of the introduction and widespread use of antibiotics and other advances in medical care [1]. In the United States and in other countries, epidemics of acute meningococcal meningitis are a common occurrence, while in parts of sub-Saharan Africa (meningitis belt) meningococcal meningitis is endemic [2]. In the United States, the overall incidence of meningitis is about 2 to 10 cases per 100,000 population per year [3–5], although the attack rates are very age-specific. The incidence is greatest in pediatric patients, especially infants, with attack rates in neonates at about 400 per 100,000, compared with 1 to 2 per 100,000 in adults and 20 per 100,000 in those less than or equal to 2 years old [6].

Specific pathogens

The relative frequency of the different causative organisms has changed in recent years. The epidemiology of bacterial meningitis has changed

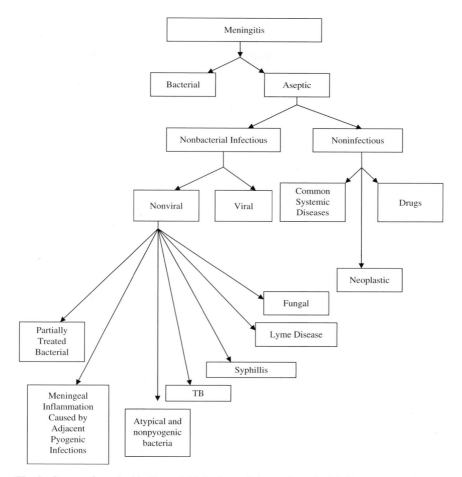

Fig. 2. Causes of meningitis. Bacterial infections of the cerebrospinal fluid (CSF) usually have a positive CSF Gram stain, positive CSF bacterial culture, and increased polymorphonuclear leukocytes in CSF. Aseptic meningitis usually has mononuclear leukocytes in CSF with a negative CSF Gram's stain and negative CSF bacterial culture. (*Courtesy of* Sharon E. Mace, MD, and Dave Schumick, of the Cleveland Clinic Center for Art and Photography; with permission.)

significantly, primarily because of widespread immunization with new vaccines. The conjugated *Haemophilus influenzae* vaccine (HIB) was introduced in the United States in the early 1990s [7], and in 2000, the *Streptococcus pneumoniae* vaccine was approved by the US Food and Drug Administration (FDA) [8]. Before the introduction of these vaccines, *H influenzae* accounted for nearly half of all bacteria meningitis cases (45%), followed by *S pneumoniae* (18%) and then *Neisseria meningitidis* (14%) [9]. After the introduction of the HIB vaccine, the most common pathogens were *S pneumoniae* (47%), *N meningitidis* (25%), group B streptococcus (12%), and *Listeria monocytogenes* (8%) (Table 1) [4]. It is likely that the most

Table 1
Pathogens responsible for bacterial meningitis

Before introduction of Haemophilus influenza type B vaccines[a]		After introduction of Haemophilus influenza type B vaccines[b]	
H influenzae	45%	Streptococcus pneumoniae	47%
Streptococcus pneumoniae	18%	Neisseria meningitidis	25%
N meningitidis	14%	Group B streptococcus (S agalactiae)	12%
Group B streptococcus (S agalactiae)	6%	Listeria monocytogenes	8%
Listeria monocytogenes	3%	H influenzae	7%
Others	14%	Others	1%
Children <5 years old (>70% H influenzae)			

[a] Percentages taken from Wenger JD, Hightower AW, Facklam RR, et al. Bacterial meningitis in the United States, 1986: report of a multistate surveillance study. The Bacterial Meningitis Study Group. J Infect Dis 1990;162(6):1316–22.
[b] Percentages taken from Schuchat A, Robinson K, Wenger JD, et al. Bacterial meningitis in the United States in 1995. Active surveillance team. New Engl J Med 1997;337(14):970–6.

recent addition of the S pneumoniae vaccine will change the specific epidemiology of bacterial meningitis again.

H influenzae was previously the most common cause of bacterial meningitis and the most common cause of acquired mental retardation in the United States [7]. S pneumoniae has supplanted H influenzae as the pathogen causing most bacterial meningitis cases in the United States [4]. S pneumoniae is the most frequent cause of bacterial meningitis in adults ages 19 to 59 years and greater than or equal to 60 years, and in infants/very young children excluding neonates (eg, age 1 to 23 months) [4].

N meningitidis was previously the third most common cause of bacterial meningitis in the United States [9] but has now moved into second place behind S pneumoniae, and it accounts for 25% of all cases of bacterial meningitis [4]. It remains to be seen whether the widespread use of the pneumococcal vaccines decreases the incidence of S pneumoniae meningitis, thereby allowing N meningitidis and L monocytogenes and other bacteria to become the prevailing pathogens causing bacterial meningitis. The widespread use of the pneumococcal vaccine beginning in infancy has decreased the incidence of invasive disease by S pneumoniae by more than 90% [10].

Clinical presentation

Signs and symptoms of meningitis include: fever, headache, stiff neck, confusion or altered mental status, lethargy, malaise, seizures, and vomiting. About 25% of adults have a classic presentation and are not a diagnostic dilemma [6]. Unfortunately, many patients have a less obvious presentation.

Furthermore, certain patients—typically the pediatric patient, especially infants; the elderly; and the immunosuppressed—may not have the classic features of meningitis. These patients often have a subtle presentation and nonspecific clinical signs/symptoms. Patients partially treated with antibiotics in addition to patients at the extremes of age (the very young and the elderly) and the immunocompromised may not have a fever.

The classic triad is fever, neck stiffness, and altered mental status. Yet in an adult study of community-acquired bacterial meningitis, less than half of the patients (44%) had the classic triad. Ninety-five percent of the patients, however, had at least two of the four symptoms of neck stiffness, fever, headache, and altered mental status [11].

A stiff neck or nuchal rigidity is caused by meningeal irritation with resistance to passive neck flexion. Although this finding is a classic sign of meningitis, it may be present only 30% of the time [12].

Positive Kernig's and Brudzinski's signs are hallmarks of meningitis, yet Kernig's and Brudzinski's signs were present in only about half of adults with meningitis [5]. With the patient supine and the thigh flexed to a 90° right angle, attempts to straighten or extend the leg are met with resistance (Kernig's sign). There are two Brudzinski's signs in patients who have meningitis. Flexion of the neck causes involuntary flexion of the knees and hips (Brudzinski's sign). Passive flexion of the leg on one side causes contralateral flexion of the opposite leg (known as Brudzinski's sign or contralateral sign or contralateral reflex).

Confusion suggests possible meningitis, as does an abnormal mental status plus fever. Meningitis also should be in the differential diagnosis when the combination of fever plus a seizure occurs. Seizures occur in 5% to 28% of adults who have meningitis [1,13,14]. Seizures are the presenting symptom in one-third of pediatric patients who have bacterial meningitis [15]. In childhood meningitis, seizures occur more frequently with *S pneumoniae* and *H influenzae* B than with meningococcal meningitis [15].

Petechiae and purpura generally are associated with meningococcal meningitis, although these skin manifestations may be present with any bacterial meningitis [16].

Signs and symptoms in infants can be particularly subtle. They may have only a fever or be hypothermic, or even afebrile. They may not have a stiff neck. The chief complaint of an infant who has meningitis is often nonspecific and includes: irritability, lethargy, poor feeding, fever, seizures, apnea, a rash, or a bulging fontanelle [17].

In geriatric patients, frequently the only presenting sign of meningitis is confusion or an altered mental status [18].

The onset of presentation varies with meningitis. Typically, the adult who has acute bacterial meningitis seeks medical care within a few hours to several days after illness onset. The presentation differs, however, depending on many variables, including: age, underlying comorbidity, immunocompetence, mental competence, ability to communicate, prior antibiotic therapy, and the specific bacterial pathogen. The onset of viral meningitis or viral meningoencephalitis is also generally acute over hours to days, but sometimes is preceded by a nonspecific febrile illness of a few days' duration.

Patients who have subacute or chronic meningitis present over weeks to months, and even years. Generally, the onset is more gradual, with a lower fever, and there may or may not be associated lethargy or disability. Fungal (eg, *Cryptococcus* and *Coccidoides*) and mycobacterium are typical causes of subacute and chronic meningitis.

The clinical presentation of meningitis also has been categorized as fulminant (10%) or insidious (90%). Patients who have an insidious onset often have been seen by a medical care provider and given a diagnosis of a nonspecific or viral illness days before their diagnosis of meningitis is made and frequently have been partially treated with oral antibiotics for an infection such as otitis, sinusitis, or bronchitis. The delay in diagnosis of meningitis in such patients is up to 2 weeks, with a median of 36 to 72 hours.

Risk factors for bacterial meningitis

Age and demographics

Meningitis can occur at any age and in previously healthy individuals. There are some risk factors that predispose the individual to meningitis, however (Box 1). Host risk factors can be grouped into four categories: age, demographic/socioeconomic factors, exposure to pathogens, and immunosuppression. Patients at the extremes of age: the elderly (age over 60 years) and pediatric patients (young children age younger than 5 years, especially infants/neonates) have an increased susceptibility to meningitis [16,18]. Demographic and socioeconomic factors include: male gender, African American race, low socioeconomic class, and crowding (eg, military recruits and college students in dormitories) [19].

Immunocompromised patients

There is an association between immunosuppression and an increased risk for bacterial meningitis. Immunosuppressive conditions include: diabetes, alcoholism, cirrhosis/liver disease, asplenia or status postsplenectomy, hematologic disorders (eg, sickle cell disease, thalassemia major), malignancy, immunologic disorders (complement deficiency, immunoglobulin deficiency), HIV, and immunosuppressive drug therapy (Table 2) [19,20].

Mechanism of entry into the central nervous system

There are several mechanisms by which organisms gain entry to the CSF, most commonly by means of hematogenous spread, but also by contiguous

---

Box 1. Risk factors for meningitis

Age
- Extremes of age: elderly (age >60 years); young children (age <5 years), especially infants/neonates

Demographic/socioeconomic
- Male gender
- African American ethnicity
- Low socioeconomic status
- Crowding: military recruits, crowded dormitories

Exposure to pathogens
- Recent colonization
- Household/close contact with meningitis patient
- Contiguous infection: sinusitis, mastoiditis, otitis media
- Bacterial endocarditis
- Intravenous drug abuse
- Dural defect: status post neurosurgery, central nervous system (CNS) trauma, congenital defect
- Ventriculoperitoneal shunt, other CNS devices
- Cochlear implants

Immunosuppression
- Status post splenectomy
- Hematologic disorders: sickle cell disease, thalassemia major
- Malignancy
- Diabetes
- Alcoholism/cirrhosis
- Immunologic disorder: complement deficiencies, immunoglobulin deficiency
- HIV
- Immunosuppressive drug therapy

---

spread and infrequently by direct entry. Factors that aid the organism in gaining entry to the CSF include:

- Recent colonization
- Close contact with a patient who has meningitis
- Contiguous infection (eg, sinusitis, mastoiditis, otitis media)
- Hematogenous seeding of the CSF (eg, intravenous drug abuse, bacterial endocarditis)
- Disruption of dura,
- Status post neurosurgery
- Penetrating CNS trauma
- Congenital defects

Table 2
Common bacterial pathogens and empiric therapy based on age, clinical setting, and risk factors

Age pediatric	Common pathogens	Empiric therapy	Alternative empiric therapy
Neonate (≤30 days)	Group B streptococcus Gram negatives: (*Escherichia coli, Klebsiella*) *Listeria*	Ampicillin + third generation cephalosporin (cefotaxime)	Ampicillin + aminoglycoside (gentamicin)
Children 1–23 months	*Streptococcus pneumoniae* *Neisseria meningitidis* Group B streptococcus *Haemophilus influenzae* *Escherichia coli*	Third generation cephalosporin (cefotaxime or ceftriaxone) + vancomycin[a]	Meropenem (carbapenem) + vancomycin[a]
Children 2–18 years	*S pneumoniae* *N meningitidis*	Third generation cephalosporin (cefotaxime or ceftriaxone) + vancomycin[a]	Carbapenem (meropenem) + vancomycin[a]
Age adult			
Young and middle-aged adults (18–50 years)	*S pneumoniae* *N meningitidis*	Third generation cephalosporin (cefotaxime or ceftriaxone) + vancomycin[a]	Carbapenem (meropenem) ± vancomycin[a]
Age >50 years (includes elderly)	*S pneumoniae* *N meningitidis* *Listeria monocytogenes*	Third-generation cephalosporin (cefotaxime or ceftriaxone) + vancomycin[a] + ampicillin	Third generation cephalosporin (cefotaxime or ceftriaxone) + vancomycin[a] + trimethoprim-sulfamethoxazole
Special considerations			
Impaired immunity (such as HIV)	*S pneumoniae* Gram-negative bacilli *L monocytogenes*	Third generation cephalosporin (ceftazidime) + vancomycin[a] + ampicillin	Carbapenem (meropenem) + vancomycin[a] + trimethoprim-sulfamethoxazole

Status post neurosurgery or penetrating trauma	*Staphylococcus aureus* Coagulase-negative staphylococci Aerobic gram-negative bacilli (eg, *Pseudomonas aeruginosa*)	Fourth generation cephalosporin (cefepime) ± vancomycin[a]	Third generation cephalosporin (ceftazidime) + vancomycin[a] or carbapenem (meropenem) + vancomycin[a]
Cerebrospinal fluid leak or basilar skull fracture	*S pneumoniae* Streptococci (various) *H influenzae*	Third generation cephalosporin (cefotaxime or ceftriaxone) + vancomycin[a]	Carbapenem (meropenem) + vancomycin[a]
Cerebrospinal fluid shunt (eg, VP shunt)	Coagulase-negative staphylococci *Staphylococcus aureus* Aerobic gram-negative bacilli (eg, *P aeruginosa*, *Propionibacterium acnes*)	Fourth generation cephalosporin (cefepime) + vancomycin[a]	Third generation cephalosporin (ceftazidime) + vancomycin[a]

[a] Some recommend the addition of rifampin when vancomycin and dexamethasone are coadministered.

- CSF shunts (eg, ventricular shunts)
- Other devices (eg, epidural catheters, Ommaya reservoirs, intracranial monitoring devices, external ventricular drains)

Postoperative neurosurgical patients and patients who have penetrating head trauma are at risk for meningitis caused by staphylococci [21]. Bacterial meningitis in patients who have a ventriculoperitoneal shunt commonly is caused by staphylococci, especially coagulase-negative strains, and gram-negative organisms [21–23]. Patients who have a cochlear implant have a greatly increased risk (greater than 30-fold) of pneumococcal meningitis [24].

Neonatal meningitis

Neonatal (age less than or equal to 1 month) meningitis is caused by the same organisms that cause bacteremia and sepsis in newborns: commonly; group-B β-hemolytic streptococci, gram-negative enteric bacteria, and *L monocytogenes*. After the first few weeks of life, *S pneumoniae* and *H influenzae* emerge as common pathogens also. The pathogenesis of neonatal meningitis probably results from a maternal–fetal infection, either by direct inoculation during the birth process or hematogenously (transplacental). There are predisposing maternal and infant risk factors for neonatal meningitis. Infant factors are prematurity and low birth weight. Maternal factors include: prolonged rupture of membranes, maternal urinary tract infection, chorioamnionitis, and endometritis [25]. Neonatal meningitis is frequently a component of a sepsis syndrome whereby bacteremia seeds the CSF.

Neonates do not have a completely functional immune system, which predisposes them to infections. Multiple factors cause impaired functioning of the polymorphonuclear neutrophils (PMNs), including decreased chemotactic ability of PMNs, decreased adhesion of PMNs to surfaces, and impaired mobility of PMNs. Newborns receive an incomplete range of antibody transmitted across the placenta. Although some IgG is received transplacentally, there is only a small amount of antibody to gram-negative bacteria and no IgM. Under conditions of stress, preliminary data suggest there is decreased phagocytosis of gram-negative bacteria and decreased killing of group B streptococci and *Escherichia coli*. In addition to impaired function of PMNs, most newborns have a functional deficiency of the alternate pathway of the complement system [26].

Geriatric meningitis

The elderly have many risk factors that predispose patients to infections. Numerous chronic illnesses and comorbid conditions, and polypharmacy and immunosuppressive medications, are associated with aging [27]. The decline in immune system function that occurs in the elderly includes a decrease in both T lymphocyte function and cell-mediated immunity [28]. Environmental factors, such as incontinence, indwelling catheters, and impaired mental status predispose to aspiration and ulcers, which lead to infections that can progress to bacteremia and hematogenous seeding of the meninges [29]. Nursing home residents can be a reservoir for antimicrobial-resistant pathogens including methicillin-resistant *Staphylococcus aureus* (MRSA) and vancomycin-resistant *Enterococcus* (VRE) [29,30].

The elderly often have a subtle clinical presentation of meningitis [18]. The geriatric patient who has meningitis is less likely to have neck stiffness and meningeal signs, and more likely to have mental status changes, seizures, neurologic deficits, and even hydrocephalus [31,32]. The elderly patient who has meningitis may not have a high fever and may even be afebrile. The mental status changes that can occur in geriatric patients who have meningitis frequently are ascribed to other conditions from delirium to psychosis, senility, a transient ischemia attack, or a stroke. Fever, when present, may be mistakenly attributed to pneumonia, a urinary tract infection, viral illness, bronchitis, bacteremia, or sepsis, especially because classic signs and symptoms of meningitis are often lacking in the elderly patient.

Conversely, the geriatric patient also may have false-positive findings of meningitis. Signs and symptoms of meningeal irritation such as nuchal rigidity or a positive Kernig's sign or Brudzinski's sign may be found in healthy elderly people [33]. This false-positive finding is attributed to the presence of limited neck mobility and cervical spine disease. Thus, classic signs and symptoms of meningeal irritation are unreliable in the elderly and make the diagnosis of meningitis more difficult [32–34]. Meningitis in the elderly, as in neonates, (eg, in the extremes of age) frequently is associated with a delay in diagnosis and has a high mortality rate [25,26,32,34].

Pathophysiology

Pathogens enter the CNS either by hematogenous spread (the most common method) or by direct extension from a contiguous site (Fig. 3). Most organisms that cause meningitis are able to colonize the upper respiratory tract by attaching to the host's nasopharyngeal mucosal epithelium. The next step is to evade the host's complement system, which allows invasion into the neighboring intravascular space. The pathogens then cross the blood–brain barrier to enter the CSF. Because the host defense mechanisms within the CSF are poor, the pathogens can proliferate. In attempt to defend against the invading organisms, a cascade of inflammatory events is set into motion by the body's immune defense mechanisms.

The bacteria that cause meningitis have properties that enhance their virulence, which accounts, at least partly, for their ability to cause meningitis. The bacteria: *H influenza, N meningitidis,* and *S pneumoniae,* all make immunoglobulin A proteases. Such proteases inactivate the host's immunoglobulin A by cleaving the antibody. This destruction of immunoglobulin

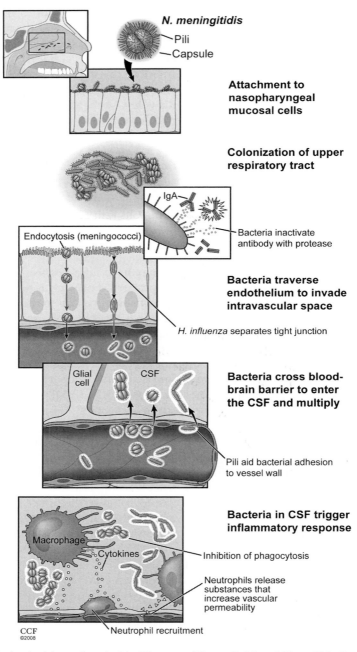

Fig. 3. Pathophysiology of meningitis. (*Courtesy of* Sharon E. Mace, MD, and Mr. Dave Schumick, of the Cleveland Clinic Center for Art and Photography; with permission.)

A antibody inactivates the host's local antibody defense, which allows bacterial adherence to the nasopharyngeal mucosa and colonization. Adhesion to the host's nasopharyngeal mucosal epithelial cells by *N meningitidis* occurs by means of fimbria or pili. When the ciliated cells of the host are damaged, as occurs from a viral upper respiratory infection or with smoking, their ability to prevent mucosal adhesion by invading bacteria is limited. The pathogens enter the intravascular space by various mechanisms. Meningococci by the process of endocytosis traverse the endothelium in membrane bound vacuoles. *H influenzae* separates the apical tight junctions between epithelial cells to invade the mucosa and gain access to the intravascular space.

Encapsulated bacteria, (eg, *S pneumoniae, H influenzae,* and *N meningitidis*) avoid destruction by their host once they are in the bloodstream, because their polysaccharide capsule inhibits phagocytosis and complement-mediated bactericidal activity.

Once the bacteria are in the bloodstream, bacterial adhesion to structures of the blood–brain barrier are aided by structural qualities of the bacteria such as the fimbria with some *E coli strains*, and the pili and fimbria with *N meningitidis*.

Because of poor host defenses in the CSF, the bacteria quickly multiply after gaining entry to the CSF. Multiple factors account for inadequate host defense mechanisms within the CSF, including: low complement levels, low immunoglobulin levels, and decreased opsonic activity, all of which result in the host's inability to destroy the bacteria by phagocytosis.

Bacterial components in the CSF trigger an inflammatory cascade in the host. Proinflammatory cytokines—interleukin (IL)-1, tumor necrosis factor (TNF), and others—are released by various cells including macrophages, microglia, meningeal cells, and endothelial cells. Cytokines, in turn, promote the migration of neutrophils into the CSF by several mechanisms. Cytokines increase the binding affinity of leukocytes for endothelial cells, and induce adhesion molecules that interact with leukocyte receptors.

Once they are in the CSF, neutrophils release substances (eg, prostaglandins, toxic oxygen metabolites, matrix metalloproteinases) that increase vascular permeability and even may cause direct neurotoxicity. The inflammatory cascade leads to abnormalities in cerebral blood flow and cerebral edema. The forces leading to cerebral edema include: vasogenic edema from increased permeability of the blood–brain barrier, cytotoxic edema caused by cellular swelling from the toxic substances released by bacteria and neutrophils, and occasionally from obstruction to CSF outflow at the arachnoid villi. Early in meningitis, cerebral blood flow increases, but later decreases, which can cause further neurologic damage. Local vascular inflammation or thrombosis can cause localized cerebral hypoperfusion. Autoregulation of cerebral blood flow can be impaired. Herniation of the brain and death can result from the increased intracranial pressure.

Management

After stabilization of the patient (including airway, breathing, circulation), the priority in the treatment of acute bacterial meningitis is the prompt administration of an appropriate bactericidal antibiotic(s) that has rapid entry into the subarachnoid space. In the emergency department, the specific pathogen usually is not known, so empiric therapy is the rule. In some cases, an anti-inflammatory agent (eg, dexamethasone, which suppresses the body's usual inflammatory reaction) also is given (see section on adjuvant therapy). Administration of antibiotics should not be delayed. If any delay, however, is expected for any reason, including a CT scan, then blood cultures should be obtained and empiric antibiotics given (see Table 2, Table 3).

Complications

Acute complications are common with bacterial meningitis (Box 2, Fig. 4). Patients may have an altered mental status or even be comatose. They may present in shock. About 15% of pediatric patients who had pneumococcal meningitis presented in shock [35]. Shock and/or disseminated intravascular coagulation (DIC) frequently are associated with meningococcal meningitis. Apnea and/or respiratory failure/distress can occur with bacterial meningitis, especially in infants.

Seizures occur in about one-third of patients who have bacterial meningitis [16]. Seizures that persist (longer than 4 days) or begin late tend to be associated with neurologic sequelae. Focal seizures carry a worse prognosis than generalized seizures. Focal seizures should raise concern for complications such as subdural empyema, brain abscess, or increased intracranial pressure, and suggest a need for neuroimaging. Subdural effusions, which are common (occurring in one-third of pediatric patients), are generally asymptomatic, resolve spontaneously, and have no permanent neurologic sequelae. The syndrome of inappropriate antidiuretic hormone (SIADH) can occur, so the electrolytes and fluid status should be monitored closely.

All of these complications—shock, DIC, altered mental status to coma, respiratory distress, seizures, increased intracranial pressure, SIADH, and other symptoms—should be managed with the usual therpay.

Diagnostic evaluation

Lumbar puncture

CSF is essential to confirm the diagnosis and institute specific antibiotic therapy (Table 4). In most patients who have acute bacterial meningitis, a lumbar puncture (LP) can be done safely without prior neuroimaging studies. The concern is that an LP, in a patient who has increased intracranial pressure, can have adverse effects even death [36]. If a patient presents with an acute fulminating febrile illness consistent with bacterial meningitis, early antibiotic therapy is warranted, because early therapy is thought to improve the prognosis and decrease morbidity and mortality. When confronted with such a patient, the recommendation is either: immediate LP, then give the initial antibiotic dose; or administer empiric antibiotics, obtain head CT scan, then do the LP. Criteria have been suggested for obtaining a head CT scan prior to the LP in suspected bacterial meningitis. The criteria are:

- Head trauma
- Immunocompromised state
- Recent seizure (within the last 7 days)
- Abnormal level of consciousness
- Focal weakness, abnormal speech
- Abnormal visual fields or gaze paresis
- Inability to follow commands or answer questions appropriately
- A history of any of the following: mass lesions, focal infection, or stroke [37]

An absolute contraindication to an LP is the presence of infection in the tissues near the puncture site. A relative contraindication to an LP is increased intracranial pressure (ICP) from a space-occupying lesion, especially when progressive signs of herniation such as unilateral cranial nerve III palsy or lateralizing signs (hemiparesis), are present [38]. The risk of herniation appears to be greater if the patient has a brain abscess [39,40]. A reduction in pressure in the spinal canal has been associated with seizures, stupor, cardiorespiratory collapse, and even sudden death in patients who have impending herniation [38].

If the procedure is essential (as with suspected meningitis), and because platelet transfusion (for thrombocytopenia) and replacement of clotting factors (for hemophilia and other disorders) can be done prior to the LP, the presence of a coagulopathy is only a relative contraindication [41]. If the patient has a coagulopathy, some experts recommend that the LP be done by experienced clinicians who are less likely to have a difficult or complicated LP that results in localized trauma to the dura. A study in children who had thrombocytopenia secondary to acute lymphoblastic leukemia documented the safety of LP in thrombocytopenic patients (without platelet transfusion prior to the LP), although less than 1% of patients had a platelet count less than or equal to 10×10^9 [42].

Of course, cardiorespiratory instability of the patient is another contraindication, although the ABCs should be dealt with before the LP. Evidence of spinal cord trauma and/or spinal cord compression would be another contraindication to an LP.

When considering bacterial meningitis, CSF should be sent for: Gram's stain and cultures, cell count with differential, glucose, and protein, and other studies as indicated. If an organism can be identified on the Gram's stain then empiric therapy can be based on this finding (see Table 3). CSF findings suggestive of bacterial meningitis are:

- Positive Gram's stain (organism identified on slide)
- Glucose less than 40 mg/dL or ratio of CSF/blood glucose less than 0.40

Table 3
Likely bacterial pathogen and antibiotic of choice based on cerebrospinal fluid Gram's stain results

Gram stain					
Positive/negative	Appearance				
Gram-positive					
±	Shape	Appearance	Bacterial pathogen	Antibiotic of choice	Dose
+	Cocci	Paired diplococci	*Streptococcus pneumoniae*	Penicillin G (if sensitive) or chloramphenicol + vancomycin + rifampin	Penicillin: adult 4 million units every 6 h; pediatric 100,000 U/kg every 6 h Chloramphenicol: 50 mg/kg every 6 h (maximum 1 g dose) Vancomycin: adult 1 g every dose; pediatric 15 mg/kg every 8-12 h (maximum 1 g every dose, 4 g/d) Rifampin: adult 600 mg/d; pediatric 5-10 mg/kg every dose given once or twice daily
+	Cocci	Single, doubles, tetrads, clusters	Staphylococci	Nafcillin or oxacillin (if methicillin-sensitive) or vancomycin (if methicillin-resistant)	Nafcillin or oxacillin: adult 1-2 g every 6 h; pediatric 25-50 mg/kg every 6 h (maximum 12 g/d) Vancomycin: adult 1 g every dose; pediatric 15 mg/kg every 8-12 h (maximum 1 g every dose, 4 g/d)

Gram stain		Organism	Appearance	Treatment	Dosing
+	Cocci	Other streptococci (β hemolytic streptococci)	Pairs and chain	Penicillin G (if sensitive) or ampicillin	Penicillin: adult 4 million units every 6 h; pediatric 100,000 U/kg every 6 h Ampicillin: 100 mg/kg 6 hrs (maximum 2 g per dose)
+	Rods	Listeria monocytogenes	Single or chains	Ampicillin + gentamycin or trimethoprim-sulfamethoxazole	Ampicillin: 100 mg/kg every 6 h (maximum 2 g per dose) Gentamycin: adult 1–2 mg/kg every 8 h; pediatric 2.5 mg/kg every 8–12 h (max 1 g q dose, 4g qd) Trimethoprim-sulfamethoxazale: 5 mg/kg every 12 h (based on trimethoprim component)
Gram-negative −	Cocci	Neisseria meningitidis	Kidney or coffee bean appearance cocci or paired diplococci	Penicillin G (if sensitive) or chloramphenicol	Penicillin: adult 4 million units every 6 h; pediatric 100,000 U/kg every 6 h Chloramphenicol: 50 mg/kg every 6 h (maximum 1 every dose)
−	Coccobacilli	Haemophilus influenzae	Coccobacilli or pleomorphic bacilli	Ceftriaxone or cefotaxime + meropenem or chloramphenicol	Ceftriaxone: 50 mg/kg every 12 h Cefotaxime: 50 mg/kg every 6 h Meropenem: 40 mg/kg every 8 h (maximum 2 g every dose) Chloramphenicol: 50 mg/kg every 6 h (maximum 1 g every dose)

(continued on next page)

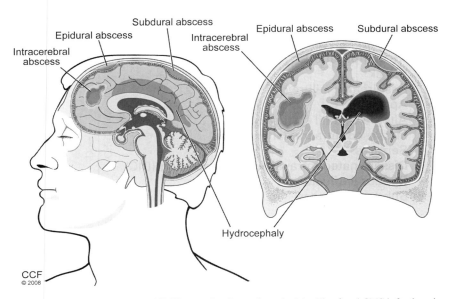

Fig. 4. Central nervous system (CNS) complications of meningitis. Also focal CNS infections in the differential diagnosis for meningitis. (*Courtesy of* Sharon E. Mace, MD, and Mr. Dave Schumick, of the Cleveland Clinic Center for Art and Photography; with permission.)

One caveat to remember is that the CSF findings in bacterial meningitis may not always yield the classic results. Reasons for a lack of classic CSF findings in bacterial meningitis include:

- Partially treated meningitis (eg, prior antibiotics)
- Time of LP (is it early in course of the disease before the patient mounts a response, or late in the course?)
- The patient's condition (is the patient able to mount a response to the invading organism or is the patient immunosuppressed or has an overwhelming infection?)

Thus, the typical CSF findings may not be present in every patient who has bacterial meningitis and may even show a normal WBC in the CSF and/or lymphocyte predominance, especially if early in the disease (see Table 4) [43]. Therefore, if there is any concern that the clinical diagnosis is meningitis, it is better to treat for bacterial meningitis (specifically, give parental antibiotics and admit for close observation while awaiting culture [CSF and blood] results) [44]. In the past, repeat LP was done routinely to follow the course of bacterial meningitis and to document sterilization of the CSF, but now repeat LP is done only if there is a specific concern or indication [45], such as when a hospitalized patient who has bacterial meningitis on appropriate antibiotics is not improving.

Additional CSF studies may be useful in selected patients. For example, in patients who have partially treated meningitis, bacterial antigen tests,

Table 4
Cerebrospinal fluid results

	Bacterial meningitis	Viral meningitis	Normal adult	Normal child	Normal term infant	Normal preterm infant
Gram's Stain	+	–	–	–	–	–
White blood cell (WBC) (per μL)	>1000	<1000	<5	0–7	8 (0–22 range)	9 (0–25 range)
WBC type	>80% polys	1% to 50% polys	All monos	0% polys	61% polys	57% polys
Glucose (mg/dL)	<40	>40	>40	40–80	52 mean (34–119 range)	50 mean (24–63 range)
Glucose ratio cerebrospinal fluid/blood	<0.4	>0.4	>0.4	>0.5	0.44–1.28	0.55–1.05
Protein (mg/dL)	<200	<200	<50	5–40	90 mean (20–170 range)	115 mean (65–150 range)

Abbreviations: Monos, mononuclear leukocytes; Polys, polymorphonuclear leukocytes.

such as counterimmunoelectrophoresis (CIE), ELISA, or PCR tests on CSF can help identify the pathogen. The sensitivity of different detection tests varies and is in the 60% to 90% range. Newer antigen detection tests are being designed, however, and older ones are being improved, so these tests, especially PCR, may become more useful and widely available in the future [46,47].

When viral meningitis is suspected, testing for viruses by PCR or viral cultures may be done. Similarly when fungal meningitis is a consideration, testing for fungal pathogens by India ink and fungal cultures and antigen testing may be done. Mixing India ink with CSF or other biologic fluids remains a quick and efficacious technique for identifying *Cryptococcus*, although clinical experience is necessary to recognize the encapsulated yeast. A positive India ink test occurs in over 80% of patients who have AIDS and half of non-AIDS patients who have cryptococcal meningitis, according to one author [48], while others report only about a 50% yield [49]. By comparison, cryptococcal antigen is positive in over 90% of patients in the CSF or serum [48–50].

If leptomeningeal meningitis is a possibility, CSF should be sent for cytology. Although it is nonspecific, CSF lactic acid has been used when a patient has had prior antibiotic therapy, which likely makes the CSF culture- and gram stain-negative. With bacterial or fungal meningitis, the CSF lactic acid is elevated, while it is generally normal (normal CSF lactic acid less than 35 mg/dL) with viral infections [51]. Seizures alone generally do not cause abnormalities in the CSF, so abnormal findings on CSF should not automatically be attributed to a seizure [52].

Laboratory studies

Laboratory studies other than CSF include: complete blood cell count (CBC), glucose, electrolytes, serum urea nitrogen (BUN,) creatinine, and blood cultures. The white blood cell (WBC) generally is elevated, and the differential usually has a leftward shift, although patients at the extremes of age (geriatric patients, infants) and the immunosuppressed may have a normal or depressed WBC. The serum glucose is useful to compare with the CSF glucose (CSF/blood glucose ratio). Renal function tests (BUN, creatinine) are useful as indicators of renal perfusion/function and when dosing medications. Electrolyte abnormalities (especially hyponatremia), dehydration, and SIADH may occur in meningitis. Blood cultures may be positive when the CSF is negative, so blood cultures are recommended in all patients who have suspected bacterial meningitis.

A chest radiograph can be valuable in identifying comorbidity (such as heart failure) and may detect a pneumonia, which could suggest a causative organism. About half of patients who have pneumococcal meningitis have pneumonia on radiograph. The urinalysis may reveal a urinary tract infection that led to bacteremia and meningitis, as well as yielding information on the patient's state of hydration and renal function. In seriously ill patients, urine output should be monitored. An EKG may assist in diagnosing comorbidity and complications from heart failure to septic shock with cardiac dysfunction and dysrhythmias. Other studies, such as an arterial blood gas, an electroencephalogram (EEG), or echocardiogram, depend on the patient's clinical presentation.

Empiric antibiotic therapy

Empiric antibiotic therapy with a broad-spectrum antibiotic that can rapidly enter the subarachnoid space is administered when the specific etiologic agent is unknown. When the exact organism cannot be identified on a Gram's stain smear of CSF, empiric therapy based on the most likely pathogen is given. The likelihood of a given pathogen is determined from clinical clues, such as the patient's age, comorbidity, immunologic status, and the history/physical examination (see Table 2). For example, based on the likely pathogen, what are the empiric antibiotics for meningitis in: a febrile military recruit who has a petechial rash, an elderly confused febrile patient who has a recent urinary tract infection, an HIV patient, or a febrile newborn (see Table 2)?

Most empiric therapy regimens include a third- or fourth-generation cephalosporin plus vancomycin [53,54]. Ampicillin is added in special situations where *Listeria* may be a pathogen (such as the elderly, those who have impaired immunity including patients who have HIV, and newborns). Meropenem is an alternative drug for the cephalosporins, while trimethoprim-sulfamethoxazole is an alternative drug for ampicillin (excluding newborns). If a cephalosporin cannot be administered (for example, with a true allergy), alternative antibiotics are a carbepenem (eg, meropenem) or chloramphenicol plus vancomycin (see Table 2).

Vancomycin penetration into the CNS is mainly dependent upon meningeal inflammation. Dexamethasone, probably because it decreases meningeal inflammation, significantly lowers therapeutic drug levels in the CSF [55,56], which has led to clinical treatment failures in adults [57]. Thus, a concern has been raised regarding vancomycin efficacy when given with dexamethasone, so some recommend adding rifampin whenever there is concurrent administration of vancomycin and dexamethasone.

Rifampin has good CSF penetration and in vitro activity against many meningeal pathogens, but when used alone, resistance develops quickly. Therefore, rifampin must be used in combination with other antimicrobial drugs [58]. When dexamethasone is given in the treatment of bacterial meningitis, rifampin generally also is given along with other antimicrobial drugs [58]. This is because of studies indicating dexamethasone is associated with a higher therapeutic failure rates and may decrease the CSF levels of various antibiotics, such as vancomycin (see Tables 2 and 4, and the adjuvant therapy section) [57,58].

Unfortunately, in the emergency department, the specific bacterial pathogen is generally unknown, so empiric therapy is the rule. The CSF Gram's stain, however, may yield an important early clue to the specific pathogen before the CSF culture results are back. The likely pathogen based on the Gram's stain and the current antibiotics of choice are listed in Table 3.

Other empiric therapy for aseptic (nonbacterial) infectious meningitis includes: acyclovir for herpes (HSV-1) meningoencephalitis (usually the CSF shows lymphocytic pleocytosis, increased number of erythrocytes, elevated protein, normal glucose), and amphotericin B and flucytosine for fungal meningitis (eg, cryptococcal meningoencephalitis).

Antibiotic resistance

Antibiotic sensitivity testing of the causative bacterial pathogen is key, so that antibiotic coverage can be tailored to provide optimal narrow coverage. Antibiotic sensitivity testing is also critical because of increasing pathogen resistance to various antibiotics.

There has been an increase in infections with antibiotic resistant strains in recent years. With the pneumococci, resistance to penicillin has occurred. In one series of patients who had pneumococcal meningitis, 25% of isolates were resistant to penicillin, and 9% were resistant to cefotaxime [59]. In other reports, up to about one-third of pneumococci tested had intermediate (14% to 22%) or high resistance (3% to 14%) to penicillin [4,60,61].

With the pneumococci, resistance to cephalosporins is starting to emerge. In the United States, in the prevaccine era, over 40% of *S pneumoniae* isolates were nonsusceptible to penicillin G, and about half of these isolates also were nonsusceptible to a third-generation cephalosporin (ceftriaxone or cefotaxime). These penicillin-nonsusceptible strains also have increased rates of resistance to trimethoprim-sulfamethoxazole, clindamycin, and particularly high resistance to macrolides (greater than 50% resistance). Increased rates of macrolide resistance (greater than 10% resistance) also are noted with the penicillin-susceptible strains [8]. Another study found *S pneumoniae* isolates had 0% to 45% penicillin resistance, 18% to 33% clindamycin resistance, and 33 to 50% erythromycin resistance. This study also noted that antibiotic resistance for *S pyogenes* isolates was 14% to 34% for erythromycin and 0% to 28% for clindamycin [62]. *S pneumoniae* organisms that cause meningitis remain susceptible to vancomycin and moxifloxacin, although decreased susceptibility to penicillin and cefotaxime was noted in some isolates [63].

Many experts recommend adding vancomycin to a third-generation cephalosporin when treating pneumococcal meningitis until the sensitivities are known [53,54,64]. Because of its poor penetration of the blood–brain barrier, monotherapy with vancomycin is not recommended [57].

Resistance to ampicillin has been noted in up to 39% of *H influenzae* isolates, and 36% produced a β-lactamase [65]. Fortunately, so far, *H influenzae* resistance to third-generation cephalosporins (eg, ceftriaxone or cefotaxime) is rare [66]. Likewise, meningococcus is sensitive to the cephalosporins, and there have been few reports of β-lactamase producing meningococcus in the United States.

Increased resistance to antibiotics has been noted with staphylococci (MRSA), enterococci (vancomycin-resistant enterococci, VRE), pneumococcus (penicillin- and cephalosporin-resistant pneumococci), and *Haemophilus* (ampicillin resistance). Resistance mechanisms to β-lactams, which consists mainly of extended-spectrum β-lactamase (ESBL), have been reported in gram-negative organisms: *Pseudomonas aeruginosa, E coli, Klebsiella pneumoniae,* and *Enterobacter cloacae.* The emergence of ESBL-producing pathogens may decrease the effectiveness of the cephalosporins against gram-negative bacilli [67,68].

Some experts are recommending that serious methicillin-susceptible Staphylococcus aureus (MSSA) infections including meningitis be treated with a β-lactamase resistant (BLR) β-lactam antimicrobial agent, such as oxacillin or nafcillin rather than vancomycin. This is because most *Staphylococcus aureus* strains produce β-lactamase enzymes and are resistant to penicillin and ampicillin. Oxacillin and nafcillin have been recommended for MSSA infections to decrease the possible emergence of vancomycin- or clindamycin-resistant strains. For MRSA, vancomycin is the drug of choice, with some experts adding rifampin or gentamicin [69].

Recently, polymicrobial infections and multiantibiotic resistance also have been identified [21,70]. Because the sensitivities to antibiotics are evolving, new antimicrobials are being developed, and the incidence of various pathogens as causative agents of meningitis is changing, the physician should be aware of and consider local/hospital trends regarding antibiotics, their sensitivities, and pathogens when considering antibiotic therapy for acute bacterial meningitis. The recommendations in Tables 2 and 3 are based on current reports; they may need modifications in the future as sensitivities/pathogens evolve.

Adjunctive dexamethasone therapy

Clinical trials

The role of corticosteroids in acute bacterial meningitis is controversial. The best answer to whether corticosteroids should be used in acute bacterial meningitis is "it depends" or "sometimes." The likely bacterial pathogen and the patient's age are key considerations in determining whether corticosteroids (specifically, dexamethasone) are given. The time of administration of dexamethasone is also critical.

The pathogenesis of bacterial meningitis and animal studies support the use of corticosteroids [71,72], while the results of clinical trials are mixed [73–80]. Animal studies of corticosteroids in experimental pneumococcal meningitis resulted in decreased cerebral edema, lowered CSF pressure, and decreased CSF lactate levels [72]. Bactericidal antibiotics given to patients who have septic meningitis results in the killing of the invading bacteria and the release of bacterial cell wall components, which in turn leads to the production of proinflammatory cytokines, such as IL-1 and TNF by macrophages and microglial cells in the subarachnoid space. Dexamethasone has several anti-inflammatory effects including: inhibition of the synthesis of IL-1 and TNF, and stabilizing the blood–brain barrier.

The reason why it is recommended that dexamethasone be given 15 to 20 minutes before administering antibiotics is that dexamethasone inhibits the release of IL-1, TNF, and other inflammatory cytokines by microglia and macrophages only if it is given before these cells are activated by the endotoxins released from the killing of bacteria. Once these cells have been induced to produce these inflammatory cytokines, dexamethasone does not affect cytokine (IL-1, TNF, others) production by the body's cells (macrophages, glial cells, and others) [48,81].

The findings regarding corticosteroids as adjunctive therapy in acute bacterial meningitis from various clinical trials are mixed and somewhat dependent on the bacterial pathogen and on the patient's age (pediatric patients versus adults). Two randomized double-blind, placebo-controlled studies of childhood bacterial meningitis documented a lower incidence of long-term hearing loss in infants/children given dexamethasone and a cephalosporin antibiotic versus those given just the antibiotic [73]. A meta-analysis of 11 studies of dexamethasone in infants/children who had bacterial meningitis found:

- With *H influenzae* meningitis, dexamethasone significantly decreased severe hearing loss irrespective of when it was given (eg, before or after antibiotic therapy)
- With pneumococcal meningitis, dexamethasone was effective in reducing hearing loss only if given before antibiotics
- For all pathogens combined, the only benefit of dexamethasone was a decrease in hearing loss with no protection against any other neurologic deficits [79]

Several other studies of dexamethasone in childhood bacterial meningitis noted similar results [74–76].

In adults who had bacterial meningitis, a randomized placebo-controlled, double-blind trial that compared dexamethasone versus placebo in addition to antibiotics found that dexamethasone decreased the incidence of unfavorable outcomes including death [77]. The reduction in unfavorable outcomes was 25% to 15% ($P = .03$) and in mortality was 15% to 7% ($P = .04$). The absolute risk reduction was 10%. Dexamethasone was given either 15 minutes before or simultaneously with antibiotics and continued every 6 hours for 4 days. Benefits were present with pneumococcal meningitis but not with any other bacterial pathogen (including *N meningitidis*) [77].

A study of neonatal (age less than or equal to 30 days) meningitis in which *K pneumoniae* was the main bacterial pathogen showed negative results with dexamethasone [80]. Therefore, dexamethasone is not recommended in this age group.

Currently, adjunctive dexamethasone is recommended in infants/children older than 6 weeks with *H influenzae* B meningitis and is considered in infants/children older than 6 weeks who have pneumococcal meningitis, and in adults who have proven or suspected pneumococcal meningitis [58]. According to the Red Book, dexamethasone may be beneficial for the treatment of *H influenzae* B meningitis in infants and children if given before or concurrently with the first dose of antibiotics [7]. The dexamethasone dose in children and adults is 0.15 mg/kg per dose intravenously every 6 hours for 2 to 4 days, with the first dose given before or concurrently with the first dose of antibiotics.

Empiric adjunctive dexamethasone therapy?

Because the organism usually is not known definitively when the patient who has bacterial meningitis is in the emergency department, empiric antibiotics are frequently the rule. Similarly, the question of empiric administration of dexamethasone in the emergency department could be argued, with some advocates for [82] and some against [83].

Several concerns regarding the use of dexamethasone have been raised. There is also the logistical necessity of administering dexamethasone either just before or at the same time as the antibiotic. There is concern that clinical signs and symptoms may be masked in the presence of dexamethasone, making it difficult to evaluate the adequacy or inadequacy of the response to therapy [83]. Gastrointestinal (GI) bleeding has been noted to occur in the 1% to 2% of patients with bacterial meningitis who received dexamethasone [83]. A decreased learning ability and decreased spatial memory, and increased hippocampal neuronal apoptosis were noted in two recent animal studies [84,85].

First, the narrow window of opportunity for drug administration should not be an issue if prospectively discussed with nursing/pharmacy/other involved hospital or department personnel, and a mechanism is put into place for rapidly obtaining and giving the medications.

Next, a significant difference in the incidence of GI bleeding between those receiving dexamethasone and those not receiving dexamethasone has not been noted, although the incidence of GI bleeding may be too small (1% to 2%) to detect a difference. One study in adults noted a higher incidence of GI bleeding in the placebo group (5 of 144 patients = 0.03%) versus the dexamethasone group (2 of 157 patients = .01%) [77], while a study in children that monitored for possible adverse effects found no abnormalities [74]. A systematic review of steroids in adults who had acute bacterial meningitis found that adverse events were distributed equally between both groups (eg, steroids versus nonsteroids). They noted a significant decrease in mortality ($P = .002$) and in neurologic sequelae ($P = .05$) with steroid treatment. They recommended "routine steroid therapy with the first dose of antibiotics" in most adults who had community-acquired bacterial meningitis [82].

An increased number of the therapeutic failures has been noted in some studies when dexamethasone is given with various antibiotics [57]. The therapeutic failures occurring with concomitant dexamethasone administration are a concern. This may, at least in part, be related to a decreased CSF level of antibiotics. The mechanism for this is not entirely clear. It may be that antibiotic therapy failures occur because dexamethasone impairs antibiotic penetration across the blood–brain barrier [57,86]. Another possibility is that dexamethasone decreases the level of antibiotic (eg, vancomycin, ceftriaxone, and rifampin) in the CSF [83]. Several studies did demonstrate decreased level of antibiotics in the CSF when dexamethasone was given in several animal studies [55,56,86], and in a study of adults who had bacterial meningitis receiving vancomycin [57]. Another animal study noted therapeutic failures when dexamethasone was given with ceftriaxone, although the antibiotic pharmacokinetics, including CSF drug levels, were not different between the animals receiving dexamethasone or not receiving dexamethasone.

Negative effects of dexamethasone were reported in a study of neonatal bacterial meningitis. Therefore, coadministration of dexamethasone with antibiotics is contraindicated in neonatal bacterial meningitis.

Furthermore, the two recent studies using different animal models demonstrating decreased learning ability and impaired memory along with molecular signs of neuronal damage are particularly concerning [84,85].

The conclusion is that the various risks and benefits of administering dexamethasone in bacterial meningitis need to be determined on an individual basis until additional evidence/research is forthcoming.

Differential diagnosis

The differential diagnosis of bacterial meningitis includes all the causes of aseptic meningitis, both the infections (mostly viral but also partially treated bacterial meningitis and focal CNS infections) and noninfectious causes: neoplasm, drugs, and systemic diseases. The infectious causes of aseptic meningitis include: partially treated bacterial, viral, fungal, tuberculosis, Lyme disease, syphilis, and meningitis caused by atypical and nonpyogenic bacteria. Meningeal irritation also can be caused by adjacent bacterial infections (such as a brain abscess, subdural empyema or epidural abscess) (see Fig. 1). A CT scan can be valuable in detecting these adjacent infections. Neoplastic disease of the meninges (leptomeningeal carcinomatosis) also can cause meningeal signs and symptoms.

Aseptic meningitis is differentiated into infectious and noninfectious causes. Viral meningitis accounts for most cases of aseptic meningitis. Nonviral infectious causes of aseptic meningitis include the following: partially treated bacterial meningitis, atypical and nonpyogenic bacterial meningitis, meningitis caused by adjacent pyogenic infections, tuberculous meningitis, syphilitic meningitis, fungal meningitis, and meningitis associated with Lyme disease (see Fig. 2).

Etiologic agents of viral meningitis include: enteroviruses (most common cause: echoviruses, but also coxsackie, and infrequently polio viruses), adenoviruses, herpes simplex, varicella-zoster virus, influenza types A and B, HIV, lymphocytic choriomeningitis virus, and Epstein-Barr virus.

A multicenter study of 3295 children admitted to the hospital with CSF pleocytosis who were treated with parenteral antibiotics noted 3.7% of the patients had bacterial meningitis, and 96.3% had aseptic meningitis [87]. A bacterial meningitis scoring system was devised using the following variables:

- Positive CSF Gram's stain
- CSF absolute neutrophil count greater than or equal to 1000 cells/μL
- CSF protein greater than 80 mg/d
- Peripheral blood absolute neutrophil count greater than or equal to 10,000 cells/μL
- A history of seizure before or at the time of presentation. The risk of bacterial meningitis was very low (0.1%) in patients with none of these criteria [87]

Atypical bacteria that can cause meningitis include: tuberculosis, *Nocardia, Treponema pallidum* (syphilis) and *Borrelia burgdorferi* (Lyme disease). Fungal etiologies for meningitis are in two categories: those that cause disease in immunocompromised patients (such as HIV patients) and those endemic to certain geographic locales. Fungi associated with a specific geographic region are: *Histoplasma, Coccidoides*, and *Blastomyces*. Organisms causing meningitis in compromised hosts include

- Fungi: Candida, Cryptococcus, and *Aspergillus*
- Parasites: *Toxoplasma gondii* and cysticercosis (pork tapeworm)
- Certain viruses

There are reports of these pathogens causing meningitis in immunocompetent individuals as well.

Focal CNS infections that are in the differential for bacterial meningitis include: brain abscess and parameningeal CNS infections (subdural empyema, epidural abscess, spinal abscess) (see Fig. 4). A CT scan can be valuable in detecting these adjacent infections.

Noninfectious etiologies of aseptic meningitis can be grouped into four categories: (1) drugs, (2) carcinomatosis meningitis or leptomeningeal carcinomatosis (metastases to the meninges), (3) associated systemic diseases, and (4) inflammatory conditions that primarily affect the CNS. The systemic diseases that can cause aseptic noninfectious meningitis are generally an autoimmune hypersensitivity disease and include: systemic lupus erythematosus, sarcoidosis, Behcet's syndrome, Wegner's granulomatosis, and lead poisoning. Noninfectious CNS inflammatory processes include: granulomatous cerebral vasculitis and chemical meningitis following myelography (with water-soluble nonionic contrast), inflammation following neurosurgery, and inflammation after spinal or epidural anesthesia.

Neoplastic disease can cause meningitis with tumors that leak inflammatory materials into the CSF, with primary CNS tumors, or with metastatic carcinomatous meningitis. Some of the drugs that have been associated with drug hypersensitivity meningitis are: nonsteroidal anti-inflammatory drugs, trimethoprim-sulfamethoxazole, and OKT3 (an antibody against T cells).

Prognosis/sequelae

The annual mortality for bacterial meningitis in the United States was about 6000 prior to the routine use of pneumococcal conjugate vaccine, with about two-thirds of all cases occurring in pediatric patients less than or equal to 18 years of age [59]. A recent report notes half of all acute bacterial cases are in children and infants [4]. In the United States, the annual mortality rate for bacterial meningitis was less 1000 (708 deaths) reported in 2003 [88]. Although the overall incidence of bacterial meningitis in the United States is decreasing, especially in pediatric patients, the proportion of patients in certain high-risk groups (such as geriatric patients) is increasing [4,34]. Whether this changing age-related trend continues and if it is related to the use of the newer vaccines and widespread immunization and/or other factors including an aging population with higher acuity and increased comorbidity (including immunosuppressed patients) remain to be determined.

The case fatality rates for bacterial meningitis are reported as 4% to 10% in the pediatric population [16], 25% in adults [1], and up to 50% for geriatric patients [34]. Meningitis case fatality rates are estimated at 3% to 7% for *H influenzae* or *N meningitidis* or group B streptococci, 20% to 25% for *S pneumoniae*, and up to 30% to 40% for *L monocytogenes* [4,8,19,81]. Higher fatality rates occur in patients at the extremes of age (the elderly and the infant, especially the neonate) [16,17,32,34,89].

The prognosis varies depending on multiple factors: age, presence of co-morbidity, responsible pathogen, and the degree of severity at presentation/neurologic presentation on admission. The severity or degree of neurologic impairment at the time of presentation is a prognostic factor [81,89]. The mortality rate rises with the following clinical parameters:

- Decreased level of consciousness at admission
- Signs of increased intracranial pressure
- Seizures within 24 hours of admission
- Age (older than 50 years or infancy)
- Comorbidity
- Need for mechanical ventilation
- Delay in initiation of treatment [81]

A recent study of community-acquired acute adult bacterial meningitis (51% *S pneumoniae*, 37% *N meningitidis*) noted risk factors associated with a poor prognosis were: advanced age, presence of osteitis or sinusitis, low Glasgow Coma Scale (GCS) on admission, tachycardia, absence of rash, thrombocytopenia, elevated erythrocyte sedimentation rate, low CSF cell count, and positive blood culture [11].

The incidence of sequelae varies with the pathogen, with about 25% of survivors having moderate or severe sequelae [81]. In one report, 40% of survivors had sequelae, including hearing loss and other neurologic sequelae [89], while others cite 60% morbidity [48,59]. Sequelae of bacterial meningitis [90] include: sensorineural hearing loss (particularly common in children who have *H influenzae* infection), decreased intellectual/cognitive function, impaired memory, dizziness, gait disturbances, focal neurologic deficits including paralysis and blindness, hydrocephalus, subdural effusion, and seizures (Box 2).

Chemoprophylaxis

The incidence of transmission of *Meningococcus* among household contacts is about 5%. According to one estimate, the risk for developing meningitis after exposure to a patient with meningococcal meningitis is 500 to 800 times greater than in the general population [91]. Therefore, chemoprophylaxis is indicated for high-risk contacts of patients who have meningitis. Because up to one-third of secondary cases of meningococcal disease develop within 2 to 5 days of illness in the index (initial) case, prompt chemoprophylaxis is indicated.

Individuals considered high-risk who need prophylaxis are: household or close contacts (individuals who slept and ate in the same household with the patient) and intimate nonhousehold contacts who have had mucosal exposure to the patient's secretions (such as a boyfriend or girlfriend). Individuals who have had direct exposure to the patient's secretions through shared utensils or toothbrushes, kissing, and school/daycare contacts in the prior seven days should receive chemoprophylaxis.

Not all health care workers need chemoprophylaxis. Health care workers who are at increased risk and require chemoprophylaxis are those who have had direct mucosal contact with the patient's secretions, as for example, during mouth-to-mouth resuscitation, endotracheal intubation, or suctioning of the airway.

Chemoprophylaxis for meningococcal meningitis is provided by rifampin given in a 600 mg dose for adults, 10 mg/kg every dose for children older than 1 month, 5 mg/kg every dose for neonates (age less than or equal to 30 days) orally every 12 hours for a total of four doses. Those receiving chemoprophylaxis should be counseled to watch for fever, rash, or any other meningeal signs/symptoms. They should be hospitalized with appropriate intravenous antibiotics if signs/symptoms of active meningococcal disease

develop, because rifampin alone is not effective against invasive meningococcal disease. Alternative single-dose chemoprophylaxis regimens are ciprofloxacin 500 mg by mouth for adults and ceftriaxone 250 mg
intramuscularly (age greater than or equal to 12 years) or 125 mg intramuscularly (age less than 12 years).

Rifampin chemoprophylaxis for *H influenzae* meningitis is warranted for
nonpregnant household contacts if there are young children (age younger
than 4 years) in the household. The by mouth dose is 600 mg for adults
and 20 mg/kg for children once daily for 4 days. Chemoprophylaxis is not
given for pneumococcal meningitis.

Immunoprophylaxis

A vaccine against meningococci has been used to immunize adults. Unfortunately, this vaccine does not confer protection in children younger
than 2 years because of a poor antibody response in this age group. This
vaccine is based the polysaccharide capsule but only confers immunity
against four serogroups of meningococci (A, C, Y, W-135). The quadrivalent vaccine has been used for routine immunization by the United States
military since the 1980s, for travelers to countries where meningococcal disease is endemic, during meningococcal epidemics, and for elective immunization of college freshman. Currently, there is no licensed vaccine against
serogroup β meningococci. The quadrivalent meningococcal conjugate vaccine (MCV4) is recommended:

- For 2- to 10-year old children at increased risk for meningococcal dis-
  ease, including patients who have asplenia (functional or anatomic),
  HIV infection, and terminal complement deficiencies
- For travelers to areas where *N meningitidis* is hyperendemic or endemic
- During outbreaks caused by a serotype included in the vaccine [92–94]

A quadrivalent meningococcal conjugate vaccine was approved by the
FDA in 2005 for use in adolescents and adults 11 to 55 years of age [93,94].

Despite there being a large number of serotypes of pneumococci, effective
pneumococcal vaccines have been developed, because most clinical disease is
caused by relatively few serotypes of pneumococci. The pneumococcal vaccines have had a positive effect in decreasing the incidence of all types of invasive pneumococcal diseases including meningitis [10].

Several pneumococcal vaccines are available. A single dose of a polyvalent vaccine effective against 23 serotypes of pneumococci is recommended
for elderly or debilitated patients, especially those who have pulmonary disease, sickle cell disease, and those who have impaired splenic function such
as patients after splenectomy. Childhood immunization recommendations
include a heptavalent conjugated pneumococcal vaccine that is 90% protective with a low incidence of adverse reactions [8].

The HIB vaccine, which confers immunity against *H influenzae* type B, is also part of the childhood immunization recommendation and has been very effective in decreasing the incidence of all types of disease caused by *H influenzae* type B, from pneumonia to meningitis [7].

Summary

Despite advances in medical care including antibiotics and vaccines, meningitis still has a high morbidity and mortality rate, especially in certain high-risk patients. Early diagnosis with the administration of appropriate antibiotics remains the key element of management.

References

[1] Durand ML, Calderwood SB, Weber DJ, et al. Acute bacterial meningitis in adults: a review of 493 episodes. N Engl J Med 1993;328:21–8.

[2] Lieb SL, Tauber MG. Acute and chronic meningitis. In: Cohen J, Powderly WG, editors. Infectious diseases. 2nd edition. St. Louis (MO): Mosby; 2004. p. 251–65.

[3] Fraser DW, Geil CC, Feldman RA. Bacterial meningitis in Bernaililli County, New Mexico: a comparison with three other American populations. Am J Epidemiol 1947;100(1): 29–34.

[4] Schuchat A, Robinson K, Wenger JD, et al. Bacterial meningitis in the United States in 1995. Active surveillance team. N Engl J Med 1997;337(14):970–6.

[5] Lavoie FW, Caucier JR. Central nervous system infections. In: Marx JA, Hockberger RS, Walls RM, et al, editors. Rosen's emergency medicine concepts and clinical practice. 6th edition. Philadelphia: Mosby Elsevier; 2006. p. 1710–25.

[6] Loring KE. CNS infections. In: Tintinalli JE, Kelen GD, Stapczynski JS, editors. Emergency medicine: a comprehensive study guide. 6th edition. New York: McGraw-Hill; 2004. p. 1431–7.

[7] *Haemophilus influenzae* infections. In: Pickering LK, Baker CJ, Long SS, et al, editors. Red Book: 2006 Report of the Committee on Infectious Diseases. 27th edition. Elk Grove Village (IL): American Academy of Pediatrics; 2006. p. 310–8.

[8] Pneumococcal infections. In: Pickering LK, Baker CJ, Long SS, et al, editors. Red Book: 2006 Report of the Committee on Infectious Diseases. 27th edition. Elk Grove Village (IL): American Academy of Pediatrics; 2006. p. 525–37.

[9] Wenger JD, Hightower AW, Facklam RR, et al. Bacterial meningitis in the United States, 1986: report of a multistate surveillance study. The Bacterial Meningitis Study Group. J Infect Dis 1990;162(6):1316–22.

[10] Black S, Shinefield H, Baxter R, et al. Postlicensure surveillance for pneumococcal invasive disease after use of heptavalent pneumococcal conjugate vaccine in Northern California Kaiser Permanente. Pediatr Infect Dis J 2004;23(6):485–9.

[11] van de Beek D, de Gans J, Spanjaard L, et al. Clinical features and prognostic factors in adults with bacterial meningitis. N Engl J Med 2004;351(18):1849–59.

[12] Ziai WC. Advances in the management of central nervous systems infections in the ICU. Crit Care Clin 2006;22(4):661–94.

[13] Pfister HW, Feiden W, Einhaulp KM. Spectrum of complications during bacterial meningitis in adults. Results of a prospective clinical study. Arch Neurol 1993;50(6):575–81.

[14] Hussein AS, Shafran SD. Acute bacterial meningitis in adults. A 12-year view. Medicine (Baltimore) 2000;79(6):360–8.

[15] Kaplan SL. Clinical presentations, diagnosis, and prognostic factors of bacterial meningitis. Infect Dis Clin North Am 1999;13:579–94.

[16] Chavez-Bueno S, McCracken GH Jr. Bacterial meningitis in children. Pediatr Clin North Am 2005;52:795–810.
[17] Edwards MS. Postnatal bacterial infections. In: Martin RJ, Fanaroff AA, Walsh MC, editors. Fanaroff and Martin's neonatal-perinatal medicine: diseases of the fetus and infant. vol. 2. 8th edition. Philadelphia: Mosby Elsevier; 2006. p. 791–829.
[18] Choi C. Bacterial meningitis. Clin Geriatric Med 1992;8(4):889–902.
[19] Geiseler PJ, Nelson KE, Levin S, et al. Community-acquired purulent meningitis: a review of 1316 cases during the antibiotic era 1954–1976. Rev Infect Dis 1980;2(5):725–45.
[20] Schutze GE, Mason EO Jr, Barson WJ, et al. Invasive pneumococcal infections in children with asplenia. Pediatr Infect Dis J 2002;21:278–82.
[21] Wang KW, Chang WN, Huang CR, et al. Postneurosurgical nosocomial bacterial meningitis in adults: microbiology, clinical features, and outcomes. J Clin Neurosci 2005;12(6): 647–50.
[22] Odio C, McCracken GH Jr, Nelson JD. CSF shunt infections in pediatrics: a seven-year experience. Am J Dis Child 1984;138:1103–8.
[23] O'Neill E, Humphreys H, Phillips J, et al. Third-generation cephalosporin resistance among gram-negative bacilli causing meningitis in neurosurgical patients: significant challenges in ensuring effective antibiotic therapy. J Antimicrob Chemother 2006;57:356–9.
[24] Reefhuis J, Honein MA, Whitney CG, et al. Risk of bacterial meningitis in children with cochlear implants. N Engl J Med 2003;349:435–45.
[25] Berman PH, Banker BQ. Neonatal meningitis: a clinical and pathological study of 29 cases. Pediatrics 1996;38:6–24.
[26] Kapur R, Yoder MC, Polin RA. Developmental immunology. In: Martin RJ, Fanaroff AA, Walsh MC, editors. Fanaroff and Martin's neonatal-perinatal medicine, vol. 2. 8th edition. Philadelphia: Mosby-Elsevier; 2006. p. 761–90.
[27] Nicolle LE, Strausbaugh LJ, Garibaldi RA. Infections and antibiotic resistance in nursing homes. Clin Microbiol Rev 1996;9(1):1–17.
[28] Yung RL. Changes in immune function with age. Rheum Dis Clin North Am 2000;26(3): 455–73.
[29] Mody L. Infection control issues in older adults. Clin Geriatric Med 2007;23(3):499–574.
[30] Yoshikawa TT. Antimicrobial resistance and aging: beginning of the end of the antibiotic era? Journal of the American Geriatric Society 2002;50(7):S226–9.
[31] Gorse GJ, Thrupp LD, Nudleman KL, et al. Bacterial meningitis in the elderly. Archives of Internal Medicine 1984;144(8):1603–7.
[32] Kulchycki LK, Edlow JA. Geriatric neurologic emergencies. Emerg Med Clin North Am 2006;24(3):273–98.
[33] Puxty JA, Fox RA, Horan MA. The frequency of physical signs usually attributed to meningeal irritation in elderly patients. J Am Geriatr Soc 1983;31(10):216–20.
[34] Adedipe A, Lowenstein R. Infectious emergencies in the elderly. Emerg Med Clin North Am 2006;24:433–48.
[35] Kornelisse RF, Westerbeek CM, Spoor AB, et al. Pneumococcal meningitis in children: prognostic indicators and outcome. Clin Infect Dis 1995;21(6):1390–7.
[36] van Crevel H, Hijdra A, de Gans J. Lumbar puncture and the risk of herniation: when should we first perform CT? J Neurol 2002;249(2):129–37.
[37] Hasbun R, Abrahams J, Jekel J, et al. Computed tomography of the head before lumbar puncture in adults with suspected meningitis. N Engl J Med 2001;345(24):1727–33.
[38] Duffy GP. Lumbar puncture in the presence of raised intracranial pressure. Br Med J 1969;1: 407–9.
[39] Brewer NS, MacCarty CS, Wellman WE. Brain abscess: a review of recent experience. Ann Intern Med 1975;82:571–6.
[40] Samson DS, Clark K. A current review of brain abscess. Am J Med 1973;54:201–10.
[41] Silverman R, Kwiatkowski T, Bernstein S, et al. Safety of lumbar puncture in patients with hemophilia. Ann Emerg Med 1993;22(11):1739–42.

[42] Howard SC, Gajjar A, Ribeiro RC, et al. Safety of lumbar puncture for children with acute lymphoblastic leukemia and thrombocytopenia. JAMA 2000;284:2222–4.

[43] Freedman SB, Marrocco A, Pirie J, et al. Predictors of bacterial meningitis in the era after *Haemophilus influenzae*. Arch Pediatr Adolesc Med 2001;155(12):1301–6.

[44] Mace SE. Meningitis. In: Greenberg MI, editor. Avoiding malpractice in emergency medicine. Wayne (PA): Greenleaf Press; 1988. p. 91–142.

[45] Durack DT, Spanos A. End-of-treatment spinal tap in bacterial meningitis. Is it worthwhile? JAMA 1982;248(1):75–8.

[46] Bryant PA, Li HY, Zaia A, et al. Prospective study of a real-time PCR that is highly sensitive, specific, and clinically useful for diagnosis of meningococcal disease in children. J Clin Microbiol 2004;42:2919–25.

[47] Schuurman T, deBoer RF, Kooistra-Smid AM, et al. Prospective study of use of PCR amplification and sequencing of 16S ribosomal DNA from cerebrospinal fluid for diagnosis of bacterial meningitis in a clinical setting. J Clin Microbiol 2004;42:734–40.

[48] Tunkel AR, Scheld WM. Acute meningitis. In: Mandell GL, Bennett JE, Dolan R, editors. Mandell, Bennett & Dolin: principles & practice of infectious diseases. 6th edition. Philadelphia: Churchill & Livingtstone; 2005. p. 1083–126.

[49] Sato Y, Osabe S, Kuno H, et al. Rapid diagnosis of cryptococcal meningitis by microscopic examination of centrifuged cerebrospinal fluid sediment. Journal of Neurological Sciences 1999;164:72–5.

[50] Collazos J. Opportunistic infections of the CNS in patients with AIDS. CNS Drugs 2003; 17(12):869–87.

[51] Beaty HN, Oppenheimer S. Cerebrospinal fluid lactic dehydrogenase and its isoenzymes in infections of the central nervous system. N Engl J Med 1968;279(22):1197–2002.

[52] Wong M, Schlaggar BL, Landt M. Postictal cerebrospinal fluid abnormalities in children. J Pediatr 2001;138:373–7.

[53] Kaplan SL. Management of pneumococcal meningitis. Pediatric Infectious Disease Journal 2002;21(6):589–91.

[54] Rodriquez CA, Atkinson R, Biter W, et al. Tolerance to vancomycin in pneumococci: detection with a molecular marker and assessment of clinical impact. Journal of Infectious Diseases 2004;190(8):1481–7.

[55] Cabellos C, Martinez-Lacasa J, Tubau F, et al. Evaluation of combined ceftriaxone and dexamethasone therapy in experimental cephalosporin-resistant pneumococcal meningitis. J Antimicrob Chemother 2000;45(3):315–20.

[56] Lutsar I, Friedland IR, Jafri HS, et al. Factors influencing the anti-inflammatory effect of dexamethasone therapy in experimental pneumococcal meningitis. J Antimicrob Chemother 2003;52(4):651–5.

[57] Viladrich PF, Gudiol F, Linares J, et al. Evaluation of vancomycin for therapy of adult pneumococcal meningitis. Antimicrob Agents Chemother 1991;35(12):2467–72.

[58] Tunkel AR, Hartman BJ, Kaplan SL, et al. Practice guidelines for the management of bacterial meningitis: Infectious Disease Society of American (IDSA) guidelines. Clinical Infectious Dieseases 2004;39:1267–84.

[59] Quagliarello VJ, Scheld WM. Treatment of bacterial meningitis. N Engl J Med 1997;336(10): 708–16.

[60] Butler JC, Hofmann J, Cetron MS, et al. The continued emergence of drug-resistant *Streptococcus pneumoniae* in the United States: an update from the Centers for Disease Control and Prevention's Pneumococcal Sentinel Surveillance System. J Infect Dis 1996;174(5):986–93.

[61] Doerm GV, Brueggemann A, Golley HP Jr, et al. Antimicrobial resistance of *Streptococcus pneumoniae* recovered from outpatients in the United States during the winter months of 1994 to 1995: results of a 30-center national surveillance study. Antimicrob Agents Chemother 1996;40:1208–13.

[62] Lin K, Tierno PM, Komisar A. Increasing antibiotic resistance of *Streptococcus* species in New York City. Laryngoscope 2004;114:1147–50.

[63] Verhaegen J, Vandecasteele SJ, Vandeven J, et al. Antibiotic susceptibility and serotype distribution of 240 *Streptococcus pneumoniae* causing meningitis in Belgium. Acta Clin Belg 2003;58(1):19–26.

[64] Friedland IR, McCracken GH Jr. Management of infections caused by antibiotic resistant *Streptococcus pneumoniae*. N Engl J Med 1994;331:377–82.

[65] Doern GV, Brueggemann AB, Pierce G, et al. Antibiotic resistance among clinical isolates of *Haemophilus influenzae* in the United States in 1994 and 1995 and detection of beta-lactamase positive strains resistant to amoxicillin-clavulanate: results of a national multicenter surveillance study. Antimicrob Agents Chemother 1997;41:292–7.

[66] Schneider JI. Rapid infectious killers. Emerg Med Clin North Am 2004;22:1099–115.

[67] Lee SH, Jeong SH. Antibiotic susceptibility of bacterial strains isolated from various infections. Lett Appl Microbiol 2002;34(3):215–21.

[68] Andes D, Craig WA. Treatment of infections with ESBL-producing organisms: pharmacokinetic and pharmacodynamic considerations. Clin Microbiol Infect 2005;(11 Suppl 6):10–7.

[69] Staphylococcal infections. In: Pickering LK, Baker CJ, Long SS, et al, editors. Red book: 2006 Report of the Committee on Infectious Diseases. 27th edition. Elk Grove Village (IL): American Academy of Pediatrics; 2006. p. 598–610.

[70] Yoshikawa TT. Resistant pathogens: considerations in geriatrics and infectious disease. J Am Geriatr Soc 2002;50(7 suppl):S226–9.

[71] Saez-Llorens X, McCracken GH Jr. Antimicrobial and anti-inflammatory treatment of bacterial meningitis. Infect Dis Clin North Am 1999;13:619–36.

[72] Tauber MG, Khayem-Bashi H, Sande MA, et al. Effects of ampicillin and corticosteroids on brain water content, cerebrospinal fluid pressure, and cerebrospinal fluid lactate levels in experimental pneumococcal meningitis. J Infect Dis 1985;151:528–34.

[73] Lebel MH, Freij BJ. Dexamethasone therapy for bacterial meningitis: results of two double-blind, placebo-controlled trials. N Engl J Med 1988;319:964–71.

[74] Schaad UB, Lips U, Gnehm HE, et al. Dexamethasone therapy for bacterial meningitis in children. Swiss Meningitis Study Group. Lancet 1993;342(8869):457–61.

[75] Molyneux EM, Walsh AL, Forsyth H, et al. Dexamethasone treatment in childhood bacterial meningitis in Malawi: a randomized control trial. Lancet 2002;360(9328):211–8.

[76] Wald ER, Kaplan SL, Mason ED Jr, et al. Dexamethasone therapy for children with bacterial meningitis—Meningitis Study Group. Pediatrics 1995;95(1):21–8.

[77] deGans J, van de Beek D. Dexamethasone in adults with bacterial meningitis. N Engl J Med 2002;347(10):1549–56.

[78] Gijwani D, Kumhar MR, Singh VB, et al. Dexamethasone therapy for bacterial meningitis in adults: a double-blind placebo control study. Neurol India 2002;50(1):63–7.

[79] McIntyre PB, Berkey CS, King SM, et al. Dexamethasone as adjunctive therapy in bacterial meningitis: a meta-analysis of randomized clinical trials since 1988. JAMA 1997; 278:925–31.

[80] Daoud AS, Batieha A, Al-Sheyyab M, et al. Lack of effectiveness of dexamethasone in neonatal bacterial meningitis. Eur J Pediatr 1999;158(3):230–3.

[81] Roos KL, Tyler KL. Meningitis, encelphalitis, brain abscess, and empyema. In: Harrison's internal medicine. New York: McGraw-Hill Co; 2007. p. 2471–90.

[82] Van de Beek D, deGans J, Macintyre P, et al. Steroids in adults with acute bacterial meningitis: a systematic review. Lancet Infect Dis 2004;4:139–43.

[83] Pelton SI, Yogev R. Improving the outcome of pneumococcal meningitis. Arch Dis Child 2005;90:333–4.

[84] Leib SL, Heimgartner C, Bifrafe YD, et al. Dexamethasone aggravates hippocampal apoptosis and learning deficiency in pneumococcal meningitis in infant rats. Pediatr Res 2003; 54:353–7.

[85] Zysk G, Bruck W, Gerber J, et al. Anti-inflammatory treatment influences neuronal–apoptotic cell death in the denate gyrus in experimental pneumococcal meningitis. J Neuropathol Exp Neurol 1996;55:722–8.

[86] Scheld WM, Brodeur JP. Effect of methyprednisolone on entry of ampicillin and gentamicin into cerebrospinal fluid in experimental pneumococcal and *Escherichia coli* meningitis. Antimicrob Agents Chemother 1983;23:108–12.

[87] Nigrovic LE, Kupperman N, Macias CG, et al. Clinical prediction rule for identifying children with cerebrospinal fluid pleocytosis at very low risk of bacterial meningitis. JAMA 2007;297(1):52–60.

[88] Vital statistics. In: Gutierrez CM, Sampson DA, Cooper KB, et al, editors. Statistical abstract of the United States: 2006. Washington, DC: U.S. Census Bureau 2005; 2006. p. 85.

[89] Miller LG, Choi C. Meningitis in the older patient: how to diagnose and treat a deadly infection. Geriatrics 1997;52:43–4, 47–50, 55.

[90] Grimwood K, Anderson VA, Bond L, et al. Adverse outcomes of bacterial meningitis in school-age survivors. Pediatrics 1995;95:646–56.

[91] Analysis of endemic meningococcal disease by serogroup and evaluation of chemoprophylaxis. J Infect Dis 1976;134:20–4.

[92] Centers for Disease Control and Prevention. Meningococcal disease and college students. Recommendations of the Advisory Committee on Immunization Practices (ACEI). MMWR Recomm Rep 2000;49(RR-7):13–20.

[93] Baker CJ, Rubin LG, Bocchini JA Jr. Recommendations updated for PCV7, MCV4 vaccines. AAP News 2007;14. Available at: www.aapnews.org. Accessed March 3, 2008.

[94] Bilukha O, Messonnier N, Fischer M. Use of meningococcal vaccines in the United States. Pediatr Infect Dis J 2007;26(5):371–6.

ELSEVIER
SAUNDERS

Emerg Med Clin N Am
26 (2008) 319–343

EMERGENCY
MEDICINE
CLINICS OF
NORTH AMERICA

Evaluation and Management of Geriatric Infections in the Emergency Department

Jeffrey M. Caterino, MD[a,b,*]

[a]*Department of Emergency Medicine, The Ohio State University, 146 Means Hall,*
1654 Upham Drive, Columbus, OH 43210-1270, USA
[b]*Department of Internal Medicine, The Ohio State University, 146 Means Hall,*
1654 Upham Drive, Columbus, OH 43210-1270, USA

By 2020, patients aged 65 years old and older will constitute 16.3% of the US population [1]. Already, they account for over 15 million emergency department visits each year, and a large percentage of these visits are related to infection [2]. For example, fever is present in 10% of all elderly emergency department patients, and the elderly account for 65% of emergency department patients with sepsis [3,4]. Elderly patients are at significantly greater mortality risk for a given infection than are younger adults, with three times the mortality from pneumonia and five to ten times the mortality from urinary tract infection when compared with younger adults [5,6]. As a result, appropriate evaluation and treatment of the infected elderly is an essential skill for the emergency physician.

The elderly are at an increased risk of acquiring infection via several mechanisms. With aging comes immunosenescence, which is manifested primarily by inefficiencies of T-cell function causing deficient cell-mediated immunity. The B-cell response is also impaired, primarily through decreased activity of T-helper cells, resulting in a failure of B-cell–T-cell interaction and a decrease in humoral immunity [7,8]. Increased numbers of comorbid conditions and indwelling medical devices (eg, indwelling urinary catheters and central venous lines) also contribute to increased rates of infection. The elderly often have poor nutritional status, poor functional status, decreased barriers to infection (eg, skin breakdown or diminished cough reflex), and may be affected by polypharmacy. The patient's living environment is also directly related to the risk for and severity of infection. For

---

* Department of Emergency Medicine, The Ohio State University, 146 Means Hall, 1654 Upham Drive, Columbus, OH 43210-1270.
E-mail address: jeffrey.caterino@osumc.edu

example, residents of nursing homes are particularly susceptible to infection and are more likely to be infected with multidrug resistant (MDR) organisms [9,10].

Infections in the elderly are distinguished from those in younger adults by significant differences in epidemiology, presentation, microbiology, and empiric treatment recommendations. The goal of this article is not to provide a comprehensive overview of disease processes that are covered elsewhere in this issue but to point out unique aspects related to the emergency department care of the elderly patient with infection. The aim is to provide the emergency medicine clinician with the tools to accurately diagnose and treat infections in this patient population.

Fever and infection in the elderly emergency department patient

Elevated temperature is one of the most common complaints in the elderly and is present in approximately 10% of elderly emergency department visits [3]. When fever is present, it is infectious in etiology approximately 90% of the time [11]. Fever in elderly emergency department patients is most commonly bacterial in origin. In several studies, it has been due to a viral cause in less than 5% of cases [3,11]. A temperature greater than 37.8°C (100°F) in an elderly emergency department patient is associated with markers of serious illness over 75% of the time as determined by positive blood cultures, death within 1 month, the need for surgery or an invasive procedure, hospitalization for 4 or more days, the administration of intravenous antibiotics for 3 or more days, or a repeat emergency department visit within 72 hours [11].

Given the high risk of a bacterial cause and the association with severe infection, fever in an elderly emergency department patient should prompt an extensive search for its source. Such a search is of course patient and symptom dependent, but most patients without an obvious source of infection should have a complete evaluation. This workup should include a complete blood count with differential, urinalysis, chest radiograph, blood cultures, and urine cultures. The possibility of a device-related infection, endocarditis, or another obscure source of bacterial infection should be investigated. One should also consider the possibility of other potentially serious causes of fever which are present 10% of the time (eg, rheumatologic disease, thyroid storm, environmental exposure, medication-related events, or malignancy).

Additionally, one should consider admission for febrile elderly patients even if no source for the fever is identified. Lack of an identifiable local source does not rule out serious infection. For example, one third of emergency department elderly patients with bacteremia will not have an identified local source of infection [12]. More than three quarters of febrile elderly patients will have a complicating factor that requires inpatient admission [11]. Otherwise well patients with adequate follow-up, intact functional status (ie, the ability to adequately perform activities of daily living),

Laboratory testing also fails to provide diagnostic certainty. The WBC count is not an accurate predictor of bacteremia. Among the elderly with bacteremia, 20% to 45% will have a normal WBC count [12,25,27,28]. The specificity of the WBC count for bacteremia is also poor [12]. Consideration of left shift improves sensitivity but decreases specificity dramatically [12]. Relying on an increase in the erythrocyte sedimentation rate is also insensitive for the diagnosis of bacteremia in the elderly (71% sensitivity) [27].

Laboratory and examination findings are insufficient to rule out bacteremia in elderly emergency department patients. Given its high mortality, a high suspicion should be maintained particularly in the presence of risk factors. Bacteremia should be considered a potential diagnosis in elderly patients with unexplained altered mental status, declining functional status, or falls even in the absence of a fever and identified source of infection. The presence of such clues will occur more commonly in elderly than younger patients, particularly in the oldest old.

The etiology of bacteremia in the elderly is heavily influenced by patient-specific factors. Patients with indwelling lines are more likely to have a skin source, those with indwelling catheters a genitourinary source, and those with altered mental status or impaired gag reflexes a pulmonary source. Urinary tract sources are the most common overall, even in the absence of indwelling urinary devices. They account for 25% to 55% of bacteremia in elderly patients presenting to the emergency department [17,21,25,28,30,32,33]. Lower respiratory infection accounts for 10% to 34%, followed by an unknown source in 11% to 31%, intra-abdominal source in 9% to 20%, and skin- or catheter-related source in 9% (Table 1) [12,17,21,25,28,30,33].

Given these common sources of bacteremia, urinary and respiratory pathogens are the predominant etiologic organisms. Exact percentages vary by study, but gram-negative organisms are the cause in approximately 70% of cases, gram-positive organisms in 25%, and anaerobes in less than 10% [21,25]. Polymicrobial infections are present in 5% to 17% of patients [17,25]. In most studies, *Escherichia coli* is the most commonly isolated organism (22%–54%) [17,21,25]. Other causative gram-negative organisms include *Klebsiella pneumoniae* (8%–16%) and *Pseudomonas* (4%–14%)

Table 1
Sources of bacteremia in the elderly

Source	Percentage of cases
Genitourinary	24–55
Lower respiratory	10–34
Unknown	11–36
Intra-abdominal	9–22
Skin/soft tissue	7–10
Catheter related	3–7
Other	5–10

Data from Refs. [12,17,21,25,28,30,33].

[17,21,25]. Gram-positive organisms include *Streptococcus pneumoniae* (4%–20%), *Staphylococcus aureus* (4%–14%), *Enterococcus* (3%–9%), and *Streptococcus viridans* (4%) [17,25]. The likelihood of *Staphylococcus aureus* bacteremia is increased in residents of long-term care facilities, particularly residents with nursing home–associated pneumonia or skin and soft-tissue infections. It is less common in patients dwelling in the community [34].

Bacteremia in the elderly is associated with high mortality rates. Overall rates have been 20% to 37% in most studies [21,25,28,32,33,35]. Mortality rates in individual patients depend on multiple factors, including functional status, presenting symptoms, the presence of shock, immunosuppression, and causative organism [20,21,29,34,36]. The presence of decreased functional status and gram-positive bacteremia are both associated with increased mortality [37]. The mortality rate in cases of *S aureus* bacteremia has ranged from 15% to as high as 60% [34,36]. Bacteremia due to lower respiratory and intra-abdominal infections is associated with increased mortality when compared with genitourinary sources [21]. Nosocomial bacteremia may also have particularly high mortality rates (21% at 7 days and 45% at 30 days), although studies are mixed [21,35,37].

Pneumonia

There are over 900,000 episodes of community-acquired pneumonia among the elderly yearly in the United States [38,39]. These cases result in 600,000 hospitalizations and almost 60,000 deaths [39–41]. As a result, pneumonia is the fifth leading cause of death among the elderly in the United States [40]. The disease particularly affects the oldest old, occurring in 1 of every 20 elderly persons aged 85 years and over each year [39].

The high incidence of pneumonia in the elderly population can be attributed to age-related immunosenescence combined with an increasing presence of risk factors for development of the disease [9,39,42–44]. Several factors contribute to an increased risk of introducing pathogens into the lower respiratory tract, including neurologic disease (eg, altered mental status, dementia, or past stroke), swallowing abnormalities, decreased functional status, malnutrition, and the use of sedative medications [39,42,44,45]. A witnessed aspiration is a particularly strong risk factor for developing pneumonia [45]. Comorbidities that suppress immune function also increase the risk. Chronic lung disease (eg, chronic obstructive pulmonary disease or asthma), structural lung disease, tobacco use, congestive heart failure, and residence in a nursing home have all been shown to be independent risk factors for the development of pneumonia in the elderly [9,42,43].

Diagnosis of pneumonia is complicated by the frequent absence of classic symptoms, such as fever, leukocytosis, or sputum production (Table 2) [46,47]. For example, only 26% of the elderly have fever compared with

Table 2
Symptoms of pneumonia in the elderly, including community acquired and nursing home populations

Symptom	Percentage of patients
Fever by history	53–60
Fever by measurement	12–32
Fatigue	84–88
Cough	63–84
Dyspnea	58–74
Productive sputum	30–65
Pleuritic chest pain	8–32
Hemoptysis	3–13
Tachypnea	65–68
Tachycardia	37–40
Symptom complexes	
Cough and fever	35
Cough or fever or dyspnea	56
Absence of pneumonia symptoms	10

Data from Refs. [16,46,48–50].

57% of younger patients [16]. Only 44% will have cough, fever, or dyspnea by history [48]. The absence of classic symptoms is particularly seen in residents of nursing homes, who are less likely to present with symptoms of pneumonia than elderly patients with community-acquired pneumonia [16]. Nursing home patients are less likely to have a productive cough or pleuritic pain but much more likely to have altered mental status [49,50]. In one study, elderly patients with nursing home–acquired pneumonia presented with altered mental status over half the time, whereas those from the community had altered mental status only 10% of the time [49]. Nearly one third of the time elderly patients with nursing home–acquired pneumonia will present with neither cough nor fever [32]. Importantly, altered mental status, lack of fever, lack of hypoxia, and increasing age have all been associated with a delay to antibiotic therapy in adults with pneumonia [51,52].

The in-hospital mortality rate for elders with community-acquired pneumonia is approximately 10% [53]. Nursing home–associated pneumonia has even greater mortality rates, as high as 53% in one study [49,50,54]. Studies have been mixed regarding the independent effect of age on mortality. It is unclear whether the increased mortality is due to advanced age itself or a result of the multiple comorbidities present in elderly patients [9,50,53,55]. Regardless, the increased mortality associated with pneumonia in elderly patients should prompt aggressive evaluation and therapy.

The most common system to identify the severity of pneumonia and risk-stratify patients is the Pneumonia Severity Index (PSI), a prognostic scoring system derived and validated on large cohorts of hospitalized patients [56]. The PSI divides patients into five classes, with successively increasing classes associated with increasing mortality. It is based on age, nursing home residence, co-existing illness, physical examination findings, laboratory studies, and radiographic findings. By definition, patients aged 50 years or more cannot be considered to be class I (lowest mortality) [56]. Patients in risk classes I and II are considered at low risk of mortality and appropriate for outpatient therapy [38,56]. The CURB-65 score is an additional scoring system that may be applied to elderly patients [38]. It has been shown to be equivalent to the PSI in a population with a mean age of 67 years, but it has not been tested in as large a population as the PSI [38,57].

The PSI has been studied in several elderly populations. In the initial derivation group, 85% of patients were over 50 years of age [56]. The usefulness of the PSI has also been demonstrated in nursing home patients [58]; however, some authorities question its accuracy in elderly patients. The PSI is heavily weighted by age, with patients receiving 1 point for every year of age. The result in some studies has been an overestimation of pneumonia severity and mortality in the elderly, with specificity for need for admission as low as 15% among the highest risk groups [59]. As a result, many patients requiring admission based on high PSI scores do not require admission on clinical grounds. Because age is the most significant determinant of PSI score, the majority of elderly patients with pneumonia will reach class III [1]. Selected class IV and V patients from assisted-living facilities have been successfully treated as outpatients in their facilities with parenteral antibiotics [58,60].

Conversely, a significant number of lower risk elderly patients as measured by PSI class I through III are admitted to the hospital for therapy, up to 40% in some studies [60–63]. Reasons for the admission of these patients have included hypoxemia, outpatient social service needs (eg, the need for aid with medication administration, checking services), failure of outpatient therapy, and the presence of other comorbid diseases [56,63,64]. Such factors are generally more likely to be present in the elderly and should also be considered in the admission decision.

In several studies, decreased functional status has been an important predictor of outcome in elderly patients with pneumonia [60]. The studies have demonstrated the importance of decreased functional status as a marker for increasing mortality in elderly patients. In some studies, it has also been seen as a superior predictor when compared with the PSI [53,59,60,65,66]. Although a good general guide and well studied in elderly populations, admission decisions should not be based exclusively on the PSI because it may not always capture the most appropriate disposition for an elderly emergency department patient with pneumonia. In particular, declining functional status should raise a flag that admission may be warranted.

Given the high associated mortality rates, rapid appropriate antibiotic therapy is essential in elderly patients with pneumonia. Studies that have demonstrated a decrease in mortality associated with rapid antibiotic administration have been conducted primarily in elderly patients [49,67]. For example, among Medicare patients with community-acquired pneumonia and no previous antibiotics, therapy within 4 hours of hospital arrival decreased in-hospital mortality (6.8% versus 7.4%; adjusted OR, 0.85, 0.74–0.98) [67].

Of particular concern in the elderly is the association of the absence of clinical symptoms with antibiotic delay. Altered mental status, lack of fever, lack of hypoxia, and increasing age have all been associated with a delay to antibiotic therapy in adults with pneumonia [51,52]. Given the possible lack of these symptoms in the elderly, extra vigilance for the presence of pneumonia and rapid administration of antibiotics are extremely important.

Perhaps the most important decision point for the emergency physician caring for an elderly patient with pneumonia is determining the likely causative organisms, which allows for initiation of appropriate antibiotic therapy. The primary distinction to be made is between community-acquired and health care–associated pneumonia (HCAP). The spectrum of patients considered to have HCAP is wider than many believe. Due to a significantly different microbiologic profile, there are significant differences in recommended empiric antibiotic therapy for patients with HCAP.

Community-acquired pneumonia in the elderly

The etiology of community-acquired pneumonia in the elderly is similar to that in younger patients. *Streptococcus pneumoniae* is the most common etiologic agent, accounting for approximately 50% of identified cases [42,68,69]. *Haemophilus influenzae* and *Moraxella catarrhalis* are also relatively common [42]. Atypical agents such as *Chlamydia pneumoniae, Mycoplasma,* and *Legionella pneumophila* are seen approximately 15% of the time in community-dwelling elderly persons, a lesser percentage than in younger patients [42]. Enteric gram-negative rods and *Staphylococcus aureus* are rarer pathogens and are more likely to be seen in the most severely ill patients. Community-acquired pneumonia developing after viral influenza has an increased chance of being caused by *S aureus* [42].

Empiric treatment of community-acquired pneumonia in the elderly is similar to that in younger patients and is based on the 2007 Infectious Disease Society of America (IDSA)/American Thoracic Society (ATS) Consensus Guidelines on the Management of Community-Acquired Pneumonia in Adults [38]. The guidelines do not contain any age-specific recommendations for antibiotic management. For patients treated in an outpatient setting, a macrolide or doxycycline is recommended; however, patients with certain comorbid diseases are at risk for drug-resistant *Streptococcus pneumoniae*. These conditions include "chronic heart, lung, liver, or renal disease; diabetes mellitus; alcoholism; malignancies; immunosuppressing conditions or drugs; use of antimicrobials within the previous 3 months; or other risk factors" [38]. In these patients, a respiratory fluoroquinolone is the preferred agent due to an increased risk of drug-resistant *S pneumoniae* [38]. Given the greater presence of such comorbidities in patients with increasing age, many elderly patients are most appropriately treated with a respiratory fluoroquinolone. Recommendations for inpatient and ICU treatment are the same in elderly and younger patients [38].

Elderly patients with community-acquired pneumonia must be distinguished from those with nursing home–acquired pneumonia (NHAP) or HCAP because there are significant differences in the etiologic organisms, recommended therapies, and outcomes. It is imperative that emergency physicians appropriately classify elderly patients with pneumonia. Many elderly patients will actually have an HCAP due to place of residence, comorbid disease process, or recent contact with the health care system. These patients require different antimicrobial coverage than those with community-acquired pneumonia.

Nursing home–and other health care–associated pneumonias

NHAP is clinically distinct from community-acquired pneumonia in the elderly. It is associated with increased comorbidity, poorer functional status, and greater mortality. The mortality rate is 19% to 53% in NHAP as compared with 8% to 14% in community-acquired pneumonia [49,50,54,70]. As measured by the PSI, NHAP is more severe than community-acquired pneumonia [56].

NHAP had previously been considered a subset of community-acquired pneumonia for the purposes of determining appropriate antimicrobial

---

Box 1. Definition of health care–associated pneumonia

1. Hospital-acquired pneumonia (HCAP): pneumonia not present at admission that develops 48 hours or more after hospitalization
2. Ventilator-associated pneumonia (VAP): pneumonia occurring 48 to 72 hours after endotracheal intubation
3. Health care–associated pneumonia (HCAP): pneumonia occurring in the presence of any of the following:
   Residence in a nursing home or long-term care facility
   Receipt of intravenous antibiotics, chemotherapy, or wound care within the preceding 30 days
   Hospitalization in an acute care hospital for 2 or more days in the preceding 90 days
   Attendance at a hospital or hemodialysis clinic

Data from American Thoracic Society, Infectious Disease Society of America. Guidelines for the management of adults with hospital-acquired, ventilator-associated, and health care–associated pneumonia. Am J Respir Crit Care Med 2005;171:388–416.

treatment [70–73]; however, the 2005 IDSA/ATS Guidelines for the Management of Adults with Hospital-Acquired, Ventilator-Associated, and Healthcare-Associated Pneumonia identified NHAP as an HCAP requiring significantly expanded antimicrobial coverage (Box 1) [10]. This position has been reiterated in the 2007 consensus guidelines on the management of community-acquired pneumonia which state that "pneumonia in non-ambulatory residents of nursing homes and other long-term care facilities epidemiologically mirrors hospital-acquired pneumonia and should be treated according to the HCAP guidelines" [38].

The rationale for this recommendation is that pneumonia in elderly nursing home patients is caused by a very different spectrum of microorganisms than in the community-dwelling population, one similar to that in other HCAPs. S pneumoniae is still the most common organism; however, enteric gram-negative rods, anaerobes, and Staphylococcus aureus are much more common in these patients. Studies of residents of long-term care facilities or admitted nursing home patients have demonstrated rates of Streptococcus pneumoniae of 0% to 39%, gram-negative rods of 0% to 70%, and Staphylococcus aureus of 0% to 47% [10,34,74–78]. Pseudomonas rates have generally been 4% to 25% but were as high as 52% in one multicenter study of hospitalized patients with NHAP [10,74,75,79]. Haemophilus influenzae (0%–19%), Moraxella catarrhalis (0%–5%), Chlamydia pneumoniae, and atypical agents are much rarer than in the community-dwelling population [42,44,75]. Atypical agents such as Legionella and Chlamydia pneumoniae have been associated with epidemic outbreaks in long-term care facilities [74].

A similar microbiologic pattern is present in other HCAPs. The complete spectrum of HCAP includes patients with classic hospital-acquired and ventilator-associated pneumonia. It also includes patients hospitalized in an acute care hospital for 2 or more days in the previous 90 days as well as residents of long-term care or nursing facilities, attendees of hospital or hemodialysis clinics, and those who have received intravenous antibiotics, chemotherapy, or wound care within the previous 30 days [10]. As a result, a large number of elderly emergency department patients should be considered as having HCAP with empiric antibiotic coverage directed at potential organisms.

Once the presence of an NHAP is determined, empiric antimicrobial therapy is selected based on the risk for the presence of MDR organisms. If there are no risk factors, coverage for antibiotic-sensitive Streptococcus pneumoniae, Haemophilus influenzae, Staphylococcus aureus, and gram-negative rods (other than Pseudomonas) is recommended. Suggested regimens include ceftriaxone, a respiratory fluoroquinolone, ampicillin/sulbactam, or ertapenem [10].

Patients at risk for MDR organisms require broader empiric coverage which should be initiated in the emergency department. Risk factors include residence in a nursing home or extended care facility. Other risk factors include antimicrobial therapy in the preceding 90 days, a high frequency of antibiotic resistance in the community, hospitalization for 2 or more days in the preceding 90 days, home infusion therapy, dialysis therapy, home wound care, a family member with a known MDR pathogen, and immunosuppressive disease or therapy [10]. Patients at risk for an MDR organism should receive empiric coverage for the organisms listed previously as well as for resistant *Pseudomonas*, *Klebsiella*, *Acinetobacter*, and *Staphylococcus* sp [10].

Appropriate antibiotic regimens to adequately cover MDR organisms include two drugs for gram-negative coverage as well as a drug for methicillin-resistant *S aureus* (MRSA) if there are risk factors or high local incidence [10]. The first gram-negative drug should be an anti-pseudomonal cephalosporin (cefepime or ceftazidime), an anti-pseudomonal carbapenem (imipenem or meropenem), or an anti-pseudomonal beta-lactam/beta-lactamase inhibitor (eg, piperacillin-tazobactam). The second gram-negative drug should be an aminoglycoside (eg, amikacin, gentamicin, or tobramycin) or an anti-pseudomonal fluoroquinolone (eg, ciprofloxacin or levofloxacin). If MRSA is a concern, vancomycin or linezolid is recommended [10]. The optimum antibiotic choice should always be based on patient factors as well as local microorganism incidence and resistance patterns.

The recommendation for considering NHAP as an HCAP with the resulting broad-spectrum empiric antibiotic coverage has generated some controversy. The best studies identifying pathogens responsible for NHAP were undertaken in intubated ICU patients from whom a reliable sputum sample could be obtained [10,80,81]. There is broad agreement that critically ill elderly patients with NHAP should be treated as if they have HCAP [70]; however, some investigators have pointed out that the evidence base identifying likely pathogens in less ill patients with NHAP is less robust. For example, many studies performed in patients did not ensure adequacy of the sputum samples, raising the possibility of oropharyngeal contamination [70,75]. As a result, they question the need for empiric broad-spectrum antibiotics in less severely ill patients with NHAP [70] based on the lack of any prospective, controlled trials of such regimens in these patients. It has also been observed that a large number of patients who have NHAP are treated successfully without hospitalization and presumably without multiple parenteral antibiotics [70,75]. Nevertheless, the recently published 2007 IDSA/ATS Community-Acquired Pneumonia Guidelines do specifically state that residents of long-term care facilities should be treated as having HCAP.

It can be agreed that elderly patients with NHAP or HCAP and severe illness require empiric therapy with multiple antibiotics to cover potentially resistant pathogens. Despite a lack of prospective, controlled trials in less severely ill patients, strict reading of the IDSA/ATS guidelines leads one to conclude that all NHAP patients should receive such therapy. This interpretation is supported by the specific exclusion of nonambulatory residents of long-term care facilities from the 2007 IDSA/ATS Community-Acquired

Pneumonia Guidelines [38]. This empiric therapy should include two drugs effective against gram-negative rods with the possible addition of an antibiotic to cover MRSA.

Urinary tract infection

Urinary tract infection is another common infection in emergency department elderly patients. Emergency department diagnosis and treatment are complicated by atypical clinical presentations, greater than expected adverse outcomes, and difficulties in choosing an empiric antibiotic regimen due to the frequent presence of resistant bacteria. Genitourinary infection puts elderly patients at significant risk due to its association with high rates of bacteremia and mortality. Among emergency department elderly patients, approximately 17% of urinary tract infections are associated with bacteremia [82]. Among patients admitted from the emergency department with a urinary tract infection, the in-hospital mortality rate is 6% [82].

Classic urinary tract infection symptoms are often not present, and atypical presentations often occur. In one study, presenting symptoms among elderly patients diagnosed with a urinary tract infection in the emergency department were as follows: urinary symptoms (26%), mental status changes (26%), temperature greater than 37.7°C or less than 35°C (17%), tachycardia (30%), systolic blood pressure less than 90 mm Hg (7%), and WBC count greater than 11,000 or less than 5000/mm^3 (43%) [82]. The presence of classic lower urinary tract symptoms in elderly patients may also not be diagnostic because they may actually be related to an anatomic abnormality or other aging-associated process rather than acute infection [83].

Laboratory diagnosis of urinary tract infection in elderly emergency department patients is complicated by several factors. A positive urine culture is generally considered the gold standard for diagnosis but will only be available to the emergency department physician if obtained at some time before the current visit. The cutoff for a positive urinary culture in the elderly is generally considered to be less than the traditional 100,000 cfu/mL standard defined initially for young women with acute pyelonephritis or multiple positive urine cultures. For elderly patients, many experts now recommend 10,000 cfu/mL as the cutoff for a positive culture obtained from a clean catch specimen and 100 cfu/mL as the cutoff for a specimen obtained by clean catheterization [84]. Because elderly patients are also frequently infected by more than one organism, each organism with sufficient colony counts should be considered a potential pathogen [85].

The most common screening method in the emergency department is the use of a reagent strip to identify the presence of nitrites or leukocyte esterase; however, the examination of reagent strips has demonstrated poor test characteristics and generally poor correlation with positive cultures [84,86,87]. The presence of nitrites alone has poor sensitivity but high specificity (>90%), with test characteristics much worse when there are low bacterial colony counts [84,86]. Leukocyte esterase has good sensitivity (62%–98%) and specificity (55%–96%) and is not affected by colony counts, but its test characteristics are not sufficient to definitively guide therapy and diagnosis [84].

Reagent test characteristics are particularly poor in elderly populations. In one study of 200 emergency department patients aged 65 years or older, 30% of reagent strips with positive cultures were negative for both nitrites and leukocyte esterase. Additionally, over 50% of strips positive for either nitrites or leukocyte esterase were associated with a negative urinary culture [82,86]. This study divided patients into those with vague non-urinary symptoms and those presenting to the emergency department for a specific non-infectious complaint (eg, cardiac problems, dyspnea, stroke). Even in symptomatic patients, reagent strip testing (positive nitrite or leukocyte esterase or both) had a sensitivity of only 74% and specificity of 70%. The positive likelihood ratio was 2.8 and negative likelihood ratio 0.3, indicating only a weak predictive ability for the reagent strips in predicting urinary tract infection in elderly emergency department patients [86].

In at least one study in adults in an emergency department, microscopy for white blood cells did not improve diagnostic accuracy over the use of reagent strips [87]. Gram stain of urine for bacteria also lacks sensitivity, and its performance is highly dependent on colony counts of the infecting organism. Patients with infection and low bacterial colony counts (a situation particularly common in the elderly) are more likely to have falsely negative urine Gram stains. Nevertheless, a urine Gram stain can help identify the causative organism [84].

Further complicating diagnosis is the high prevalence of asymptomatic bacteriuria in elderly patients. Asymptomatic bacteriuria is present in 15% to 50% of all long-term care facility patients and 5% to 20% of all community-dwelling elders [85,88–91]. The challenge for the emergency physician is determining when vague symptoms in an elderly patient associated with positive urine testing are due to a urinary infection or another cause. A positive urine reagent test or microscopy should not dissuade the physician from searching for other causes of vague symptoms in the elderly. Even a positive urinary culture may not prove that the urinary tract is the source of the patient's symptoms. In one study of nursing home residents with a fever but no localizing symptoms, the positive predictive value of a positive urine culture was only 12%, suggesting that a large number of patients had some other source as the cause of the fever [92]. Between 32% and 75% of patients with fever and bacteriuria had some other source of infection [92]. This finding was confirmed in the study of elderly emergency department patients discussed previously [86]. In that study, 14% of patients who were in the emergency department for an unrelated noninfectious issue such as chest pain had a positive urine culture in comparison with 19% of patients in the group with vague symptoms [86]. This rate occurred even with a restrictive definition of positive urine cultures; therefore, even if fever is present in the setting of positive urine testing, the high rates of asymptomatic bacteriuria present in the elderly population make consideration of other sources of infection necessary [90].

As is true in younger patients, *Escherichia coli* remains the most common cause of genitourinary infection in the elderly (30%–60% of cases); however, other etiologies are more common than in younger patients, including *Proteus mirabilis*, *Klebsiella pneumoniae*, *Enterococcus*, and *Pseudomonas* [82,93]. The risk of these non–*Escherichia coli* organisms is also greater in patients with complicated urinary tract infections or residents of long-term care facilities [85,91,93,94].

Choosing an antibiotic and duration of therapy depends on the presence or absence of complicating factors, the likelihood of an MDR organism, and the presence of systemic symptoms. A complicated urinary tract infection is generally defined as the presence of any of the following: diabetes, indwelling catheter or device, structural or functional genitourinary abnormalities, nephrolithiasis, immunosuppression, renal transplant, renal failure, recent genitourinary instrumentation, benign prostatic hypertrophy, or renal tumor [91,93,94]. Some authorities consider urinary tract infection in the elderly to be, by definition, complicated because it is generally due to an abnormality of the genitourinary tract [94].

Assessing the likelihood of a resistant organism has an important role in determining appropriate empiric antibiotic therapy because resistance rates are high among elderly patients with urinary tract infection. Studies are mixed as to whether age independently predisposes to infection with resistant organisms [91,95–97]. Nevertheless, there is agreement that the presence of certain factors places elderly patients at increased risk of resistant genitourinary bacteria. These factors include residence in a long-term care facility, recent antibiotic use, the presence of an indwelling catheter or structural genitourinary abnormality, and baseline decreased functional status [91,95–99]. In one study of emergency department patients aged 65 years and over, Wright and colleagues [95] found that 45% were infected with an MDR organism, 46% with an organism resistant to trimethoprim-sulfamethoxazole (TMP-SMX), and 11% to fluoroquinolones. In the subset of patients presenting from long-term care facilities, rates were even higher. Sixty-one percent had an MDR organism, 68% an organism resistant to TMP-SMX, and 41% an organism resistant to fluoroquinolones.

Treatment of uncomplicated community-acquired urinary tract infection in the elderly is generally with a fluoroquinolone which possesses good genitourinary penetration or with amoxicillin-clavulanate. Due to the increased rates of resistance, TMP-SMX is not preferred as an empiric first-line agent [91,100]. Alternative intravenous therapies include a fluoroquinolone, gentamicin plus or minus ampicillin, or a third-generation cephalosporin plus or minus an aminoglycoside [100]. The optimal duration of therapy for uncomplicated urinary tract infections in the elderly is unclear. Single-dose therapy is not recommended [101]. In one review, short courses of 3 to 6 days had equivalent outcome to longer 7- to 14-day courses [101].

Selecting the optimum treatment for urinary tract infections acquired in a long-term care facility or in the presence of other complicating factors is more difficult due to the high prevalence of resistant organisms. A fluoroquinolone should generally be considered although only cautiously used as monotherapy due to increased rates of resistance in these patient populations [95]. In these cases, empiric fluoroquinolone monotherapy may be may be less preferred than combination therapy. Alternative or additional therapies may include aminoglycosides plus or minus ampicillin, antipseudomonal beta-lactams, or an anti-pseudomonal carbapenem [91]. Beta-lactams may be ineffective in the presence of organisms producing extended-spectrum beta-lactamases [91]. Because the resistance patterns for individual patients are generally not available in the emergency department, the choice of antibiotic should be based on patient characteristics, past patient culture results, and local resistance patterns. Patients who have an increased risk of drug-resistant organisms or who are moderately to severely ill should be strongly considered for initial two-drug therapy to ensure effectiveness of the empiric regimen. In patients with urinary tract infections associated with chronic indwelling catheters, replacement of the catheter is associated with improved clinical outcomes and should be undertaken in the emergency department [102].

Asymptomatic bacteriuria in nursing home residents, even in the presence of a positive urine culture, should not be treated because there is no proven benefit but increases in costs, adverse drug effects, and development of drug-resistant organisms [85].

Influenza

Although it affects all age groups, influenza causes the most severe disease in the aged. Advancing age is associated with increased rates of influenza-related hospitalization [103]. Ninety percent of deaths related to influenza occur in patients aged 65 years and over [104]. As is true for bacterial pneumonia, the elderly may fail to demonstrate the classic signs of influenza. For example, many will not have fever or cough [105]. Secondary bacterial pneumonia may occur and is most commonly caused by *Streptococcus pneumoniae*, *Staphylococcus aureus*, and *Haemophilus influenzae* [106].

For the treatment of influenza, oseltamivir and zanamivir are recommended [107]; however, zanamivir is inhaled and may cause bronchospasm in patients with underlying lung disease. Oseltamivir is given in the usual adult dosage of 75 mg orally twice daily for 5 days. Oseltamivir should be renally dosed for patients with creatinine clearance less than 30 mL/min, with a recommended once daily regimen for those with clearance of 10 to 30 mL/min [107]. Amantadine and rimantadine are not recommended due to the emergence of viral resistance as well as increased side effects in the elderly, particularly central nervous system side effects with amantadine [107]. Due to the severe systemic effects (fatigue, myalgias, and decline in functional status) and the severity of the respiratory illness, many elderly patients with influenza will require admission. For those being discharged, close follow-up is essential.

The occurrence of two or more cases of influenza in a nursing home or other institutional setting should trigger prophylaxis of residents with antiviral agents. It is recommended that these agents be administered even to facility patients who have been vaccinated [105,108]. The emergency department diagnosis of influenza in an elderly patient from a long-term care facility should prompt notification of that facility so that appropriate measures may be taken.

Yearly influenza vaccination is recommended for all adults aged 50 years and older [109]. Influenza vaccination of the community-dwelling elderly is associated with a 27% reduction in the risk of hospitalization and 48% reduction in the risk of death [110]. Only the trivalent inactivated vaccine is approved for elderly patients; the live attenuated intranasal vaccine should only be used in healthy persons aged 5 to 49 years [109]. The only contraindications are previous anaphylaxis to eggs or components of the vaccine. Vaccine-related Guillain-Barre syndrome and moderate-to-severe febrile illnesses are relative contraindications. Patients with illness associated with mild or no fever may receive the vaccine [109]. Pneumococcal and influenza vaccination programs have been successfully implemented in the emergency department setting [111]. Given the proven benefits, emergency department physicians should consider offering vaccination to all appropriate patients.

Sepsis

More than 60% of the 750,000 patients in whom sepsis or severe sepsis develops in the United States each year are aged 65 years or older [112,113]. Among emergency department patients, a similar age distribution holds, with 65% of septic emergency department patients aged 65 years or older [4]. Increasing age brings with it an increasing incidence of sepsis. There are less than five cases of sepsis per 100,000 population in persons aged less than 65 years. This rate increases to 26 cases per 100,000 population yearly in persons aged 85 years and older [112,113]. Elderly patients also die at higher rates from sepsis than do younger patients, although studies are mixed as to whether this is due to an independent effect of age or to comorbidities and other patient factors that are more common in the elderly [7,113]. Factors that have been identified as increasing the risk for sepsis in the elderly include the presence of comorbid disease, malnutrition, decreased functional status, the presence of indwelling medical devices, and residence in a long-term care facility [7].

The presenting signs and symptoms of sepsis in the elderly may be different from those in younger patients. In general, the differences already discussed under specific disease processes also apply to sepsis. In one study, patients 75 years of age or older with sepsis were more likely to have tachypnea or altered mental status than younger patients and were less likely to have tachycardia or hypoxemia [114].

Sepsis in the elderly is most commonly due to a respiratory source, with genitourinary sources the second most common cause. Elderly patients are more likely to have respiratory or genitourinary sources of sepsis than are younger patients [113,115]. As a result, elderly patients also have a different spectrum of causative microorganisms than younger patients. The elderly are more likely to have gram-negative sepsis, particularly residents of long-term care facilities, because such residence is associated with gram-negative colonization of the oropharynx [115]. The increased rates of antimicrobial resistance in long-term care facilities make elderly residents particularly susceptible to serious gram-negative infection with drug-resistant organisms [7]. Other risk factors include recent hospitalizations, comorbidities, and immunocompromised states [7]. Initial empiric antimicrobial agents should be selected with consideration for the possibility of such MDR organisms.

Treatment of severe sepsis or septic shock in the elderly should be as aggressive as in younger patients and in compliance with current guidelines. All patients with severe sepsis or septic shock should have antibiotics started within 1 hour of recognition of the disease entity [116]. Initial therapy should be directed by likely sources of infection, patient characteristics, and local resistance patterns. Antibiotics should be broad spectrum to cover all potential organisms, with possible double coverage if resistant organisms are of concern. Failure to choose empiric antibiotics effective against the causative organisms has been associated with significantly increased rates of mortality [116]. Such choices are particularly important in the elderly given the more severe disease burden, absence of physiologic reserve, and increased likelihood of resistant organisms.

In addition to rapid institution of appropriate antibiotic therapy, several other interventions are suggested for patients with severe sepsis or septic shock. Interventions proven effective include rapid restoration of organ perfusion and the administration of drotrecogin alfa to select patients [116]. Due to the high percentage of elderly patients in the septic population, in most studies of sepsis, patients have had an average age of approximately 60 to 65 years [7,116–119]. As a result, elderly patients are well represented in these studies, and the results can be applied directly to an elderly emergency department population. It is recommended that, in general, therapy be as aggressive in elderly patients with severe sepsis as in younger patients within the constraints of living wills, code status [7].

Rapid restoration of adequate end organ perfusion includes restoration of effective circulating volume, maintenance of mean arterial pressure, and provision of adequate oxygen delivery to end organs. End organ oxygen delivery is monitored through the use of central venous oxygen saturation monitoring. The most commonly applied protocol is early goal-directed therapy as described by Rivers and colleagues [116,117,120]. The average age of subjects in the initial early goal-directed therapy study was 67.1 years [117]; therefore, the findings are applicable to elderly emergency department patients. In the protocol, intravenous fluids are administered to restore effective circulating volume with a goal central venous pressure of 8 to 12 mm Hg (> 12 mm Hg in intubated patients). Mean arterial pressure should be supported by vasopressors such as norepinephrine or dopamine. Once volume has been restored and adequate mean arterial pressure established, adequacy of end organ oxygen delivery should be monitored by measurement of central venous oxygen saturation. In patients with central venous oxygen saturation less than 70% (indicative of inadequate oxygen delivery), further support through the use of transfusion to a hematocrit of 30% with or without dobutamine infusion should be instituted.

Although, there may be a tendency to be less aggressive in resuscitating elderly patients with sepsis due to concerns over side effects such as volume overload, arrhythmia from drug infusion, or complications of central line placement, such concerns should not deter the emergency physician from the implementation of these proven interventions, which have been used successfully in patients 65 years of age and older. Given their increased risk of mortality, elderly patients are the most likely group to benefit from aggressive therapy. The use of interventions proven to decrease mortality should be pursued as aggressively in emergency department elderly patients as in younger patients.

Elderly patients also qualify as being appropriate for other therapies with proven benefit in sepsis. The use of intravenous corticosteroids has been recommended for patients who have a persistent vasopressor requirement after adequate fluid resuscitation [116,121]. However, the use of corticosteroids for septic shock recently has been called into question in a high quality randomized trial that demonstrated no mortality benefit but potential harm from steroid use caused by increased rates of superinfection [122].

Drotrecogin alfa may safely be used in elderly patients when appropriate criteria are met. Although most commonly administered in the ICU, there are increasing reports of emergency department use. In a retrospectively defined subgroup analysis of the PROWESS trial, patients 75 years of age or older with severe sepsis who were treated with drotrecogin alfa had an absolute risk reduction in 28-day mortality of 15.5% with similar results for in-hospital mortality [123]. This mortality benefit was maintained over a 2-year follow-up period and when controlling for differences between the treatment and placebo groups. There was no increased risk of severe bleeding, and age was not related to bleeding rates [123]. The researchers cautioned that rigorous entry criteria should be maintained. Patients excluded from the study were those with recent (< 3 months) stroke, intracranial pathology, or the need for systemic anticoagulation, all conditions more commonly present in elderly patients. Other studies have demonstrated decreased resource use as well as cost effectiveness for drotrecogin alfa in elderly patients with sepsis

[124,125]. Assuming proper protocols are in place in the emergency department to ensure safe administration to appropriate patients, drotrecogin alfa may be administered to elderly patients.

Summary

Evaluation and management of the elderly patient with infection in the emergency department presents several challenges to the emergency physician. Elderly patients often present without classic signs and symptoms of infection, requiring vigilance in the face of nonspecific symptoms such as confusion or decreased functional status. These patients are at higher risk of poor outcomes than are younger adults. They are also in many cases at greater risk of infection with resistant organisms, necessitating the empiric use of broad-spectrum antimicrobial agents. Consideration of these unique aspects of the infected elderly patient will aid the emergency physician in providing optimal care to this at-risk patient population.

References

[1] High KP. Why should the infectious diseases community focus on aging and care of the older adult? Clin Infect Dis 2003;37(2):196–200.
[2] McCaig LF, Nawar EW. National hospital ambulatory medical care survey: 2004 emergency department summary. Adv Data 2006;372:1–29.
[3] Keating HJ III, Klimek JJ, Levine DS, et al. Effect of aging on the clinical significance of fever in ambulatory adult patients. J Am Geriatr Soc 1984;32(4):282–7.
[4] Strehlow MC, Emond SD, Shapiro NI, et al. National study of emergency department visits for sepsis, 1992 to 2001. Ann Emerg Med 2006;48(3):326–31.
[5] High K, Bradley S, Loeb M, et al. A new paradigm for clinical investigation of infectious syndromes in older adults: assessing functional status as a risk factor and outcome measure. J Am Geriatr Soc 2005;53(3):528–35.
[6] Yoshikawa TT. Epidemiology and unique aspects of aging and infectious diseases. Clin Infect Dis 2000;30(6):931–3.
[7] Girard TD, Opal SM, Ely EW. Insights into severe sepsis in older patients: from epidemiology to evidence-based management. Clin Infect Dis 2005;40(5):719–27.
[8] Grubeck-Loebenstein B, Wick G. The aging of the immune system. Adv Immunol 2002;80: 243–84.
[9] Koivula I, Sten M, Makela PH. Risk factors for pneumonia in the elderly. Am J Med 1994; 96(4):313–20.
[10] American Thoracic Society, Infectious Disease Society of America. Guidelines for the management of adults with hospital-acquired, ventilator-associated, and health care-associated pneumonia. Am J Respir Crit Care Med 2005;171(4):388–416.
[11] Marco CA, Schoenfeld CN, Hansen KN, et al. Fever in geriatric emergency patients: clinical features associated with serious illness. Ann Emerg Med 1995;26(1):18–24.
[12] Caterino JM, Scheatzle MD, Forbes ML, et al. Bacteremic elder emergency department patients: procalcitonin and white count. Acad Emerg Med 2004;11(4):393–6.
[13] Castle SC, Norman DC, Yeh M, et al. Fever response in elderly nursing home residents: are the older truly colder? J Am Geriatr Soc 1991;39(9):853–7.
[14] Norman DC. Fever in the elderly. Clin Infect Dis 2000;31(1):148–51.

[15] Norman DC, Yoshikawa TT. Fever in the elderly. Infect Dis Clin North Am 1996;10(1): 93–9.

[16] Marrie TJ, Haldane EV, Faulkner RS, et al. Community-acquired pneumonia requiring hospitalization: is it different in the elderly? J Am Geriatr Soc 1985;33(10):671–80.

[17] Fontanarosa PB, Kaeberlein FJ, Gerson LW, et al. Difficulty in predicting bacteremia in elderly emergency patients. Ann Emerg Med 1992;21(7):842–8.

[18] Gagliardi JP, Nettles RE, McCarty DE, et al. Native valve infective endocarditis in elderly and younger adult patients: comparison of clinical features and outcomes with use of the Duke criteria and the Duke Endocarditis Database. Clin Infect Dis 1998;26(5):1165–8.

[19] McBean M, Rajamani S. Increasing rates of hospitalization due to septicemia in the US elderly population, 1986–1997. J Infect Dis 2001;183(4):596–603.

[20] Brun-Buisson C, Doyon F, Carlet J. Bacteremia and severe sepsis in adults: a multicenter prospective survey in ICUs and wards of 24 hospitals. French Bacteremia-Sepsis Study Group. Am J Respir Crit Care Med 1996;154(3 Pt 1):617–24.

[21] Khayr WF, CarMichael MJ, Dubanowich CS, et al. Epidemiology of bacteremia in the geriatric population. Am J Ther 2003;10(2):127–31.

[22] Whitelaw DA, Rayner BL, Willcox PA. Community-acquired bacteremia in the elderly: a prospective study of 121 cases. J Am Geriatr Soc 1992;40(10):996–1000.

[23] Sinclair D, Svendsen A, Marrie T. Bacteremia in nursing home patients: prevalence among patients presenting to an emergency department. Can Fam Physician 1998;44:317–22.

[24] Bahagon Y, Raveh D, Schlesinger Y, et al. Prevalence and predictive features of bacteremic urinary tract infection in emergency department patients. Eur J Clin Microbiol Infect Dis 2007;26(5):349–52.

[25] Lee CC, Chen SY, Chang IJ, et al. Comparison of clinical manifestations and outcome of community-acquired bloodstream infections among the oldest old, elderly, and adult patients. Medicine (Baltimore) 2007;86(3):138–44.

[26] Gleckman R, Hibert D. Afebrile bacteremia: a phenomenon in geriatric patients. JAMA 1982;248(12):1478–81.

[27] Chassagne P, Perol MB, Doucet J, et al. Is presentation of bacteremia in the elderly the same as in younger patients? Am J Med 1996;100(1):65–70.

[28] Windsor AC. Bacteraemia in a geriatric unit. Gerontology 1983;29(2):125–30.

[29] Deulofeu F, Cervello B, Capell S, et al. Predictors of mortality in patients with bacteremia: the importance of functional status. J Am Geriatr Soc 1998;46(1):14–8.

[30] Bentley DW, Bradley S, High K, et al. Practice guideline for evaluation of fever and infection in long-term care facilities. Clin Infect Dis 2000;31(3):640–53.

[31] Chi RC, Jackson LA, Neuzil KM. Characteristics and outcomes of older adults with community-acquired pneumococcal bacteremia. J Am Geriatr Soc 2006;54(1):115–20.

[32] Muder RR, Brennen C, Swenson DL, et al. Pneumonia in a long-term care facility: a prospective study of outcome. Arch Intern Med 1996;156(20):2365–70.

[33] Esposito AL, Gleckman RA, Cram S, et al. Community-acquired bacteremia in the elderly: analysis of one hundred consecutive episodes. J Am Geriatr Soc 1980;28(7):315–9.

[34] Bradley SF. Staphylococcus aureus infections and antibiotic resistance in older adults. Clin Infect Dis 2002;34(2):211–6.

[35] Setia U, Serventi I, Lorenz P. Bacteremia in a long-term care facility: spectrum and mortality. Arch Intern Med 1984;144(8):1633–5.

[36] Bader MS. Staphylococcus aureus bacteremia in older adults: predictors of 7-day mortality and infection with a methicillin-resistant strain. Infect Control Hosp Epidemiol 2006; 27(11):1219–25.

[37] Gavazzi G, Escobar P, Olive F, et al. Nosocomial bacteremia in very old patients: predictors of mortality. Aging Clin Exp Res 2005;17(4):337–42.

[38] Mandell LA, Wunderink RG, Anzueto A, et al. Infectious diseases society of America/ American Thoracic Society consensus guidelines on the management of community-acquired pneumonia in adults. Clin Infect Dis 2007;44(Suppl 2):S27–72.

[39] Jackson ML, Neuzil KM, Thompson WW, et al. The burden of community-acquired pneumonia in seniors: results of a population-based study. Clin Infect Dis 2004;39(11): 1642–50.

[40] Pneumonia and influenza death rates–United States, 1979–1994. MMWR Morb Mortal Wkly Rep 1995;44(28):535–7.

[41] Kochanek KD, Smith BL. Deaths: preliminary data for 2002. Natl Vital Stat Rep 2004; 52(13):1–47.

[42] Ferrara AM, Fietta AM. New developments in antibacterial choice for lower respiratory tract infections in elderly patients. Drugs Aging 2004;21(3):167–86.

[43] Farr BM, Bartlett CL, Wadsworth J, et al. Risk factors for community-acquired pneumonia diagnosed upon hospital admission: British Thoracic Society Pneumonia Study Group. Respir Med 2000;94(10):954–63.

[44] Loeb M, McGeer A, McArthur M, et al. Risk factors for pneumonia and other lower respiratory tract infections in elderly residents of long-term care facilities. Arch Intern Med 1999;159(17):2058–64.

[45] Vergis EN, Brennen C, Wagener M, et al. Pneumonia in long-term care: a prospective case-control study of risk factors and impact on survival. Arch Intern Med 2001;161(19): 2378–81.

[46] Metlay JP, Schulz R, Li YH, et al. Influence of age on symptoms at presentation in patients with community-acquired pneumonia. Arch Intern Med 1997;157(13):1453–9.

[47] Starczewski AR, Allen SC, Vargas E, et al. Clinical prognostic indices of fatality in elderly patients admitted to hospital with acute pneumonia. Age Ageing 1988;17(3):181–6.

[48] Harper C, Newton P. Clinical aspects of pneumonia in the elderly veteran. J Am Geriatr Soc 1989;37(9):867–72.

[49] Meehan TP, Fine MJ, Krumholz HM, et al. Quality of care, process, and outcomes in elderly patients with pneumonia. JAMA 1997;278(23):2080–4.

[50] Lim WS, Macfarlane JT. A prospective comparison of nursing home acquired pneumonia with community acquired pneumonia. Eur Respir J 2001;18(2):362–8.

[51] Waterer GW, Kessler LA, Wunderink RG. Delayed administration of antibiotics and atypical presentation in community-acquired pneumonia. Chest 2006;130(1):11–5.

[52] Fine JM, Fine MJ, Galusha D, et al. Patient and hospital characteristics associated with recommended processes of care for elderly patients hospitalized with pneumonia: results from the Medicare quality indicator system pneumonia module. Arch Intern Med 2002; 162(7):827–33.

[53] Conte HA, Chen YT, Mehal W, et al. A prognostic rule for elderly patients admitted with community-acquired pneumonia. Am J Med 1999;106(1):20–8.

[54] Marrie TJ, Blanchard W. A comparison of nursing home-acquired pneumonia patients with patients with community-acquired pneumonia and nursing home patients without pneumonia. J Am Geriatr Soc 1997;45(1):50–5.

[55] Kaplan V, Angus DC. Community-acquired pneumonia in the elderly. Crit Care Clin 2003; 19(4):729–48.

[56] Fine MJ, Auble TE, Yealy DM, et al. A prediction rule to identify low-risk patients with community-acquired pneumonia. N Engl J Med 1997;336(4):243–50.

[57] Ewig S, de RA, Bauer T, et al. Validation of predictive rules and indices of severity for community acquired pneumonia. Thorax 2004;59(5):421–7.

[58] Mylotte JM, Naughton B, Saludades C, et al. Validation and application of the pneumonia prognosis index to nursing home residents with pneumonia. J Am Geriatr Soc 1998;46(12): 1538–44.

[59] Naito T, Suda T, Yasuda K, et al. A validation and potential modification of the pneumonia severity index in elderly patients with community-acquired pneumonia. J Am Geriatr Soc 2006;54(8):1212–9.

[60] Torres OH, Munoz J, Ruiz D, et al. Outcome predictors of pneumonia in elderly patients: importance of functional assessment. J Am Geriatr Soc 2004;52(10):1603–9.

[61] Atlas SJ, Benzer TI, Borowsky LH, et al. Safely increasing the proportion of patients with community-acquired pneumonia treated as outpatients: an interventional trial. Arch Intern Med 1998;158(12):1350–6.

[62] Marrie TJ. Community-acquired pneumonia in the elderly. Clin Infect Dis 2000;31(4): 1066–78.

[63] Arnold FW, Ramirez JA, McDonald LC, et al. Hospitalization for community-acquired pneumonia: the pneumonia severity index vs clinical judgment. Chest 2003;124(1):121–4.

[64] Goss CH, Rubenfeld GD, Park DR, et al. Cost and incidence of social comorbidities in low-risk patients with community-acquired pneumonia admitted to a public hospital. Chest 2003;124(6):2148–55.

[65] Marrie TJ, Majumdar SR. Management of community-acquired pneumonia in the emergency room. Respir Care Clin N Am 2005;11(1):15–24.

[66] Mehr DR, Binder EF, Kruse RL, et al. Predicting mortality in nursing home residents with lower respiratory tract infection: the Missouri LRI Study. JAMA 2001;286(19): 2427–36.

[67] Houck PM, Bratzler DW, Nsa W, et al. Timing of antibiotic administration and outcomes for Medicare patients hospitalized with community-acquired pneumonia. Arch Intern Med 2004;164(6):637–44.

[68] Loeb M. Pneumonia in older persons. Clin Infect Dis 2003;37(10):1335–9.

[69] Neralla S, Meyer KC. Drug treatment of pneumococcal pneumonia in the elderly. Drugs Aging 2004;21(13):851–64.

[70] Mylotte JM. Nursing home-acquired pneumonia: update on treatment options. Drugs Aging 2006;23(5):377–90.

[71] Guidelines for the management of community-acquired pneumonia in adults admitted to hospital: the British Thoracic Society. Br J Hosp Med 1993;49(5):346–50.

[72] Zimmer JG, Hall WJ. Nursing home-acquired pneumonia: avoiding the hospital. J Am Geriatr Soc 1997;45(3):380–1.

[73] Mandell LA, Bartlett JG, Dowell SF, et al. Update of practice guidelines for the management of community-acquired pneumonia in immunocompetent adults. Clin Infect Dis 2003;37(11):1405–33.

[74] Muder RR, Aghababian RV, Loeb MB, et al. Nursing home-acquired pneumonia: an emergency department treatment algorithm. Curr Med Res Opin 2004;20(8):1309–20.

[75] Muder RR. Pneumonia in residents of long-term care facilities: epidemiology, etiology, management, and prevention. Am J Med 1998;105(4):319–30.

[76] Yakovlev SV, Stratchounski LS, Woods GL, et al. Ertapenem versus cefepime for initial empirical treatment of pneumonia acquired in skilled-care facilities or in hospitals outside the intensive care unit. Eur J Clin Microbiol Infect Dis 2006;25(10):633–41.

[77] Loeb M. Epidemiology of community- and nursing home-acquired pneumonia in older adults. Expert Rev Anti Infect Ther 2005;3(2):263–70.

[78] Dempsey CL. Nursing home-acquired pneumonia: outcomes from a clinical process improvement program. Pharmacotherapy 1995;15(1 Pt 2):33S–8S.

[79] Kollef MH, Shorr A, Tabak YP, et al. Epidemiology and outcomes of health care-associated pneumonia: results from a large US database of culture-positive pneumonia. Chest 2005;128(6):3854–62.

[80] El-Solh AA, Sikka P, Ramadan F, et al. Etiology of severe pneumonia in the very elderly. Am J Respir Crit Care Med 2001;163(3 Pt 1):645–51.

[81] El-Solh AA, Pietrantoni C, Bhat A, et al. Microbiology of severe aspiration pneumonia in institutionalized elderly. Am J Respir Crit Care Med 2003;167(12):1650–4.

[82] Ginde AA, Rhee SH, Katz ED. Predictors of outcome in geriatric patients with urinary tract infections. J Emerg Med 2004;27(2):101–8.

[83] Raz P. Urinary tract infection in elderly women. Int J Antimicrob Agents 1998;10(3):177–9.

[84] Wilson ML, Gaido L. Laboratory diagnosis of urinary tract infections in adult patients. Clin Infect Dis 2004;38(8):1150–8.

[85] Nicolle LE. Urinary tract infection in long-term care facility residents. Clin Infect Dis 2000; 31(3):757–61.

[86] Ducharme J, Neilson S, Ginn JL. Can urine cultures and reagent test strips be used to diagnose urinary tract infection in elderly emergency department patients without focal urinary symptoms? CJEM 2007;9(2):87–92.

[87] Lammers RL, Gibson S, Kovacs D, et al. Comparison of test characteristics of urine dipstick and urinalysis at various test cutoff points. Ann Emerg Med 2001;38(5):505–12.

[88] Raz R. Asymptomatic bacteriuria: clinical significance and management. Nephrol Dial Transplant 2001;16(Suppl 6):135–6.

[89] Aguirre-Avalos G, Zavala-Silva ML, Diaz-Nava A, et al. Asymptomatic bacteriuria and inflammatory response to urinary tract infection of elderly ambulatory women in nursing homes. Arch Med Res 1999;30(1):29–32.

[90] Nicolle LE. Urinary tract infection in geriatric and institutionalized patients. Curr Opin Urol 2002;12(1):51–5.

[91] Nicolle LE. Resistant pathogens in urinary tract infections. J Am Geriatr Soc 2002; 50(Suppl 7):S230–5.

[92] Orr PH, Nicolle LE, Duckworth H, et al. Febrile urinary infection in the institutionalized elderly. Am J Med 1996;100(1):71–7.

[93] Nicolle LE. A practical guide to antimicrobial management of complicated urinary tract infection. Drugs Aging 2001;18(4):243–54.

[94] Nicolle LE. Urinary tract pathogens in complicated infection and in elderly individuals. J Infect Dis 2001;183(Suppl 1):S5–8.

[95] Wright SW, Wrenn KD, Haynes M, et al. Prevalence and risk factors for multidrug resistant uropathogens in ED patients. Am J Emerg Med 2000;18(2):143–6.

[96] Sotto A, De Boever CM, Fabbro-Peray P, et al. Risk factors for antibiotic-resistant Escherichia coli isolated from hospitalized patients with urinary tract infections: a prospective study. J Clin Microbiol 2001;39(2):438–44.

[97] Terpenning MS, Bradley SF, Wan JY, et al. Colonization and infection with antibiotic-resistant bacteria in a long-term care facility. J Am Geriatr Soc 1994;42(10):1062–9.

[98] Wiener J, Quinn JP, Bradford PA, et al. Multiple antibiotic-resistant Klebsiella and Escherichia coli in nursing homes. JAMA 1999;281(6):517–23.

[99] Wingard E, Shlaes JH, Mortimer EA, et al. Colonization and cross-colonization of nursing home patients with trimethoprim-resistant gram-negative bacilli. Clin Infect Dis 1993; 16(1):75–81.

[100] Warren JW, Abrutyn E, Hebel JR, et al. Guidelines for antimicrobial treatment of uncomplicated acute bacterial cystitis and acute pyelonephritis in women: Infectious Diseases Society of America (IDSA). Clin Infect Dis 1999;29(4):745–58.

[101] Lutters M, Vogt N. Antibiotic duration for treating uncomplicated, symptomatic lower urinary tract infections in elderly women. Cochrane Database Syst Rev 2002;(3):CD001535.

[102] Raz R, Schiller D, Nicolle LE. Chronic indwelling catheter replacement before antimicrobial therapy for symptomatic urinary tract infection. J Urol 2000;164(4):1254–8.

[103] Thompson WW, Shay DK, Weintraub E, et al. Mortality associated with influenza and respiratory syncytial virus in the United States. JAMA 2003;289(2):179–86.

[104] Thompson WW, Shay DK, Weintraub E, et al. Influenza-associated hospitalizations in the United States. JAMA 2004;292(11):1333–40.

[105] Harper SA, Fukuda K, Uyeki TM, et al. Prevention and control of influenza: recommendations of the Advisory Committee on Immunization Practices (ACIP). MMWR Recomm Rep 2005;54(RR-8):1–40.

[106] Stamboulian D, Bonvehi PE, Nacinovich FM, et al. Influenza. Infect Dis Clin North Am 2000;14(1):141–66.

[107] Dumyati G, Falsey AR. Antivirals for influenza: what is their role in the older patient? Drugs Aging 2002;19(10):777–86.

[108] Bradley SF. Prevention of influenza in long-term care facilities: Long-Term Care Committee of the Society for Healthcare Epidemiology of America. Infect Control Hosp Epidemiol 1999;20(9):629–37.

[109] Fiore AE, Shay DK, Haber P, et al. Prevention and control of influenza: recommendations of the Advisory Committee on Immunization Practices (ACIP), 2007. MMWR Recomm Rep 2007;56(RR-6):1–54.

[110] Nichol KL, Nordin JD, Nelson DB, et al. Effectiveness of influenza vaccine in the community-dwelling elderly. N Engl J Med 2007;357(14):1373–81.

[111] Rimple D, Weiss SJ, Brett M, et al. An emergency department-based vaccination program: overcoming the barriers for adults at high risk for vaccine-preventable diseases. Acad Emerg Med 2006;13(9):922–30.

[112] Angus DC, Linde-Zwirble WT, Lidicker J, et al. Epidemiology of severe sepsis in the United States: analysis of incidence, outcome, and associated costs of care. Crit Care Med 2001; 29(7):1303–10.

[113] Martin GS, Mannino DM, Moss M. The effect of age on the development and outcome of adult sepsis. Crit Care Med 2006;34(1):15–21.

[114] Hazinski MF, Iberti TJ, MacIntyre NR, et al. Epidemiology, pathophysiology and clinical presentation of gram-negative sepsis. Am J Crit Care 1993;2(3):224–35.

[115] Martin GS, Mannino DM, Eaton S, et al. The epidemiology of sepsis in the United States from 1979 through 2000. N Engl J Med 2003;348(16):1546–54.

[116] Dellinger RP, Carlet JM, Masur H, et al. Surviving sepsis campaign guidelines for management of severe sepsis and septic shock. Intensive Care Med 2004;30(4):536–55.

[117] Rivers E, Nguyen B, Havstad S, et al. Early goal-directed therapy in the treatment of severe sepsis and septic shock. N Engl J Med 2001;345(19):1368–77.

[118] Bernard GR, Vincent JL, Laterre PF, et al. Efficacy and safety of recombinant human activated protein C for severe sepsis. N Engl J Med 2001;344(10):699–709.

[119] Graham TA. Evidence-based emergency medicine/systematic review abstract: do corticosteroids decrease mortality in sepsis? Ann Emerg Med 2005;45(3):330–2.

[120] Nguyen HB, Rivers EP, Abrahamian FM, et al. Severe sepsis and septic shock: review of the literature and emergency department management guidelines. Ann Emerg Med 2006;48(1): 28–54.

[121] Annane D, Sebille V, Charpentier C, et al. Effect of treatment with low doses of hydrocortisone and fludrocortisone on mortality in patients with septic shock. JAMA 2002;288(7): 862–71.

[122] Sprung CI, Annane D, Keh D, et al. Hydrocortisone therapy for patients with septic shock. N Engl J Med 2008;358(2):111–24.

[123] Ely EW, Angus DC, Williams MD, et al. Drotrecogin alfa (activated) treatment of older patients with severe sepsis. Clin Infect Dis 2003;37(2):187–95.

[124] Alexander SL, Ernst FR. Use of drotrecogin alfa (activated) in older patients with severe sepsis. Pharmacotherapy 2006;26(4):533–8.

[125] Manns BJ, Lee H, Doig CJ, et al. An economic evaluation of activated protein C treatment for severe sepsis. N Engl J Med 2002;347(13):993–1000.

ELSEVIER
SAUNDERS

Emerg Med Clin N Am
26 (2008) 345–366

EMERGENCY
MEDICINE
CLINICS OF
NORTH AMERICA

Infections Related to Pregnancy

Diane L. Gorgas, MD

*Department of Emergency Medicine, The Ohio State University Medical Center,
164 Means Hall, 1654 Upham Drive, Columbus, OH 43210, USA*

Urinary tract infection is a common complication of pregnancy, occurring in as many as 15% of pregnant women. More concerning is the predisposition of the patient to sustain pyelonephritis. Twenty percent to forty percent of pregnant women with asymptomatic bacteriuria will experience pyelonephritis [1]. Conversion of bacteriuria to pyelonephritis will most likely occur in multiparous women during the second trimester of pregnancy [2], and women with a history of antenatal urinary tract infections are particularly at risk [3]. This risk has led to a debate over the screening and treating of asymptomatic bacteriuria in pregnant patients [4–6]. Factors that predispose to bacteriuria and its complications include normal physiologic changes in the pregnant woman's anatomy, including impaired emptying of the urinary bladder, relative stasis of urine within the ureters, an increased vesiculoureteral reflux, and an increased pH of urine [7].

Diagnosis

The purpose of diagnosing a urinary tract infection in pregnancy is multifactorial concerning fetal health. In addition to the maternal dangers of acute pyelonephritis, there are independent risks to the fetus, including congenital abnormalities, premature rupture of membranes, and low birth weight infants [8]. Socioeconomic status, personal hygiene, education level, pregnancy duration, contraceptive use, and the use of underclothing have no significant bearing on the risk for urinary tract infection [9]. The only independent risk is a history of previous urinary tract infection.

Etiologic agents for urinary tract infection in the pregnant patient mirror those in nonpregnant cohorts. The most common isolated bacteria are *Escherichia coli*; other organisms less commonly seen are *Enterobacter*, *Staphylococcus*, or group B streptococcus [10,11]. Despite obvious logistical

E-mail address: diane.gorgas@osumc.edu

limitations in collecting a clean catch midstream or in obtaining a sample in a gravid woman, similar colony counts have been proposed to define "bacteriuria." Two consecutive positive cultures with colony counts greater than 10^5 colony forming units defines significant bacteriuria [6,9].

Treatment

The antibiotic choice in pregnancy should consider the likely pathogens in conjunction with fetal and maternal safety based on gestational age. Recommended antibiotics in pregnancy should be US Food and Drug Administration category B. These drugs include cephalosporins and penicillins. Other common agents used to treat urinary pathogens may have untoward effects in pregnancy. Antibiotics that can have deleterious effects near term are the sulfonamides, which can increase the risk of neonatal kernicterus, and nitrofurantoin, which can cause hemolysis in an infant with glucose-6-phosphate dehydrogenase deficiency [2,5]. First trimester antibiotic untoward effects occur from the use of tetracyclines, which can cause bone and teeth dysplasia; from trimethoprim, which inhibits folate metabolism and may predispose the fetus to neural tube defects; from aminoglycosides, which can cause eighth cranial nerve palsies; and from fluoroquinolones, which have been associated with cartilaginous abnormalities [12].

The duration of treatment has received significant attention in the literature. Although general agreement is found regarding the duration of treatment for pyelonephritis (minimum of 7–10 days), several conflicting studies can be found regarding the duration of treatment for uncomplicated lower urinary tract infections [13]. The current literature has espoused the efficacy and safety of single dose oral treatment of cystitis in pregnant patients [14,15]. Limitations of this therapeutic practice in the emergency department are thought to be related to unreliable follow-up.

Although it may be prudent to obtain urine cultures for all pregnant women, the literature does not spell out this recommendation as routine practice [16]. Certainly all pregnant women with a urinary tract infection that is resistant to therapy, recurrent, or associated with pyelonephritis should have a culture performed routinely. In the United States, no studies have been published specifically looking at the development of antibiotic resistance in pregnant patients, but pathogens tend to mirror those in nonpregnant populations [17].

Chorioamnionitis

Chorioamnionitis is an infection of the chorioamniotic membranes and amniotic cavity that occurs most commonly in the third trimester. It is not an uncommon infection associated with pregnancy, occurring in 1% to 10% of all pregnancies [18]. The incidence of the condition increases significantly with preterm labor.

The etiology in most cases is an ascending vaginal infection through the cervical os [19], most commonly seen in cases of premature rupture of membranes and prolonged labor [20]. The condition can be acquired hematogenously or transabdominally from amniocentesis. It has also been reported in association with other obstetric procedures including cerclage placement.

Diagnosis

The diagnosis of chorioamnionitis is a clinical one characterized by fever, uterine tenderness, foul smelling amniotic fluid on rupture of membranes, and maternal and fetal tachycardia. Of these symptoms, fever is found most commonly and is present in 85% to 100% of cases [21]. Laboratory adjuncts in diagnosing the infection include a maternal white blood cell count which is usually elevated with a left shift. The most sensitive and specific laboratory finding is the presence of leukoattractants in the amniotic fluid. These proteins act as markers for subsequent leukocyte migration and activation [22]. Because leukoattractant assays are not readily available in the emergency setting, other amniotic fluid tests that may point toward the diagnosis are the microscopic presence of bacteria and leukocytes. Some studies have proposed the presence of amniotic fluid leukocyte esterase, low glucose, and elevated C-reactive protein as suggestive findings [23]. Fluid culture can be helpful in tailoring therapy and is recommended.

It has been unclear in studies whether chorioamnionitis represents a polymicrobial infection, or whether the majority of cases are caused by single etiologic agents. The most commonly identified organism is *Ureaplasma urealyticum* [24], but *Mycoplasma hominis, Gardnerella vaginalis, Bacteroides bivius, Escherichia coli*, group B streptococci, anaerobic streptococci, and aerobic gram-negative rods have also been implicated. Bacterial vaginitis has been associated with the condition as well, but most sources believe this is a correlation and not a causative relationship.

Although prevention of chorioamnionitis is not absolute, there are predictable risk factors for the development of the condition. Major risk factors for disease include an increased number of vaginal examinations, the duration of ruptured membranes and of total labor, and the use of internal fetal monitors. Minor risk factors for the condition include coitus during pregnancy, bacterial colonization, particularly vaginal group B streptococci colonization, premature rupture of membranes or premature labor, or any invasive procedures, but particularly endovaginal procedures [25]. It is unclear at what duration premature rupture of membranes becomes a significant risk factor, but there has been no proven difference in the rate of chorioamnionitis development between 12 hours and 72 hours [26].

The presence of chorioamnionitis during labor and in the puerperal period can have significant manifestations in maternal and fetal care. Chorioamnionitis significantly increases the risk of maternal and fetal bacteremia, with estimates being 10% in both populations [27]. From a delivery perspective, the presence of chorioamnionitis can cause slow cervical dilatation, prolonged labor, and decreased responsiveness to oxytocin. From a fetal perspective, increased mortality is associated with early gestational age, low birth weight, or an infection with *Escherichia coli* or group B streptococci. Fetal mortality also increases exponentially with the delay in maternal antibiotic treatment. The early philosophy in the treatment of chorioamnionitis was to withhold maternal antibiotic treatment until after the infant was delivered and the cord clamped to allow for unadulterated cultures to be obtained from the infant. This practice has largely been abandoned in favor of early and aggressive maternal treatment. In cases of mild chorioamnionitis, there is a 2.6-fold increase in fetal mortality; in moderate to severe cases, a 4.1-fold increase is noted [21]. Long-term fetal morbidity is associated with lower developmental scores and a higher rate of neurologic abnormalities.

Treatment

Once the condition is suspected, treatment should be initiated with intravenous antibiotics, although no standard of therapy regarding antibiotic choice has been established. Treatment suggestions in the literature include cefoxitin, piperacillin, or combination therapy with ampicillin plus an aminoglycoside. It has been suggested that clindamycin should be added if *Bacteroides* sp are suspected, or if the patient will be delivered by cesarean section, although this is controversial [28]. Intravenous antibiotic treatment, once initiated, should be continued for at least 48 hours after the patient becomes afebrile. Continued oral therapy should be completed for an additional 7 to 10 days. The question of when and how to deliver an infant in a chorioamniotic environment is unsettled. Conflicting opinions regarding emergent versus urgent delivery and cesarean section versus vaginal delivery have been debated in the literature, but, largely, the specifics of the case determine the course of action [25].

Endometritis

Endometritis, or a generalized uterine infection also called endomyometritis or endoparametritis, is the most frequent cause of infection in the puerperal period. The risk of endometritis rises exponentially in post–cesarean section patients, particularly in nonelective high-risk patients, in whom the risk can reach 85% to 95% [29]. It is a more uncommon diagnosis post vaginal delivery, complicating 1% to 3% of uncomplicated vaginal deliveries [30]. Complicating features of endometritis such as pelvic thrombophlebitis and pelvic abscess are also proportionately more likely to occur post cesarean (4%–9%) than with vaginal deliveries (<2%) [31]. Bacteremia is also more common in the post–cesarean section patient (20%) when compared with vaginal delivery cases of endometritis (4%) [32]. Other risk factors for the development of endometritis include prolonged labor, prolonged rupture of membranes, increased frequency of vaginal examinations, and the use of internal fetal monitoring.

Diagnosis

The pathogenesis of endometritis appears to be a mixed polymicrobial ascending infection from the lower genital tract. Anaerobic organisms are found in 80% of uterine isolates and aerobic organisms in 70% of late (3–6 days) postpartum infections [33]. Common isolates include gram-positive anaerobes such as group B streptococci, *Enterococcus*, and *Gardnerella* sp; gram-negative aerobes such as *Escherichia coli* and *Enterobacter*; and other anaerobes such as *Bacteroides* and *Peptostreptococcus*. Post–cesarean section infections are thought to be derived in a similar ascending fashion, but the increased risk is believed to be due to increased uterine manipulation, the presence of devitalized tissue at the suture sites, and the possibility of bacterial contamination through the incision.

The classic triad found in endometritis is fever, lower abdominal pain and uterine tenderness, and foul smelling lochia [29]. Other sources of infection must be ruled out to confirm the diagnosis of endometritis. The work-up of patients with suspected endometritis should include a complete blood count, urinalysis, and blood cultures because of the high rate of concomitant bacteremia. Cervical cultures, although not particularly useful in the initial management of these cases, may help direct therapy for treatment failures and help identify *Chlamydia* as an etiologic agent; therefore, they are recommended.

Treatment

Treatment of postpartum endometritis includes broad-spectrum intravenous antibiotic therapy, the gold standard of which has been clindamycin and gentamicin [34]. After initiation of treatment, a response should be seen within 48 hours, and therapy should be continued for an additional 48 hours after defervescence. No proven utility of continued oral antibiotic therapy after discharge has been noted. Treatment failures at 48 hours should prompt consideration of *Enterococcus* as an etiologic agent, particularly if antibiotics (usually a cephalosporin) were administered peripartum in cases of cesarean section delivery [35]. The addition of ampicillin to the treatment regimen is usually associated with a positive therapeutic response.

Persistent treatment failures should lead to continued diagnostic work-up for complications of endometritis, including septic thrombophlebitis, ovarian vein thrombosis, or pelvic abscess.

Group B streptrococcal infection

Group B streptococci have been a leading cause of maternal and neonatal mortality. The first set of national consensus guidelines was published in

1996. Since then, there has been a 70% reduction in early neonatal infection but no significant impact on the rates of late group B streptococcal neonatal infection [32].

Diagnosis

Multiple studies have reported rates of group B streptococcal maternal colonization of 10% to 30%, with repeated screenings during gestation resulting in higher positive culture rates [36,37]. Both rectal and vaginal colonization rates have been studied. Although vaginal colonization is more common, rectal growth of group B streptococci occurs frequently enough for many studies to recommend swabs of both areas to determine the presence of the bacterium. These infections can be separated into four different categories: chronic (36%), transient (20%), intermittent (15%), and acute (29%) [36]. Streptococcal carriage has been noted to be significantly less in patients aged 20 years old or older and in multiparous patients (four pregnancies or greater) [36]. Risk factors for colonization include African American race [38]. It is unclear whether Latino American descent places patients at increased or decreased risk, because study findings are conflicting. Maternal colonization leads to invasive disease in 1 to 2 cases per 1000 total births [39]. Ultimately, the risk of fetal loss or group B streptococcal disease in the infant occurs in 28% of maternal cases [38]. Neonatal group B sepsis occurred in 1.6 to 2.6 of 1000 live births (dependent on when group B streptococci was cultured, that is, 23 versus 26 weeks) [40]. An independent risk factor for development of disease in the neonate is the amount of maternal colonization, with heavy colonization being more likely to cause neonatal infection. Neonatal infection is only one complication of maternal colonization; preterm delivery and low birth weight infants are more frequently seen in heavily colonized mothers [41]. Current recommendations regarding the screening of term, otherwise healthy pregnant (35–37 weeks' gestation) patients include obtaining vaginal and rectal swabs between 35 and 37 weeks or at the time of labor.

Treatment

Treatment should be initiated in all women with positive cultures during the 35- to 37-week screening, and in any woman who has had an infant infected with group B streptococci in the neonatal period or with a positive group B streptococcal urine culture (regardless of the colony count). Other groups that should be treated empirically include all patients with labor at less than 37 weeks' gestation unless a negative screen has been obtained within the last 5 weeks. Additional scenarios in which treatment is recommended include fever during labor and premature rupture of membranes for greater than 18 hours [41]. Group B streptococci–associated chorioamnionitis is reported in most (88%) cases in which neonatal infection occurred despite intrapartum maternal antibiotic therapy [42].

Intrapartum chemoprophylaxis of group B streptococci colonization has resulted in a significant reduction of neonatal infection [43]. Because of the now routine outpatient treatment of patients with positive cultures, antibiotic resistance is becoming more common. Traditional treatment called for penicillin or, as alternatives in a penicillin-allergic patient, oral clindamycin or erythromycin [44]. This treatment regimen has traditionally been very effective at preventing group B streptococcal neonatal colonization. Recent studies have shown a virtual eradication of positive group B streptococcal neonatal skin cultures if antibiotics are given 6 hours before delivery [45], with slightly lower rates if they are given intrapartum [46]. In vitro resistance to clindamycin and erythromycin is increasing, with recent (1990) numbers approaching resistance rates of 5% and 18%, respectively [47]. Empiric treatment of the neonate should take place in high-risk cases. These cases include infants of mothers with group B streptococci bacterium, mothers with previous deliveries complicated with early onset group B streptococcal disease, and all mothers with chorioamnionitis. This empiric treatment in the neonate should continue until the infant's screening cultures are negative [42].

An alternative approach is immunoprophylaxis of the mother against group B streptococci with a type III polysaccharide vaccine. This treatment can impart vertical immunity to the newborn and may eventually obviate the need for antibiotic treatment entirely [48,49].

Septic abortion

Although it is an infrequently seen complication since the advent of legalized pregnancy termination, septic abortion still can occur. Although this has largely become obsolete in developed nations, the World Health Organization estimates that one in eight pregnancy-related deaths world-wide is directly attributable to unsafe abortion practices [50]. The mechanism of septic abortion is most commonly associated with substandard nonsterile techniques and inadvertent retained products of conception after incomplete uterine evacuation. This mechanism translates into 68,000 deaths per year, almost exclusively in developing countries [51]. The clinical presentation of a septic abortion is similar to endometritis and is characterized by fever, abdominal pain, and uterine tenderness. The presentation of disease can vary from minor fever and discomfort to fulminant septic shock with pulmonary edema, adult respiratory distress syndrome, disseminated intravascular coagulation, pulmonary embolism, and subsequent cardiovascular collapse and death [52].

Etiologic agents in cases of septic abortion are nearly uniformly polymicrobial and are caused by ascending infections through an open cervical os. Common isolates are *Escherichia coli, Bacteroides* sp, anaerobic gram-negative rods, group B beta-hemolytic streptococci, and staphylococcus. Sexually transmitted disease may also be implicated, including gonorrhea and infection with *Chlamydia* and *Trichomonas* [21]. Pre-procedural screening for sexually transmitted diseases before pregnancy termination may help prevent infection in selected cases.

Diagnosis

Although largely a clinical diagnosis, laboratory adjuncts for the diagnosis should include arterial blood gases, lactate levels, a Gram stain of the cervix with cultures of the endocervix, blood, and urine, and screening for disseminated intravascular coagulation (coagulation profile with fibrin, fibrinogen, and fibrin split products). Plain radiographic examination of the abdomen may reveal free air or retained post-procedural foreign bodies and may be helpful. Similarly, pelvic ultrasound may suggest surgical complications, including retained products of conception or retained surgical foreign bodies [53].

Treatment

Treatment of septic abortion should focus on removal of any inciting agents (products of conception or foreign bodies) and is usually accomplished through dilatation and curettage of the uterine cavity. This procedure removes the source of the endotoxin. Although theoretically curative in these cases, it is rarely held as an isolated therapeutic approach. Antibiotic therapy is almost always instituted and should be started concomitantly with uterine evacuation. Parenteral administration of triple antibiotic therapy is the standard of care. Suggested regimens include (1) gram-positive anaerobic and aerobic coverage with penicillin, ampicillin, or a cephalosporin; (2) gram-negative aerobic coverage with an aminoglycoside; and (3) gram-negative anaerobic coverage with clindamycin or metronidazole [21]. Tetanus toxoid should also be considered.

HIV in pregnancy

Entire texts have been and still will be written regarding HIV infection in pregnancy. This section attempts to review salient information regarding testing, maternal management, and, most importantly, limiting vertical transmission of the disease. The rate of HIV infection in the United States has appeared to reach a plateau or steady state, with roughly 40,000 new cases developing yearly [54]. Recent Centers for Disease Control guidelines have given special emphasis to the role of the emergency physician in surveillance and treatment with regards to HIV, because the emergency department represents the only source of medical care for many patients and may serve a primary care role for many at-risk populations. In underdeveloped countries, notably throughout the continent of Africa, rates of HIV infection are steadily increasing yearly. Efforts are now being made to protect newborns from the development of disease, but the first barrier in this crusade has been knowledge of the maternal HIV status. There are many obstacles in determining this status, not the least of which is the consideration of the impact of a positive test on these women and their families. Women who test positive may receive a disproportionately more difficult time from society, partners, and their families than do their male counterparts [55]. This realization has led to an opinion that women should be tested before pregnancy so informed reproductive choices can be made; however, prenatal testing imposes an unfair burden on women in cultures, either globally or locally, when support structures do not exist to aid in post diagnosis. Other strategies proposed to ease the burden of prenatal testing include provider initiated testing and counseling with a right to refuse (opt out), group pretest counseling, rapid HIV testing, and community and male involvement for support [56].

The consequences of undiagnosed HIV in pregnancy are sobering. High rates of infant mortality, usually secondary to overwhelming infection, are common (25%), and the majority of infants have long-term neurologic sequelae (65%) [57]. When HIV infection occurs intrauterine as opposed to during delivery, the fetus can develop growth failure, microcephaly, and craniofacial abnormalities [58].

Prevention of vertical transmission has fallen into two different and complementary strategies. One focuses on the timing and route of delivery and the second on a pharmacologic approach to peripartum care. Regarding the route and timing of delivery, two studies published in 1999 demonstrated that cesarean section before the initiation of labor and rupture of membranes (also known as elective cesarean section) reduced the risk of vertical transmission by up to 50% to 70% [59,60]. One study showed a 1.8% incidence of HIV transmission (3 of 170) versus 10.5% (21 of 200) with vaginal deliveries [60]. Based on these results, current recommendations from the American College of Obstetricians and Gynecologists and the US Public Health Service suggest counseling of women with viral loads greater than 1000 copies/mL for elective cesarean section [61,62]. Since 1999, these recommendations have led to a dramatic increase in the numbers of cesarean sections among HIV-positive mothers. Unfortunately, this increase has resulted in an ethical conundrum, because a recent study has just shown that elective cesarean section to prevent vertical transmission in HIV-infected mothers leads to increased maternal morbidity and mortality. HIV-infected mothers undergoing elective cesarean section are more likely to develop endometritis (11.6% versus 5.8% in noninfected controls), maternal sepsis (1.1% versus 0.2%), and pneumonia (1.3% versus 0.3%), and are more likely to require postpartum transfusions (4.0% versus 2.0%). The risk of maternal mortality also increases from 0.1% in noninfected controls to 0.8% in the HIV-infected population [63]. Given these risks, it is unclear what recommendations should be made if the viral load is low (ie, <1000), or if the patient is currently taking antiretroviral agents [62].

Pharmacologic therapy is synergistic in decreasing HIV transmission along with the delivery strategies outlined previously. Antiretroviral agents should be tailored based on the maternal viral load but should, at a minimum, include zidovudine from 28 weeks; gestation; zidovudine, lamivudine, and a single dose of nevirapine during delivery; and zidovudine and lamivudine for 7 days after delivery to reduce the development of nevirapine resistance [64]. The use of zidovudine alone decreased the risk of vertical transmission 43%, and the addition of nevirapine improved that reduction to 68% [65]. Newborn infants should receive a single dose of nevirapine and 1 to 4 weeks of zidovudine. Infants undergoing this chemoprophylaxis not only have a decreased risk of contracting HIV infection but also a decreased risk of neonatal mortality (80% reduction) [65]. Currently published US standards recommend a three-part zidovudine prophylaxis regimen (prenatal, intranatal, and neonatal) even for mothers with a viral load less than 1000 copies/mL [62]. This strategy has ultimately led to a risk of vertical transmission of less than 1% [66]. An alternative strategy of just using single dose nevirapine has been studied as well which, in and of itself, can lead to a decrease in maternal transmission to 10% to 15% [67].

Safety profiles for any drug given during pregnancy are a concern. Protease inhibitors have been associated with an increased risk of maternal glucose intolerance, preeclampsia, and preterm birth [68]. Any pregnancy exposed to antiretroviral agents should be registered with the Antiretroviral Pregnancy Registry to better understand the risk of birth defects. Neonatal treatment with antiretrovirals seems to be well tolerated, but a concern over persistent mitochondrial dysfunction resulting in increased cancer development rates has been raised [69].

Although peripartum prophylaxis has been the mainstay of therapy, there are significant concerns regarding vertical transmission for breastfeeding infants as well. Although somewhat less studied, vertical transmission through breastfeeding accounts for 50% of all neonatal and infant HIV cases worldwide and carries a transmission risk of 15% when continued beyond the first year [69]. Studies are underway to examine methods to decrease this risk, including early intensive breastfeeding only plans with rapid weaning at 3 to 6 months, treatments of expressed milk to inactivate the virus, and antiretroviral therapy for the mother and infant during breastfeeding periods [70].

Pneumonia in pregnancy (non-varicella type)

Before the 1960s, pneumonia was a common scourge to obstetricians, affecting 6 to 8 women per 1000 deliveries. These figures reached a nadir in the 1970s and 1980s, decreasing to a rate of 0.4 to 0.8 women per 1000 deliveries, but have recently increased in incidence, thought to be a product of higher numbers of infertility pregnancies and the emergence of chronically ill women becoming pregnant at higher rates when compared with the general population [71]. Nevertheless, there does not appear to be an appreciable increased risk of developing pneumonia in pregnancy.

Risk factors for the development of pneumonia do not appear to be influenced by maternal age or parity. The incidence is lowest in the first trimester and increases steadily throughout pregnancy, most likely owing to mechanical limitations of the growing uterus on pulmonary function [72]. Maternal comorbidities, including anemia and asthma, have been postulated as risk factors [73] and in combination impart a fivefold risk for developing pneumonia [74]. Independent iatrogenic risk factors for the development of pneumonia are the use of antepartum corticosteroids to enhance fetal lung maturity and tocolytics to induce labor.

Diagnosis

The diagnosis of pneumonia in pregnancy is commonly more difficult than in nonpregnant matched cohorts, and the disease is frequently misdiagnosed on initial presentation. The most common misdiagnoses noted are pyelonephritis, appendicitis, and preterm labor [71]. The diagnosis can be confounded by attributing symptoms of the disease state to normal physiologic changes in pregnancy. These symptoms include dyspnea, chest discomfort, and fatigue. Some distinguishing features that help define pathology are the presence of cough and dyspnea at rest [71]. Pregnancy-specific diagnoses that can be mistaken for pneumonia and that present with similar symptoms and a positive chest radiograph include noncardiogenic pulmonary edema in preeclampsia and eclampsia or secondary to tocolytic agents or aspiration pneumonia. Rarely, choriocarcinoma with pulmonary metastases can occur and be mistaken for pneumonia.

Common pathogens of pneumonia in pregnant patients tend to parallel that in nonpregnant age-matched cohorts. *Streptococcus pneumoniae* is the most common organism identified, followed by *Haemophilus influenzae* [75,76]. *Legionella* has been reported as well. Pathogens associated with aspiration pneumonia in pregnancy are believed to mirror pathogens in nonpregnant patients, but no confirmatory studies have been done. Anaerobes such as the gram-positive cocci, *Peptostreptococcus*, and *Peptococcus* sp and the gram-negative bacilli *Fusobacterium* and *Bacteroides* sp predominate in two thirds of cases. The pregnant patient in the third trimester is at increased risk of aspiration due to several features, including relaxation of the gastroesophageal sphincter, delayed gastric emptying, and increased intra-abdominal pressure. Patients undergoing cesarean section, especially under general anesthetic, have even higher risks of aspiration [77]. Other pathogenic organisms are theoretically more likely to be seen in pregnancy because of changes in cellular immunity, but no surveillance studies have demonstrated definitively higher incidence rates [77]. These organisms include fungi leading to infections, including coccidioidomycosis. When it occurs, coccidioidomycosis tends to be associated with a higher rate of dissemination and systemic illness when contracted in the third trimester.

Treatment

Treatment options, although not specifically studied for efficacy in pregnant patients, must be considered from a fetal safety point of view. Penicillins, macrolides (including newer ones), and cephalosporins have good safety records in pregnancy and should be efficacious. Quinolones, tetracyclines, chloramphenicol, and sulpha compounds should generally be avoided unless dictated use is mandated by culture and sensitivity [71].

Varicella infections in pregnancy

Although chickenpox is a relatively uncommon disease in adults, with only 7% of cases occurring within the child-bearing age period of 14 to 45 years, it receives a significant amount of attention because of the morbidity and mortality associated with it [78]. Overall, the incidence of the disease is between 0.5 to 3 cases per 1000 pregnancies, although as many as 10% of pregnant women are susceptible to infection based on a lack of antibody titers [79].

Historically, the mortality rate associated with maternal varicella infection has been high, up to 41% documented before 1965 [78,79]. More recent studies and advances in antimicrobial therapy in conjunction with improved ICU support of the ventilatory compromised patient have led to much improved mortality, with most studies citing mortality rates of less than 5%. Nonetheless, maternal and fetal morbidity is still a concern, and if prevention can be offered in exposed cases, primary effort at disease control should occur. The American Academy of Pediatrics has defined "close exposure" cases, those at increased risk for the development of disease, to be (1) household contacts, (2) face-to-face contact for at least 5 minutes, and (3) contact indoors with a case of chickenpox or herpes zoster for more than 1 hour [78]. These definitions do not account for the fact that 20% of infected mothers state that they have had no known chickenpox exposures. Nonetheless, current recommendations advise post-exposure treatment of pregnant women with varicella-zoster immune globulin (VZIG) within 72 hours of exposure, although some benefit is inferred if treatment is initiated within 10 days of exposure [80]. The administration of VZIG has been proven beneficial to maternal morbidity and mortality, and some evidence has shown that it may have some protective properties against fetal varicella syndrome [78].

Diagnosis

The timing of a varicella infection in pregnancy can help predict consequences. Infection within the first 20 weeks of pregnancy has a 1% risk of embryopathy, most notably manifesting as limb abnormalities diagnosed in subsequent ultrasound fetal interrogation [78]. Virus is not uncommonly found in amniotic fluid and cord blood post infection, but levels do not correlate with any definable disease state within the fetus; therefore, amniocentesis and cordocentesis are not recommended.

Varicella pneumonitis during pregnancy manifests in two clinical stages, early and late. The early phase is characterized by the onset of respiratory symptoms 1 to 6 days after the onset of a rash, a dry cough associated with exertional dyspnea, and mild hypoxemia. Patients within the early phase typically have normal lung sounds, no cyanosis, and frequently have a normal chest radiograph. Pneumonia without a rash has not been reported. In the late phase, respiratory symptoms progress, with dyspnea at rest noted and resting cyanosis. The cough can become productive and blood streaked. Physical findings show basilar crepitance and moderate-to-severe hypoxia [78]. The chest radiograph in late phases is not characterized by consolidation but by diffuse, sometimes nodular, infiltrates [81].

Risk factors have been identified for the acquisition of varicella pneumonia and the severity of the clinical presentation. These factors include non–pregnancy-related features such as maternal smoking, pre-existing chronic obstructive pulmonary disease, a mother who is immunocompromised (including steroid use), and certain characteristics of the rash, such as the initial extent of the eruption and a hemorrhagic rash [78]. Exposure in late pregnancy also infers a higher risk for varicella pneumonitis and predicts a more virulent course of illness [82]. It is unclear whether this risk is attributable to immunosuppressive or other biochemical changes inherent in pregnancy or because of mechanical changes in pulmonary function brought on by decreased diaphragmatic excursion as the uterus enlarges. Overall, there is debate as to whether the severity of illness in pregnancy is as serious as once believed [83]. Mortality rates in nonpregnant versus pregnant patients in whom pneumonitis develops have been reportedly similar (15%–40% versus 2%–35%), although tremendous variability can be found from case series to case series [78]. General rates of developing pneumonitis are between 5% and 14%. Although some data support the supposition that varicella pneumonia is a more serious illness in pregnancy, this cannot be uniformly supported.

Once a diagnosis of varicella pneumonia has been made, assessing the severity of the illness is paramount. Criteria for hospitalization have been set forth as follows: (1) chest symptoms, (2) neurologic symptoms other than headache, (3) hemorrhagic rash or bleeding or a dense rash with mucous membrane involvement, and (4) significant immunosuppression [78]. Factors that should be considered in predicting maternal and fetal morbidity are pregnancy approaching term, a history of obstetric complications, a smoking history or chronic obstructive pulmonary disease, or poor social supports.

Treatment

Treatment considerations for varicella in pregnancy should begin when a patient presents with a rash whose duration is 24 hours or less. If the patient is in her second half of pregnancy, the consensus opinion is that she should receive a course of oral acyclovir [80]. This recommendation largely stems from the increased pulmonary morbidity found in late pregnancy. No consensus opinion has been published regarding acyclovir administration in patients who present 24 hours to 10 days after rash onset, although acyclovir may be beneficial up to 10 days post symptom onset. Also, no consensus has been reached on early pregnancy exposure or disease development. Although no studies have been specifically designed to test for the safety of acyclovir in early pregnancy, the drug appears to have low teratogenicity and untoward fetal effects [84].

Treatment issues for varicella pneumonia that are unique in pregnancy focus on fetal health and growth. The severe hypoxia that can develop in cases of advanced maternal pneumonitis can be difficult to treat and the deleterious effects of hypoxia magnified in a developing fetus. Case reports of extracorporeal membrane oxygenation suggest this may be helpful in prolonged maternal hypoxia despite maximal ventilator support [85]. Maternal nutrition should be observed closely as well, because fetal intrauterine growth is closely linked to maternal nutrition. Acyclovir administration for varicella pneumonitis treatment should begin with intravenous dosing for rapid establishment of plasma peak concentrations. Appropriate dosing is 10 mg/kg three times a day with the intravenous route maintained for at least 5 days [82,86]. Oral acyclovir is poorly, incompletely, and slowly absorbed, making it less than ideal as a primary therapy. Concurrent bacterial sepsis can occur, as well as secondary consolidated bacterial pneumonia. The most common causative bacterial organisms are *Streptococcus pneumoniae, Staphylococcus aureus*, and *Haemophilus influenzae* [87]. No concrete recommendations have been published regarding the routine use of antibacterial agents in varicella pneumonia, but with the high risk of secondary infection and slow response to antiviral therapy, early institution of antibiotic therapy is reasonable.

Fetal infection can occur via three routes: (1) transplacental viremia, (2) ascending infection via vaginal or external genitalia lesions during birth, or (3) respiratory droplets or direct contact with lesions after birth. The most virulent of these exposures occurs when an infant is born to a mother who develops the rash up to 4 days pre- or 2 days postpartum. These infants have a 20% risk of developing varicella infection and a subsequent 20% to 30% mortality rate; therefore, they should all be treated [88]. Maternal chickenpox 5 to 21 days pre-delivery generally results in benign neonatal chickenpox [89]. The difference between these two clinical scenarios is that the likelihood of transplacental antibodies imparting some immunity to the fetus rises exponentially within the 4- to 7-day window. Although this suggests the idea of passive immunity in newborns, and although it is known that 90% of cord blood is varicella zoster virus antibody positive, there have been cluster cases of primary varicella infection in newborns less than 8 weeks of age [78]. Maternal shingles at birth imparts no increased risk to the fetus because it is not associated with viremia.

Mastitis

Mastitis is a spectrum of illnesses ranging from mild breast redness and warmth in a lactating mother to an extremely painful condition associated with systemic toxicity, high fevers, and complications including abscess [90]. It is a common post partum, with incidences between 1% and 30% depending on the reporting source [91–93]. Together with urinary tract infection, mastitis accounts for over 80% of postpartum infections [94]. It generally occurs within the first 3 months post partum, with a peak occurrence in the second and third postpartum week, and has a 4% to 8% recurrence rate within the 3-month period [93]. A debate in the literature exists as to whether this condition represents a variant of normal lactation physiology or a true disease state [95]. For the purposes of this article, it will be treated as a pathologic condition.

Predictable risk factors for the infection include a history of mastitis in the past, the presence of cracked, sore nipples, ineffective breastfeeding techniques leading to incomplete breast emptying and persistent breast engorgement, and the use of a manual breast pump [95]. A past medical history of any immunocompromising disease process, including diabetes or steroid use, as well as previous alterations in breast anatomy, such as a previous lumpectomy with radiotherapy or the presence of breast implants, increases the risk. Maternal risks that may be altered that increase the risk include employment outside the home, wearing tight-fitting bras or clothing, and the presence of stress or fatigue [95]. Features that are somewhat protective for mastitis are maternal smoking during pregnancy, supplementation with water in the first month, the use of a pacifier on a daily basis within the first month, and a feeding frequency less than 10 times per day. The duration of breastfeeding is not associated with risk [93].

Diagnosis

Mastitis is a clinical diagnosis and can present with a wide spectrum of symptoms. Minor cases may be characterized by slight warmth, redness, and tenderness within the breast and some pain with nursing. Systemic symptoms in more severe cases can be malaise, myalgia, fever, and chills [93]. Other localized breast findings consistent with mastitis are decreased milk output, a localized hard-wedge shaped area of the breast, a breast mass near the nipple, and possibly enlarged axillary nodes or sinus tract formation in granulomatous mastitis [96].

Table 1
Summary of infectious complications associated with pregnancy

Diagnosis	Timing	Causative organisms	Treatment
Urinary tract infection	All trimesters, more likely second and third	*Escherichia coli*; other organisms less commonly seen are *Enterobacter*, *Staphylococcus*, or group B streptococcus	Cephalosporins, penicillins
Chorioamnionitis	Third trimester	*Ureaplasma urealyticum*, *Mycoplasma hominis*, *Gardnerella vaginalis*, *Bacteroides bivius*, *Escherichia coli*, group B streptococcus, anaerobic streptococci, and aerobic gram-negative rods	Cefoxitin, piperacillin, or combination therapy with ampicillin plus an aminoglycoside
Endometritis	24 Hours to 2 weeks post delivery	Gram-positive anaerobes: group B streptococcus, *Enterococcus*, and *Gardnerella* sp; gram-negative aerobes: *Escherichia coli*, *Enterobacter*, *Bacteroides*, and *Peptostreptococcus*	Clindamycin and gentamicin ± ampicillin
Septic abortion	8 Hours to 1 week post procedure	*Escherichia coli*, *Bacteroides* sp, anaerobic gram-negative rods, group B beta-hemolytic streptococci, and *Staphylococcus* Consider gonorrhea and chlamydia	Check for retained products of conception/foreign bodies; use triple antibiotic therapy (ampicillin or cephalosporin, aminoglycoside, clindamycin or metronidazole

Infection	Timing	Organism	Treatment
HIV	Peripartum through lactation, fetal risk of vertical transmission	HIV	? Elective cesarean section; zidovudine from 28 weeks; gestation; lamivudine at delivery and for 10 days post partum; single dose nevirapine at delivery
Pneumonia (non-varicella type)	Any (third trimester risk from respiratory mechanics)	*Streptococcus pneumoniae, Haemophilus influenzae, Legionella*	Penicillins, macrolides, cephalosporins
Pneumonia (varicella type)	Any (risk of vertical transmission, peripartum greatest)	Varicella	Acyclovir at 20 weeks or greater
Mastitis	Within 3 months post partum	*Staphylococcus aureus*, coagulase-negative staphylococci, group A and B-hemolytic streptococci, *Escherichia coli*, and *Bacteroides* sp	Warm compresses, frequent nursing; dicloxacillin, cloxacillin treatment failure: cephalosporin, Augmentin; penicillin allergic: erythromycin or clindamycin

[26] Shalev E, Peleg D, Eliyahu S, et al. Comparison of 12- and 72-hour expectant management of premature rupture of membranes in term pregnancies. Obstet Gynecol 1995;85(5 Pt 1):766–8.

[27] Lee W, Clark SL, Cotton DB, et al. Septic shock during pregnancy. Am J Obstet Gynecol 1988;159(2):410–6.

[28] McGregor JA. Chlamydial infection in women. Obstet Gynecol Clin North Am 1989;16(3): 565–92.

[29] Cox SM, Gilstrap LC III. Postpartum endometritis. Obstet Gynecol Clin North Am 1989; 16(2):363–71.

[30] Druelinger L. Postpartum emergencies. Emerg Med Clin North Am 1994;12(1):219–37.

[31] Yonekura ML. Treatment of postcesarean endomyometritis. Clin Obstet Gynecol 1988; 31(2):488–500.

[32] Gibbs RS. Clinical risk factors for puerperal infection. Obstet Gynecol 1980;55(Suppl 5): 178S–84S.

[33] Gibbs RS. Infection after cesarean section. Clin Obstet Gynecol 1985;28(4):697–710.

[34] Faro S, Phillips LE, Baker JL, et al. Comparative efficacy and safety of mezlocillin, cefoxitin, and clindamycin plus gentamicin in postpartum endometritis. Obstet Gynecol 1987;69(5):760–6.

[35] Hillier S, Watts DH, Lee MF, et al. Etiology and treatment of post cesarean section endometritis after cephalosporin prophylaxis. J Reprod Med 1990;35(Suppl 3):322–8.

[36] Anthony BF, Okada DM, Hobel CJ. Epidemiology of the group B streptococcus: maternal and nosocomial sources for infant acquisitions. J Pediatr 1979;95(3):431–6.

[37] McKenna DS, Iams JD. Group B streptococcal infections. Semin Perinatol 1998;22(4):267–76.

[38] Zaleznik DF, Rench MA, Hillier S, et al. Invasive disease due to group B streptococcus in pregnant women and neonates from diverse population groups. Clin Infect Dis 2000; 30(2):276–81.

[39] Glantz JC, Kedley KE. Concepts and controversies in the management of group B streptococcus during pregnancy. Birth 1998;25(1):45–53.

[40] Regan JA, Klebanoff MA, Nugent RP, et al. Colonization with group B streptococci in pregnancy and adverse outcome: VIP Study Group. Am J Obstet Gynecol 1996;174(4): 1354–60.

[41] Money DM, Dobson S, Canadian Paediatric Society Infectious Diseases Committee. The prevention of early-onset neonatal group B streptococcal disease. J Obstet Gynaecol Can 2004;26(9):826–40.

[42] Benitz WE, Gould JB, Druzin ML. Risk factors for early-onset group B streptococcal sepsis: estimation of odds ratios by critical literature review. Pediatrics 1999;103(6):1–14.

[43] Baker CJ. Group B streptococcal infections. Clin Perinatol 1997;24(1):59–70.

[44] Edwards RK, Clark P, Duff P. Intrapartum antibiotic prophylaxis 2: positive predictive value of antenatal group B streptococci cultures and antibiotic susceptibility of clinical isolates. Obstet Gynecol 2002;100(3):540–4.

[45] Lim DV, Morales WJ, Walsh AF, et al. Reduction of morbidity and mortality rates for neonatal group B streptococcal disease through early diagnosis and chemoprophylaxis. J Clin Microbiol 1986;23(3):489–92.

[46] Smaill F. Intrapartum antibiotics for group B streptococcal colonisation. Cochrane Database Syst Rev 2000;(2):CD000115.

[47] Morales WJ, Dickey SS, Bornick P, et al. Change in antibiotic resistance of group B streptococcus: impact on intrapartum management. Am J Obstet Gynecol 1999;181(2):310–4.

[48] Schuchat A. Epidemiology of group B streptococcal disease in the United States: shifting paradigms. Clin Microbiol Rev 1998;11(3):497–513.

[49] Noya FJ, Baker CJ. Prevention of group B streptococcal infection. Infect Dis Clin North Am 1992;6(1):41–55.

[50] Singh S. Hospital admissions resulting from unsafe abortion: estimates from 13 developing countries. Lancet 2006;368(9550):1887–92.

[51] Grimes DA, Benson J, Singh S, et al. Unsafe abortion: the preventable pandemic. Lancet 2006;368(9550):1908–19.

[52] Schwartz RH. Septic shock. In: Charles D, editor. Obstetric and perinatal infections. St. Louis (MO): Mosby-Yearbook; 1993. p. 118.

[53] Stubblefield PG, Grimes DA. Septic abortion. N Engl J Med 1994;331(5):310–4.

[54] Rothman RE. Current Centers for Disease Control and Prevention guidelines for HIV counseling, testing, and referral: critical role of and a call to action for emergency physicians. Ann Emerg Med 2004;44(1):31–42.

[55] de Bruyn M, Paxton S. HIV testing of pregnant women–what is needed to protect positive womenapos;s needs and rights? Sex Health 2005;2(3):143–51.

[56] Bolu OO, Allread V, Creek T, et al. Approaches for scaling up human immunodeficiency virus testing and counseling in prevention of mother-to-child human immunodeficiency virus transmission settings in resource-limited countries. Am J Obstet Gynecol 2007;197(Suppl 3):S83–9.

[57] Struik SS, Tudor-Williams G, Taylor GD, et al. Infant HIV infection despite 'universal' antenatal testing. Arch Dis Child 2007;93(1):59–61.

[58] Ellis GL, Melton J, Fikins K. Viral infections during pregnancy: a guide for the emergency physician. Ann Emerg Med 1990;19(7):802–11.

[59] The mode of delivery and the risk of vertical transmission of human immunodeficiency virus type 1–a meta-analysis of 15 prospective cohort studies. The International Perinatal HIV Group. N Engl J Med 1999;340(13):977–87.

[60] Elective caesarean section versus vaginal delivery in prevention of vertical HIV-1 transmission: a randomised clinical trial. The European Mode of Delivery Collaboration. Lancet 1999;353(9158):1035–9.

[61] Jamieson DJ, Clark J, Kourtis AP, et al. Recommendations for human immunodeficiency virus screening, prophylaxis, and treatment for pregnant women in the United States. Am J Obstet Gynecol 2007;197(Suppl 3):S26–32.

[62] Jamieson DJ, Read JS, Kourtis AP, et al. Cesarean delivery for HIV-infected women: recommendations and controversies. Am J Obstet Gynecol 2007;197(Suppl 3):S96–100.

[63] Louis J, Landon MB, Gersnoviez RJ, et al, Maternal-Fetal Medicine Units Network, National Institute of Child Health and Human Development. Perioperative morbidity and mortality among human immunodeficiency virus infected women undergoing cesarean delivery. Obstet Gynecol 2007;110(2 Pt 1):385–90.

[64] Dao H, Mofenson LM, Ekpini R, et al. International recommendations on antiretroviral drugs for treatment of HIV-infected women and prevention of mother-to-child HIV transmission in resource-limited settings: 2006 update. Am J Obstet Gynecol 2007;197(Suppl 3):S42–55.

[65] Suksomboon N, Poolsup N, Ket-Aim S. Systematic review of the efficacy of antiretroviral therapies for reducing the risk of mother-to-child transmission of HIV infection. J Clin Pharm Ther 2007;32(3):293–311.

[66] Gilling-Smith C, Nicopoullos JD, Semprini AE, et al. HIV and reproductive care: a review of current practice. BJOG 2006;113(8):869–78, Epub 2006 Jun 2.

[67] McIntyre JA. Controversies in the use of nevirapine for prevention of mother-to-child transmission of HIV. Expert Opin Pharmacother 2006;7(6):677–85.

[68] Watts DH. Treating HIV during pregnancy: an update on safety issues. Drug Saf 2006;29(6): 467–90.

[69] Kourtis AP, Jamieson DJ, de Vincenzi I, et al. Prevention of human immunodeficiency virus-1 transmission to the infant through breastfeeding: new developments. Am J Obstet Gynecol 2007;197(Suppl 3):S113–22.

[70] Fowler MG, Lampe MA, Jamieson DJ, et al. Reducing the risk of mother-to-child human immunodeficiency virus transmission: past successes, current progress and challenges, and future directions. Am J Obstet Gynecol 2007;197(Suppl 3):S3–9.

[71] Lim WS, Macfarlane JT, Colthorpe CL. Pneumonia and pregnancy. Thorax 2001;56:398–405.

[72] Goodrum LA. Pneumonia in pregnancy. Semin Perinatol 1997;21(4):276–83.

[73] Madinger NE, Greenspoon JS, Ellrodt AG. Pneumonia during pregnancy: has modern technology improved maternal and fetal outcome? Am J Obstet Gynecol 1989;161(3):657–62.

[74] Munn MB, Groome LJ, Atterbury JL, et al. Pneumonia as a complication of pregnancy. J Matern Fetal Med 1999;8(4):151–4.

[75] Benedetti TJ, Valle R, Ledger WJ. Antepartum pneumonia in pregnancy. Am J Obstet Gynecol 1982;144(4):413–7.

[76] Berkowitz K, LaSala A. Risk factors associated with the increasing prevalence of pneumonia during pregnancy. Am J Obstet Gynecol 1990;163(3):981–5.

[77] Rodrigues J, Niederman MS. Pneumonia complicating pregnancy. Clin Chest Med 1992; 13(4):679–91.

[78] Nathwani D, Maclean A, Conway S, et al. Varicella infections in pregnancy and the newborn: a review prepared for the UK Advisory Group on Chickenpox on behalf of the British Society for the Study of Infection. J Infect 1998;36(Suppl 1):59–71.

[79] Eder SE, Apuzzio JJ, Weiss G. Varicella pneumonia during pregnancy: treatment of two cases with acyclovir. Am J Perinatol 1988;5(1):16–8.

[80] Haake DA, Zakowski PC, Haake DL, et al. Early treatment with acyclovir for varicella pneumonia in otherwise healthy adults: retrospective controlled study and review. Rev Infect Dis 1990;12(5):788–98.

[81] Weinstein L, Meade RH. Respiratory manifestations of chickenpox: special consideration of the features of primary varicella pneumonia. AMA Arch Intern Med 1956;98(1):91–9.

[82] Smego RA Jr, Asperilla MO. Use of acyclovir for varicella pneumonia during pregnancy. Obstet Gynecol 1991;78(6):1112–6.

[83] Clements DA, Katz SL. Varicella in a susceptible pregnant woman. Curr Clin Top Infect Dis 1993;13:123–30.

[84] Spangler JG, Kirk JK, Knudson MP. Uses and safety of acyclovir in pregnancy. J Fam Pract 1994;38(2):186–91.

[85] Clark GP, Dobson PM, Thickett A, et al. Chickenpox pneumonia, its complications and management: a report of three cases, including the use of extracorporeal membrane oxygenation. Anaesthesia 1991;46(5):376–80.

[86] Barbosa-Cesnik C, Schwartz K, Foxman B. Lactation mastitis. JAMA 2003;289(13):1609–12.

[87] Ellenbogen C, Graybill JR, Silva J Jr, et al. Bacterial pneumonia complicating adenoviral pneumonia: a comparison of respiratory tract bacterial culture sources and effectiveness of chemoprophylaxis against bacterial pneumonia. Am J Med 1974;56(2):169–78.

[88] Weller TH. Varicella and herpes zoster: changing concepts of the natural history, control, and importance of a not-so-benign virus. N Engl J Med 1983;309(23):1434–40.

[89] Hermann KL. Congenital and perinatal varicella. Clin Obstet Gynecol 1982;25:605–9.

[90] Marchant DJ. Inflammation of the breast. Obstet Gynecol Clin North Am 2002;29(1):89–102.

[91] Foxman B, D'Arcy H, Gillespie B, et al. Lactation mastitis: occurrence and medical management among 946 breastfeeding women in the United States. Am J Epidemiol 2002;155(2): 103–14.

[92] Vogel A, Hutchison BL, Mitchell EA. Mastitis in the first year postpartum. Birth 1999;26(4): 218–25.

[93] Vogel A, Hutchinson BL, Mitchell EA. Factorsa associated with the duration of breastfeeding. Acta Paediatr 1999;88(12):1320–6.

[94] Yokoe DS, Christiansen CL, Johnson R, et al. Epidemiology of and surveillance for postpartum infections. Emerg Infect Dis 2001;7(5):837–41.

[95] Fetherston C. Mastitis in lactating women: physiology or pathology? Breastfeed Rev 2001; 9(1):5–12.

[96] Asoglu O, Ozmen V, Karanlik H, et al. Feasibility of surgical management in patients with granulomatous mastitis. Breast J 2005;11(2):108–14.

[97] Osterman KL, Rahm VA. Lactation mastitis: bacterial cultivation of breast milk, symptoms, treatment, and outcome. J Hum Lact 2000;16(4):297–302.

[98] Pouchot J, Foucher E, Lino M, et al. Granulomatous mastitis: an uncommon cause of breast abscess. Arch Intern Med 2001;161(4):611–2.

[99] Deshpande W. Mastitis. Community Pract 2007;80(5):44–5.

ELSEVIER
SAUNDERS

Emerg Med Clin N Am
26 (2008) 367–387

EMERGENCY
MEDICINE
CLINICS OF
NORTH AMERICA

HIV Infection and Complications in Emergency Medicine

Catherine A. Marco, MD, FACEP[a],*,
Richard E. Rothman, MD, PhD, FACEP[b]

[a]Department of Surgery, Division of Emergency Medicine, University of Toledo
College of Medicine, 3045 Arlington Avenue, 328 Mulford Library,
Mail Stop 1050, Toledo, OH 43614, USA
[b]Department of Emergency Medicine, Johns Hopkins University School of Medicine,
1830 E. Monument Street, Suite 6-100, Baltimore, MD 21287, USA

It is estimated that worldwide approximately 39.5 million adults and 2.3 million children were living with HIV/AIDS at the end of 2006 [1]. In the United States, most HIV/AIDS cases occur in adult men (73%) and fewer in adult women (18%) and children (1%). Most HIV infections in the United States affect patients aged 40 years and younger. There is a disproportionate rate of infection among minority groups, particularly African American and Hispanic populations. HIV infection typically is fatal within 15 years of primary HIV seroconversion, but this outcome is highly variable depending on early detection and antiretroviral therapy. Although the prevalence of HIV/AIDS has decreased recently in the United States [2], the incidence has remained relatively stable at 40,000 new cases per year.

Risk factors for HIV infection include men who have sex with men, injecting drug use, heterosexual exposure to an infected partner, and maternal-neonatal transmission. Recently, there has been a decrease in HIV seropositivity among men who have sex with men and increases in patients with injecting drug use and heterosexual risk factors.

HIV infection may be transmitted by one of several modalities. Proven transmission routes include semen, vaginal secretions, blood products, breast milk, and transplacental transmission in utero.

Disclaimer: This article is not intended to be a comprehensive review of all HIV-related disorders, particularly in light of the rapidly evolving diagnostic and therapeutic modalities available. Appropriate updated resources and infectious disease consultations should be sought whenever clinically indicated.

* Corresponding author.
E-mail address: cmarco2@aol.com (C.A. Marco).

0733-8627/08/$ - see front matter © 2008 Elsevier Inc. All rights reserved.
doi:10.1016/j.emc.2008.01.001   emed.theclinics.com

What is HIV?

The HIV virus, a human retrovirus, infects immune system cells and produces immunodeficiency. The HIV virus is extremely labile and is easily neutralized by heat or disinfecting agents (such as isopropyl alcohol, hydrogen peroxide, disinfectant, alcohol, or household bleach).

What is AIDS?

AIDS was defined by the Centers for Disease Control and Prevention (CDC) in 2003 as laboratory evidence of HIV infection and at least one of several conditions indicative of immunodeficiency or other complication (Box 1) [3].

Box 1. AIDS-defining illnesses[a]

Laboratory data
    CD4 count < 200/mm^3
Infections
    Candidiasis, esophageal or pulmonary
    Coccidioidomycosis
    Cryptococcosis
    Cryptosporidiosis
    Cytomegalovirus infection
    Herpes esophagitis
    Histoplasmosis
    Isosporiasis
    Mycobacterial disease
    Pneumocystis carinii infection
    Progressive multifocal leukoencephalopathy
    Bacterial pneumonia (recurrent)
    Salmonellosis
    Brain toxoplasmosis
Malignancies
    Cervical cancer
    Kaposi's sarcoma
    Lymphoma
Miscellaneous/other
    HIV encephalopathy
    HIV wasting syndrome

---

[a] This represents only a partial list of selected AIDS-defining illnesses. For a complete list, refer to the 1993 CDC Case Definition, available at: http://www.cdc.gov/mmwr/preview/mmwrhtml/00018871.htm.

Should HIV testing be performed in the emergency department?

HIV infection can be diagnosed by various laboratory means. HIV infection is most commonly diagnosed by HIV antibody detection. Commonly used tests include enzyme-linked immunoassay and a Western blot assay, a testing strategy that typically takes about 1 week to perform [4]. Typically, a positive enzyme-linked immunoassay is confirmed by a positive Western blot. Using this testing strategy, laboratory tests of HIV serology are more than 99.9% sensitive and specific. Other testing modalities include HIV antigen assays, viral culture, P24 assay, monoclonal antibody detection, and polymerase chain reaction. False-negative HIV tests may occur during the first few months following an acute infection, after viral transmission but before the appearance of antibodies.

Although previously, serologic testing of patients for HIV in the emergency department had been discouraged, the CDC recently issued guidelines supporting routine testing for HIV in all health care settings, including emergency departments, without separate informed consent or formal pretest counseling [5,6]. Because early recognition of HIV and early therapeutic intervention can significantly improve outcomes, routine HIV testing may lead to improved patient care and reduced opportunistic infection and other disease complications. Currently, many states still have laws requiring informed consent before testing [7]. Some barriers exist to emergency department testing, such as time constraints, financial burden, the impact on emergency department crowding, the responsibility to provide follow-up care, and lack of training with the delivery of new HIV diagnosis [8,9]. Guidelines for those persons interested in setting up HIV testing programs are available from the American Hospital Association [10]. Emergency physicians should be familiar with state laws and institutional policies regarding HIV testing in the emergency department.

Rapid point-of-care testing in the emergency department has several advantages, most notably, access to populations at risk of HIV infection, identification of infected patients, rapid patient notification, counseling, education regarding high-risk behavior, and referral for treatment [11–14]. Several rapid tests are available for emergency department testing with results available in less than 1 hour, including the single use diagnostic system (SUDS) assay (venipuncture), the OraQuick Rapid HIV-1 Antibody Test (fingerstick), Reveal (venipuncture), Uni-Gold Recombigen (venipuncture), and Determine (venipuncture). These rapid tests typically have a sensitivity of 97% to 99% and should be confirmed by Western blot.

Is HIV seropositivity reportable?

AIDS is a reportable disease in all 50 states. HIV infection is reportable in most states. As of 2007, 47 states are conducting confidential name-based HIV infection reporting based on the CDC recommendations of 2005 [15].

Thirty-three states have been conducting confidential name-based HIV infection reporting for 5 years or more.

Clinical emergency department presentations of HIV infection and AIDS

Initial evaluation

The initial emergency department evaluation should include the identification of emergent and urgent disorders. If indicated, airway, breathing, and circulation must be rapidly stabilized. Following initial assessment and stabilization, pertinent elements of the history should include the chief complaint and relevant historical elements. Past medical history should include details about HIV infection, complications, treatments, and medications. Many patients are knowledgeable about their historic laboratory data, often including the CD4 count and viral load. The physical examination should focus on the organ system of chief complaint but should also address other potential infections and disorders. The generation of an appropriate differential diagnosis is crucial, and many HIV-related disorders cannot be definitively diagnosed in the emergency department. Management priorities include the initiation of appropriate therapy and appropriate consultation and disposition.

Systemic symptoms of HIV infection

Systemic symptoms such as fever, weight loss, fatigue, and malaise are common among HIV-infected patients. The differential diagnosis is lengthy and includes infectious causes, malignancies, and drug reactions.

Primary HIV infection

The acute seroconversion syndrome resulting from HIV infection commonly occurs 2 to 6 weeks after the initial exposure and may consist of nonspecific systemic symptoms such as fever, fatigue, adenopathy, pharyngitis, diarrhea, weight loss, and rash. The fever may occur in the afternoon or evening and is generally responsive to antipyretics. Other symptoms may include rash, myopathy, or peripheral neuropathy. These systemic symptoms may be present for 1 to 3 weeks and may be misdiagnosed as a simple viral syndrome.

Fever

Fever is a common chief complaint in emergency department patients with HIV infection or AIDS. The primary focus of emergency department evaluation is to identify treatable etiologies, which may include a variety of infections, drug reactions, or other causes. Diagnostic tests should be tailored to the individual patient and may include chest radiography, a complete blood

count, electrolytes, erythrocyte sedimentation rate, liver function tests, a serologic test for syphilis, urinalysis and culture, blood cultures (aerobic, anaerobic, and fungal), blood tests for cryptococcal antigen, and serologic tests for
Toxoplasma and *Coccidioides*. If fever is accompanied by gastrointestinal
symptoms, stool culture and stool examination for ova and parasites may
be indicated. If urinary tract infection is suspected, urine culture for bacterial
pathogens, fungus, and mycobacteria should be obtained. If additional respiratory symptoms are present, sputum smear and culture for fungus and
mycobacteria may be indicated. If there are neurologic signs or symptoms,
cranial CT scan or MRI should be performed, and a lumbar puncture should
be considered. Many patients with fever or other systemic symptoms can be
managed as outpatients provided adequate medical follow-up, observation,
medications, transportation, and home assistance are available. Indications
for hospital admission include hemodynamic instability, significant dehydration, neutropenia with fever, hypoxia, or other need for urgent diagnosis and
treatment.

Neurologic symptoms

Neurologic complications have a 75% to 90% incidence among AIDS
patients. The most common AIDS-defining neurologic complications include infection with *Cryptococcus neoformans,* toxoplasmosis, HIV encephalopathy, and primary central nervous system (CNS) lymphoma. Other
CNS infections commonly occur, such as bacterial meningitis, histoplasmosis, cytomegalovirus (CMV), progressive multifocal leukoencephalopathy,
herpes simplex virus (HSV), neurosyphilis, and tuberculosis. Noninfectious
processes causing neurologic symptoms include drug adverse effects, CNS
lymphoma, cerebrovascular accident, and metabolic encephalopathy.

Clinical presentations of serious neurologic complications are often nonspecific. The most common symptoms include headache, altered mental
status, seizures, meningismus, or focal neurologic deficits. Emergency department workup should address the individual patient symptomatology
and severity of illness and may include neuroimaging and possible lumbar
puncture. Emergent lumbar puncture should be considered for patients
with CD4 cell counts less than 200 cells/mm^3 with fever and meningismus
in the absence of focal neurologic deficits. In cases of focal deficits, new seizures, or suspicion of focal lesions, immediate neuroimaging is recommended followed by lumbar puncture. For emergency department evaluation,
CT without contrast is usually adequate to identify significant mass lesions.
If there is a high suspicion of mass lesion, a contrast CT scan or MRI may
be performed.

Cryptococcus neoformans

C neoformans is a fungal CNS infection that may cause focal cerebral lesions or diffuse meningoencephalitis. It occurs in 10% of AIDS patients and

is found most commonly in those with CD4 counts less than 100 cells/mm^3. Presenting symptoms typically include fever and headache, often accompanied by nausea and vomiting. Other symptoms include visual changes, dizziness, seizures, and cranial nerve deficits. The mortality rate may be as high as 30%, particularly with delay of diagnosis and definitive treatment.

Emergent CT may be done to rule out mass lesion. Definitive diagnosis is made by a positive cerebrospinal fluid cryptococcal antigen, which is nearly 100% sensitive and specific. Other diagnostic tests may be performed, including India ink staining (60% to 80% sensitive), fungal culture (95% sensitive), and serum cryptococcal antigen (95% sensitive). Treatment of cryptococcal meningitis should be initiated with intravenous amphotericin B or another systemic antifungal agent; 5-flucytosine may be added to this regimen. Oral fluconazole may be used as initial therapy in patients with normal mental status. Decisions regarding empiric therapy should be based on clinical suspicion. If bacterial or fungal meningitis is suspected, empiric therapy should be instituted with a regimen to cover routine bacterial pathogens as well as fungal pathogens.

Toxoplasma gondii

T gondii is the most common organism causing focal intracranial mass lesions in patients with HIV infection and occurs in approximately 3% to 4% of patients. Presenting symptoms may include headache, fever, altered mental status, focal deficits, and seizures. Serologic testing is not helpful due to the widespread antibody presence among the general population. Brain CT findings typically include multiple subcortical lesions with ring enhancement seen on contrast CT. MRI is more sensitive in detecting the number and extent of lesions. Toxoplasmosis of the brain can be difficult to distinguish from other mass lesions, such as lymphoma, cerebral tuberculosis, fungi, progressive multifocal leukoencephalopathy, CMV, and Kaposi's sarcoma, and biopsy may be required.

Patients with suspected toxoplasmosis should be treated as inpatients with pyrimethamine plus sulfadiazine with folinic acid to reduce the incidence of pancytopenia. Steroids are beneficial in cases in which significant edema or mass effect is noted. Seizure prophylaxis with phenytoin may be indicated.

Primary central nervous system lymphoma

CNS lymphoma occurs typically in patients with CD4 cell counts less than 100 cells/mm^3. Clinical presentations may include altered mental status, headache, or focal neurologic deficits. Brain CT shows hyperdense or isodense round or multiple enhancing lesions, particularly in the periventricular region; biopsy is required for definitive diagnosis. The prognosis for lymphoma in the HIV-infected patient is poor, and the median survival is less than 1 month. Life expectancy may be extended to several months with brain irradiation along with corticosteroids and chemotherapy, including methotrexate and zidovudine [16].

HIV neuropathy

HIV neuropathy occurs in up to 50% of HIV infected patients and is characterized by painful sensory symptoms in the feet. The etiology is not well understood but is thought to be related to primary HIV infection. Treatment should include analgesia with agents such as nonsteroidal anti-inflammatory agents, narcotics, amitriptyline, or phenytoin.

HIV encephalopathy

HIV encephalopathy occurs in up to one third of patients with HIV, typically in patients with CD4 counts of less than 200 cells/mm^3. HIV encephalopathy is a progressive process caused by HIV infection and may cause memory impairment or cognitive deficits. Deficits become progressive and can include more obvious changes in mental status or seizures. HIV encephalopathy is a diagnosis of exclusion, and emergency department evaluation should rule out other treatable CNS processes. HIV encephalopathy may be treated with antiretroviral therapy in coordination with an infectious disease specialist or neurologist.

Ophthalmologic presentations

Retinal cotton-wool spots are the most common eye finding in AIDS patients and do not require specific intervention. Other ophthalmologic manifestations of HIV include CMV retinitis, Kaposi's sarcoma of the eyelids or conjunctiva, and a variety of other infections.

CMV retinitis is the most common cause of blindness in AIDS patients and occurs in 10% to 30% of patients. A reduced incidence of CMV retinitis has been noted following widespread treatment with highly active antiretroviral therapy (HAART) [17]. CMV retinitis may present with blurred vision, a change in visual acuity, floaters, flashes of light, photophobia, scotoma, redness, or pain [18]. It appears on ophthalmoscopy as fluffy white retinal lesions, often perivascular (although not pathognomonic). The differential diagnosis should include toxoplasmosis, syphilis, HSV infection, varicella zoster virus infection, and tuberculosis. Treatment should be initiated with ganciclovir. Other therapies may include foscarnet, intravitreal injections of fomivirsen, or ganciclovir-containing intravitreal implants.

Pulmonary symptoms

The differential diagnosis of respiratory symptoms is broad and includes bacterial infections (eg, Streptococcus pneumoniae, Haemophilus influenzae, Chlamydia pneumoniae, Mycobacterium tuberculosis), protozoal infections (eg, Pneumocystis jiroveci, Toxoplasma gondii), viral infections (eg, CMV, adenovirus), fungal infections (eg, Cryptococcus neoformans, Histoplasma capsulatum, Aspergillus fumigatus), malignancies (eg, Kaposi's sarcoma, carcinoma, lymphoma), and other disorders (eg, lymphocytic interstitial pneumonitis, pulmonary hypertension). Symptoms may include cough, dyspnea, fever, or hemoptysis.

Diagnostic tests should include chest radiography and oxygen saturation. A complete blood count and arterial blood gas analysis may be considered. Other tests may be indicated, such as serum lactic dehydrogenase, sputum culture, blood culture, Gram's stain, and special stains (Gomori, Giemsa, or acid-fast).

Chest radiography is often nonspecific. Certain patterns may be suggestive of specific disorders. A focal infiltrate suggests bacterial pneumonia. A diffuse interstitial pattern may be associated with *Pneumocystis carinii* pneumonia (PCP), CMV, tuberculosis, *Mycobacterium avium* complex, histoplasmosis, lymphoid interstitial pneumonitis, or *Mycoplasma pneumoniae*. Nodular findings may indicate Kaposi's sarcoma, *Mycobacterium tuberculosis*, *Mycobacterium avium* complex, fungal lesions, and toxoplasmosis. Hilar adenopathy with diffuse pulmonary infiltrates is suggestive of cryptococcosis, histoplasmosis, mycobacterial infection, or neoplasm.

Pneumocystis pneumonia

PCP is one of the most common opportunistic infections among AIDS patients. More than 80% of AIDS patients acquire PCP at some time during their illness. PCP pneumonia is caused by the organism *Pneumocystis jiroveci* (formerly referred to as *Pneumocystis carinii)* [19]. It is still acceptable to use the acronym PCP (pneumocystis pneumonia). The typical clinical presentation is a nonproductive cough with dyspnea that is worse on exertion. Hypoxia or an increased alveolar arterial gradient may be seen. The chest radiograph may show the classic diffuse interstitial infiltrate but may also be normal. Other findings may include asymmetry, nodules, cavitation, or bullae. Definitive diagnosis is achieved with immunofluorescence of sputum using monoclonal antibodies. Sputum may be obtained by induction but often requires bronchoscopy (bronchoalveolar lavage, brush biopsy, transbronchial biopsy). Gallium scanning has high sensitivity but relatively low specificity.

The emergency department physician should not wait for a definitive diagnosis to initiate treatment. Treatment should be initiated expeditiously with trimethoprim and sulfamethoxazole (TMP-SMX) (TMP, 15 to 20 mg/kg/day; SMX, 75 to 100 mg/kg/day) either orally or intravenously for a total of 21 days. A typical adult dose may be two Bactrim DS tablets every 8 hours. Alternatives include pentamidine isethionate, dapsone, or other agents. Steroid treatment (prednisone, 40 mg orally twice daily with a tapering dose over 3 weeks) should be initiated for patients with a PaO_2 less than 70 mm Hg or an alveolar arterial gradient of greater than 35 and has been shown to be associated with a decreased risk of respiratory and failure in these patients [20].

Mycobacterium tuberculosis

The incidence of *Mycobacterium tuberculosis* in HIV-infected patients has increased dramatically, particularly in socioeconomically disadvantaged groups, including prisoners and intravenous drug users [21]. Symptoms may include fever, cough, and hemoptysis. Radiographic abnormalities may include classic findings of upper lobe infiltrates and cavitation, adenopathy, or other atypical features [22]. Extrapulmonary disease is more common among HIV-infected patients (up to 75% of cases) and includes CNS, bone, visceral, skin, pericardial, eye, pharynx, and lymph node involvement. Multidrug-resistant tuberculosis is of increasing concern, particularly among the HIV-infected population. Diagnostic tests may include purified protein derivative skin testing, sputum stain and culture, or biopsy of affected organs.

Treatment should be determined taking into consideration local resistance as well as individual susceptibility tests. AIDS patients with tuberculosis should receive a four-drug regimen with isoniazid, rifampin, pyrazinamide, and ethambutol for 6 months [23,24]. Empiric treatment should be given for HIV-infected persons with close contact with a patient with active tuberculosis [25].

Other pulmonary complications

Fungal pulmonary disorders may include cryptococcosis, aspergillosis, histoplasmosis, coccidioidomycosis, nocardiosis, and blastomycosis [26]. CMV is the most common viral pulmonary pathogen and typically occurs in advanced immunosuppression. Kaposi's sarcoma is associated with hilar peribronchovascular thickening, lower lobe reticulonodular opacities, adenopathy, pleural effusion, or focal consolidation. Other malignancies may be seen, including non-Hodgkin's lymphoma, Hodgkin's disease, and bronchogenic carcinoma. Lymphoproliferative pulmonary disorders may include lymphocytic interstitial pneumonia, nonspecific interstitial pneumonia, and bronchiolitis obliterans.

Cardiovascular manifestations

Although cardiac involvement is frequently found at autopsy (up to 73% of deceased AIDS patients), clinically significant cardiac disease in the AIDS patient is relatively uncommon [27]. Cardiac complications may include pericardial effusion, cardiomyopathy, right or left ventricular hypertrophy, myocarditis, endocarditis, malignancy, coronary artery disease, and cardiotoxicity of medications [28,29]. Pericardial effusions, rarely clinically significant in this population, may be associated with malignancies, uremia, lymphatic obstruction, or infections, such as with *Mycobacterium tuberculosis, Streptococcus pneumoniae, Staphylococcus aureus,* or other bacterial, viral, fungal, or protozoal infections. Cardiomyopathy may be seen with primary HIV infection, viral, mycobacterial, fungal, or protozoal infection, or drug-induced, immunologic, or ischemic etiologies. Infective endocarditis occurs commonly in patients with a history of injecting drug use. Cardiac neoplasms occur rarely, typically either Kaposi's sarcoma or lymphoma.

Gastrointestinal complications

Gastrointestinal symptoms commonly include diarrhea, weight loss, malabsorption, abdominal pain, bleeding, esophageal symptoms, and hepatobiliary symptoms. These symptoms may result from HIV infection specifically or from opportunistic infections or malignancies. Nonspecific symptoms of nausea, vomiting, and abdominal pain may represent adverse effects of antiretroviral therapy and may be seen with nucleoside reverse transcriptase inhibitors, non-nucleoside reverse transcriptase inhibitors, and protease inhibitors.

Oral disease may be seen with fungal infections (oral candidiasis, histoplasmosis, cryptococcosis, penicillinosis), viral lesions (HSV, herpes zoster, CMV, hairy leukoplakia, papillomavirus), bacterial lesions (periodontal disease, necrotizing stomatitis, tuberculosis, *Mycobacterium avium* complex, bacillary angiomatosis), neoplasms (Kaposi's sarcoma, lymphoma, Hodgkin's lymphoma), and autoimmune or idiopathic lesions (eg, salivary gland disease, aphthous ulcers). Oral candidiasis, the most common diagnosis, affects more than 80% of AIDS patients. *Candida albicans* typically involves the tongue and buccal mucosa and may be asymptomatic, or may present with soreness, burning, and dysphagia. Candidiasis may appear as whitish lacy plaques which are easily scraped away from an erythematous base. Microscopic examination on potassium hydroxide smear can confirm the diagnosis. Treatment should be instituted with clotrimazole troches (10 mg orally five times daily for 14 days). Alternative regimens include nystatin vaginal tablets, which may be dissolved slowly in the mouth four times daily, or nystatin pastilles (two pastilles dissolved in the mouth five times daily). Systemic therapy may be required in some cases, such as ketoconazole, fluconazole, or itraconazole. Hairy leukoplakia is also common and typically produces white, corrugated, or filiform thickened lesions on the lateral aspects of the tongue and can be distinguished from thrush because it cannot be scraped away. Specific therapy is not necessary, but if symptomatic, treatment may be initiated with acyclovir, ganciclovir, foscarnet, or Retin-A. Other oral disorders may include HSV, *Mycobacterium avium* complex, and oral Kaposi's sarcoma.

Esophageal disorders may present with complaints of dysphagia, odynophagia, or chest pain. Esophagitis may be caused by *Candida,* HSV, or CMV infection, Kaposi's sarcoma, *Mycobacterium avium* complex, reflux esophagitis, or idiopathic entities. The recommended approach for patients with esophageal complaints is to initiate empiric therapy with systemic oral antifungal agents for 2 weeks and proceed with endoscopy for patients who fail to improve after 2 weeks [30]. In uncertain cases, endoscopy, air-contrast barium swallow, fungal stains, viral cultures, and, occasionally, biopsy may be performed to establish a definitive diagnosis.

Diarrhea is estimated to occur in 50% to 90% of patients. Diarrhea may lead to massive fluid loss with dehydration, fever, chills, and weight loss.

Antiretroviral agents have a high incidence of gastrointestinal adverse effects. Potential pathogens include parasites (*Cryptosporidium parvum, Enterocytozoon bieneusi, Isospora belli, Giardia lamblia, Entamoeba histolytica,* and others), bacteria (*Salmonella, Shigella, Campylobacter, Helicobacter pylori, Mycobacterium tuberculosis, Clostridium difficile,* and others), viruses (CMV, HSV, HIV, and others), and fungi (*Histoplasma capsulatum, Cryptococcus neoformans,* and others).

Cryptosporidium and *Isospora* infections are common causes of prolonged watery diarrhea [31]. Diagnostic tests may include acid-fast stain of stool samples, monoclonal antibody, or enzyme-linked immunoabsorbent assays. Symptomatic management includes diet modification with or without loperamide. *Cryptosporidium* infections may be treated (with variable success) with azithromycin, and *Isospora* infections may be treated with TMP-SMX.

Viruses may cause diarrhea, including CMV, adenovirus, astrovirus, rotavirus, and others. Emergency department management should include rehydration, repletion of fluid and electrolytes, and appropriate diagnostic studies. Diagnostic tests may include microscopic examination of stool for leukocytes and erythrocytes, and stool samples for bacterial culture, ova, and parasites. Colonoscopy or sigmoidoscopy may be arranged for patients who require further evaluation. Often, a definitive diagnosis is elusive in AIDS patients with diarrhea, and symptomatic management is undertaken with treatments such as attapulgite (Kaopectate), psyllium (Metamucil), diet modification, or diphenoxylate hydrochloride with atropine (Lomotil).

Hepatomegaly occurs in as many as 50% of AIDS patients and may be a result of hepatitis or other infection with opportunistic organisms such as CMV, *Mycobacterium avium-intracellulare, Mycobacterium tuberculosis,* and *Histoplasma capsulatum.*

Renal disease related to HIV infection

Renal insufficiency may result from a variety of etiologies. Prerenal azotemia is the most common abnormality, often seen in association with volume loss related to systemic or gastrointestinal infection. Correction of fluid and electrolyte abnormalities should be initiated. Acute renal failure may occur as a result of drug nephrotoxicity (eg, pentamidine, aminoglycosides, sulfa drugs, foscarnet, rifampin, dapsone, and amphotericin B). HIV-associated nephropathy is a cause of renal insufficiency, often in the late stages of immunosuppression [32]. Vasculitis, tuberculosis, or other systemic infections may also lead to renal insufficiency. Postrenal azotemia may result from obstruction due to lymphoma, stones, fungus ball, blood clot, or sloughed papilla.

Emergency department evaluation should include urinalysis, assessment of fluid status and renal function, and assays for blood urea nitrogen and creatinine. If obstruction is suspected, ultrasound or CT may demonstrate the site and degree of obstruction. Renal biopsy may be indicated for patients with undiagnosed renal disease. Treatment is based on the primary etiology. Therapies for HIV-associated nephropathy have demonstrated variable results but may include corticosteroids, angiotensin-converting enzyme inhibitors, and dialysis.

Sexually transmitted diseases

Sexually transmitted diseases (STDs) are common among HIV-infected patients. The prevalence of syphilis in general in the United States is increasing [33]. Syphilis infections have been associated with increased susceptibility to HIV seroconversion [34]. Common STDs including gonorrhea, Chlamydia, and herpes infections should be considered, and serologic testing for syphilis should be performed in all patients with suspected STD. Combined screening for HIV and STDs in the emergency department is feasible and identifies high-risk patients [35]. Empiric therapy may be instituted before laboratory proof of infection. The recommended treatment of primary or secondary syphilis of less than 12 months' duration is benzathine penicillin, 2.4 million units intramuscularly. For latent syphilis or an unknown duration of secondary syphilis, three weekly injections should be given. Patients with known or suspected syphilis should be evaluated for the presence of neurosyphilis, which has an increasing incidence among HIV-infected individuals. Neurosyphilis should be treated with 12 to 24 million units of intravenous penicillin G daily for 10 to 14 days.

Dermatologic disorders

Any preexisting dermatologic conditions may be exacerbated following HIV infection. Additionally, common skin and soft tissue infections and conditions may have an atypical or exacerbated presentation. Generalized skin disorders such as xerosis (dry skin) and pruritus are common and may be present before a significant immunocompromised state.

Kaposi's sarcoma may present in various stages from single lesions to dissemination with mucous membrane involvement. Kaposi's sarcoma typically presents with skin nodules, lymph node involvement, or involvement of the gastrointestinal tract or other organs. The typical cutaneous appearance is violaceous, pink, or red papules, plaques, nodules, and tumors. Treatments include cryotherapy, radiotherapy, and intralesional or systemic chemotherapy [36].

Varicella zoster virus is commonly seen in patients with AIDS and may involve multiple dermatomes. In the HIV-infected patient with single dermatomal zoster infection, outpatient management should be initiated with oral famciclovir, acyclovir, penciclovir, or valaciclovir. Admission and intravenous acyclovir may be indicated for patients with systemic involvement, ophthalmic zoster, or severe multidermatomal zoster.

HSV infections are also commonly seen. Both HSV-1 and HSV-2 may be seen as local infection or systemic involvement. HSV infections commonly present with symptoms of fever, adenopathy, malaise, and ulcerative lesions of mucosal and cutaneous sites. Common cutaneous sites include the oral mucosa, genitalia, and rectum. Antiviral agents such as acyclovir, famciclovir, penciclovir, or valaciclovir may be instituted. For disseminated infection or neurologic involvement, intravenous antiviral therapy should be instituted. For local infections, topical therapy with acyclovir or penciclovir may be effective.

Molluscum contagiosum manifests as small flesh-colored papules with a whitish core. Treatment is not mandatory, but if desired, cryotherapy or curettage can be employed for cosmetically significant lesions.

Scabies should be considered in patients with pruritic dermatitis with excoriations. Preferred treatment is with 5% permethrin. Sexual and household contacts as well as the living environment (eg, linens, carpets, furniture) should be treated. Norwegian scabies is a virulent variant seen in HIV-infected patients and is particularly contagious and challenging to eradicate.

Psychiatric presentations

HIV infection and AIDS are complex diagnoses with numerous integral psychologic and social issues in addition to complex physiologic, neurologic, and psychiatric abnormalities. Challenging issues may face patients, including communication with families and friends, employment issues, financial issues, insurance status, medical care, and acceptance of a diagnosis with an uncertain prognosis, often involving chronic illness, disability, or death.

It has been estimated that 60% of HIV-infected patients experience depression [37]. Patients with a previous history of depression are at increased risk. Depression may result in suicidal ideation or attempt. Therapeutic options may include antidepressant pharmacotherapy, hospitalization, or other multidisciplinary psychosocial interventions. Other psychiatric disorders may include personality disorders, addiction disorders, and adjustment disorders.

Psychosis may present with hallucinations, delusions, or other abnormal behavioral changes. Treatable disorders should be ruled out, including CNS infection, drug effects, metabolic or endocrine abnormalities, or other organic etiologies. Psychosis should be typically treated with antipsychotic agents.

Hematologic complications

Hematologic complications in HIV-infected patients may include anemia (up to 80% of patients), neutropenia, and thrombocytopenia. Hematopoiesis may be adversely affected by HIV infection, tumor, infection, or medications [38]. Coagulation disorders may be seen secondary to lupus anticoagulant, viral infections, or idiopathic causes.

Pediatric considerations

Pediatric patients with HIV or AIDs may present with failure to thrive, developmental delay, recurrent or severe bacterial infections, chronic diarrhea, candidiasis, opportunistic infections, or numerous other presentations [39]. In addition to stabilization, diagnostic tests, and institution of definitive care, close follow-up and communication with families and primary physicians are imperative.

Drug reactions

Drug reactions are common among HIV-infected patients for two reasons: (1) patients are commonly treated with a variety of drugs known to produce adverse effects, and (2) for unclear reasons, HIV-infected individuals often have more frequent or more severe reactions to medications than their cohorts. Dermatologic reactions are particularly common. Gastrointestinal effects such as nausea, vomiting, and diarrhea are also common reactions to many agents. Antimicrobial drugs are common culprits of medication reactions. Potential drug interactions should always be considered when prescribing new medications. Drug reactions should always be considered as a possible etiology of presenting symptoms. Potential drug reactions are numerous, and current pharmacologic references should be consulted when drug reactions are suspected.

Antiretroviral therapy

The use of highly active antiretroviral therapy has had dramatic effects on the clinical consequences of HIV infection since its introduction in 1996. The incidence of AIDS-defining illnesses and the death rate from AIDS have declined significantly over this time period [40]. The US Department of Health and Human Services (DHHS) published guidelines for the use of antiretroviral agents in HIV-infected adults and adolescents in 2003 [41]. In summary, the goals of antiretroviral therapy include virologic, immunologic, and clinical effects. The principal clinical goals of therapy are to prolong and improve quality of life.

There are four basic classes of antiretroviral drugs: the nucleoside reverse transcriptase inhibitors, the non-nucleoside reverse transcriptase inhibitors, the protease inhibitors, and a newer class, the fusion inhibitors (Table 1) [42].

The nucleoside reverse transcriptase inhibitors are a group of drugs that competitively inhibit the viral enzyme reverse transcriptase. Several controlled trials have shown that zidovudine (azidothymidine [AZT], Retrovir) decreases the number and severity of opportunistic infections [43]. Some important side effects of these agents include bone marrow suppression with zidovudine, distal sensory peripheral neuropathy with didanosine (Videx), stavudine (Zerit), and zalcitabine (Hivid), and pancreatitis with didanosine.

The non-nucleoside reverse transcriptase inhibitors are noncompetitive reverse transcriptase inhibitors and act by blocking RNA-dependent and DNA-dependent DNA polymerase activity. Examples of agents in this class

Table 1
Drugs for HIV infection

Class of drug	Examples of generic names	Examples of trade names
NRTI (nucleoside reverse transcriptase inhibitors)	Zidovudine	Retrovir
	Zalcitabine	Hivid
	Stavudine	Zerit
	Lamivudine	Epivir
	Didanosine	Videx
	Abacavir	Ziagen
NNRTI (non-nucleoside reverse transcriptase inhibitors)	Delavirdine	Rescriptor
	Efavirenz	Sustiva
	Nevirapine	Viramune
PI (protease inhibitors)	Amprenavir	Agenerase
	Indinavir	Crixivan
	Saquinavir	Invirase
	Fosamprenavir	Lexiva
	Darunavir	Prezista
	Atazanavir	Reyataz
	Tipranavir	Aptivus
FI (fusion inhibitor)	Enfuvirtide	Fuzeon

From Centers for Disease Control. Updated U.S. public health service guidelines for the management of occupational exposures to HBV, HCV, and HIV and recommendations for postexposure prophylaxis. MMWR 2001;50(No. RR-11):24.

are nevirapine (Viramune) and efavirenz (Sustiva). Resistance to these agents is significant; therefore, they are typically recommended for use as part of a three-drug (or more) regimen. Dermatologic reactions are common adverse effects, with Stevens-Johnson syndrome developing in a small minority of patients ($<5\%$) [44].

Protease inhibitors block the enzyme HIV protease, which activates the HIV proteins. Protease inhibitors are believed to be associated with the marked decline in mortality rates for HIV infection; however, their high cost and high incidence of adverse reactions are negative considerations. Common adverse reactions include gastrointestinal symptoms (including nausea, diarrhea, and bloating) and metabolic effects (including hyperglycemia, hyperlipidemia, and fat redistribution) [45].

Several combination products are available for patient ease in dosing multiple medications; however, these products lack flexibility in individual dosing [46,47].

Expert consensus on highly active antiretroviral therapy continues to evolve. Treatment is recommended for patients with either low CD4 counts or high HIV viral load. Selection of an appropriate combination of drugs is a complex issue and requires consideration of multiple individual factors, including clinical symptoms, the presence of opportunistic infections, cost, compliance, adverse effects, and others. DHHS federal recommendations for highly active antiretroviral therapy can be found on the National Institutes of Health Web site [48].

Precautions and postexposure prophylaxis

Precautions and exposures

Exposure to potentially contagious blood and body secretions is common in emergency medicine. Over half of emergency physicians report at least one occupational exposure during a 2-year period [49]; however, the overall risk of HIV seroconversion through occupational exposures remains extremely small. The risk of HIV transmission has been estimated at 0.3% for significant percutaneous exposure and 0.09% for mucocutaneous exposure [50]. Because HIV transmission by health care workers to patients appears to be extremely rare, routine screening of health care workers is not indicated [51].

Emergency department staff can significantly reduce their risk of exposure to blood-borne pathogens by following universal precautions. CDC guidelines for universal precautions include the use of protective barriers (gloves, gown, mask, and eye protection) for any possible exposure. Protective equipment is indicated for most emergency department procedures, including examination of the bleeding patient and other commonly performed procedures where contact with blood or body fluids is likely.

Postexposure prophylaxis

Occupational exposures

Postexposure prophylaxis has demonstrated a reduced risk of HIV transmission and seroconversion [52]. The CDC has developed guidelines for postexposure prophylaxis for occupational exposure to HIV (Table 2) [49]. Current guidelines recommend individual case determination of the risk of the exposure before decisions about postexposure prophylaxis. Recommendations are based on two factors—the type of exposure and the HIV status of the source. Higher risk exposures include deep percutaneous injuries, visible blood on a device, and injuries sustained when placing a catheter in a vein or artery; lower risk percutaneous exposures include superficial injuries or solid needles (such as suture needles). Higher risk sources include patients with acute seroconversion, high viral load, or AIDS; lower risk sources are patients with asymptomatic HIV infection or viral load of less than 1500 copies/mL [53]. When the status of the source is not known, rapid testing should be performed. Some states allow testing of source patients without informed consent in some circumstances. Current CDC guidelines recommend no postexposure prophylaxis for HIV-negative sources and a 4-week regimen of two drugs for most HIV percutaneous or mucus membrane exposures [54]. Two-drug therapy options include combination therapy such as zidovudine and lamivudine, lamivudine and stavudine, or didanosine and stavudine. For the highest risk exposures, a three-drug regimen with the addition of either a protease inhibitor (eg, indinavir or nelfinavir), a non-nucleoside reverse transcriptase inhibitor (eg, efavirenz), or

Table 2
Guidelines for postexposure prophylaxis

Exposure type	HIV-negative source	Unknown source	HIV-positive class 1 source[a]	HIV-positive class 2 source[b]
Less severe (solid needle, superficial injury)	No PEP warranted	Generally, no PEP warranted; consider two-drug PEP for suspected HIV risk factors	Recommend basic two-drug PEP	Recommend expanded three-drug PEP
More severe (large-bore hollow needle, deep puncture, visible blood on device, needle used in artery or vein)	No PEP warranted	Generally, no PEP warranted; consider two-drug PEP for suspected HIV risk factors	Recommend expanded three-drug PEP	Recommend expanded three-drug PEP

Abbreviation: PEP, postexposure prophylaxis.
[a] HIV-positive class 1: asymptomatic HIV infection or known low viral load.
[b] HIV-positive class 2: symptomatic HIV infection, AIDS, acute seroconversion, or known high viral load.
Adapted from Centers for Disease Control. Updated US Public Health Service guidelines for the management of occupational exposures to HBV, HCV and HIV and recommendations for postexposure prophylaxis. MMWR Morb Mortal Wkly Rep 2001;50(RR-1):1.

a nucleoside reverse transcriptase inhibitor (eg, abacavir) is recommended. Postexposure prophylaxis should be initiated as soon as possible after the exposure and should be continued for 4 weeks. Current guidelines suggest starting treatment within 1 to 2 hours and generally recommend therapy for those who seek treatment within 36 hours of exposure. Initial treatment should not be delayed while awaiting information regarding the final determination of the overall risk of exposure because therapy can be stopped after the first dose as new information becomes available. In addition to evaluation and management of HIV exposure risk, all patients should be tested and treated for other infectious agents such as hepatitis. Institutions should maintain policies regarding occupational exposures and postexposure prophylaxis procedures.

Nonoccupational exposure

Postexposure prophylaxis for nonoccupational exposures to blood and body fluids should also be considered, especially for certain sexual or injection drug exposures [55]. Although there is a paucity of data regarding the efficacy of this therapy in nonoccupational settings, the same principles of inhibition of viral replication would apply in these settings. Patients who may be considered for nonoccupational postexposure prophylaxis include sexual assault victims, police, emergency medical services personnel, and the sexual or needle-sharing partners of sources with suspected HIV infection.

As is true for occupational exposures, the institution of postexposure prophylaxis should be considered on an individual case basis [56]. Factors to be considered include the risk of the source, the risk of the exposure, and the risk for ongoing exposures. Baseline HIV testing of the exposed patient and the source, if available, should be performed. Patients should be informed regarding the lack of proven benefit for nonoccupational postexposure prophylaxis [57]. Potential adverse effects of medications should be weighed carefully against potential benefits, and patients should be counseled regarding these potential effects. Specifically, sexual assault victims should be counseled regarding the risks and benefits of postexposure prophylaxis.

Infectious disease consultants should be involved in postexposure prophylaxis decisions if possible. Other resources for occupational and nonoccupational exposures include the CDC/UCSF National Clinicians PEP Hotline, providing 24-hour assistance (1-888-448-4911), and UCLA's online decision making support accessed at: http://www.needlesick.mednet. ucla.edu.

Disposition

Specialty consultation should be sought when there is doubt about diagnostic or management options. Consultations with an infectious disease specialist, intensivist, neurologist, gastroenterologist, psychiatrist, AIDS specialist, or others may be indicated.

Disposition decisions should be based on a variety of factors in the individual case, such as the severity of symptoms, the potential for deterioration in status, the ability to function as an outpatient, the ability to maintain adequate oral intake, access to medical care, access to medications, and compliance with medications and outpatient visits.

References

[1] Joint United Nations Programme on HIV/AIDS. AIDS epidemic update: 2003. Available at: http://data.unaids.org/pub/EpiReport/2006/2006_EpiUpdate_en.pdf. Accessed December 11, 2003.
[2] Centers for Disease Control and Prevention. HIV/AIDS Surveillance Report, 2005, vol. 17. Rev edition. Atlanta (GA): US Department of Health and Human Services, Centers for Disease Control and Prevention; 2007.
[3] Centers for Disease Control and Prevention. 1993 Revised classification system for HIV infection and expanded surveillance case definition for AIDS among adolescents and adults. MMWR Morb Mort Wkly Rep 1993;41(RR–17):1.
[4] Franco-Paredes C, Tellez I, del Rio C. Rapid HIV testing: a review of the literature and implications for the clinician. Curr HIV/AIDS Rep 2006;3:169–75.
[5] Branson BM, Handsfield HH, Lampe MA. Revised recommendations for HIV testing of adults, adolescents and pregnant women in health-care settings. MMWR Recomm Rep 2006;55(RR14):1–17.
[6] Branson BM, Handsfield HH, Lampe MA, et al. Revised recommendations for HIV testing of adults, adolescents, and pregnant women in health-care settings. Available at: http://www.cdc.gov/mmwr/preview/mmwrhtml/rr5514a1.htm. Accessed February 11, 2007.
[7] Stobbe M. Study: majority of states bar HIV testing. Available at: http://www.forbes.com/feeds/ap/2007/10/09/ap4203309.html. Accessed October 10, 2007.

[8] Arbelaez C, Losina E, Wright E, et al. The barriers affecting health care providers' willingness to perform routine HIV testing in the emergency department. Ann Emerg Med 2007;50: S118.

[9] Irvin CB, Flagel BT, Fox JM. The emergence department is not the ideal place for routine HIV testing. Ann Emerg Med 2007;49:722.

[10] Williams TG, Reiter J, Wright CS. HIV testing in the emergency department: a practical guide. Available at: http://www.edhivtestguide.org/. Accessed November 12, 2007.

[11] Rapid tests for HIV infection. The Medical Letter on Drugs and Therapeutics 2003;45:54–5.

[12] Rothman RE. Current Centers for Disease Control and Prevention guidelines for HIV counseling, testing, and referral: critical role of and a call to action for emergency physicians. Ann Emerg Med 2004;44:31–42.

[13] Borg KT. To test or not to test? HIV, emergency departments, and the new Centers for Disease Control and Prevention guidelines. Ann Emerg Med 2007;49:573–4.

[14] McKenna M. HIV testing: should the emergency department take part? Ann Emerg Med 2007;49:190–2.

[15] Centers for Disease Control. HIV infection reporting. Available at: http://www.cdc.gov/hiv/topics/surveillance/reporting.htm. Accessed October 10, 2007.

[16] Sackoff J, McFarland J, Su S, et al. Prophylaxis for opportunistic infections among HIV-infected patients receiving medical care. J Acquir Immune Defic Syndr Hum Retrovirol 1998;19(4):387–92.

[17] Whitcup SM. Cytomegalovirus retinitis in the era of highly active antiretroviral therapy. JAMA 2000;283:653–8.

[18] Wei LL, Park SS, Skiest DJ. Prevalence of visual symptoms among patients with newly diagnosed cytomegalovirus retinitis. Retina 2002;22:278–82.

[19] Stringer JR, Beard CB, Miller RF, et al. A new name (*Pneumocystis jiroveci*) for *Pneumocystis* from humans. Emerg Infect Dis 2002;8:891–6.

[20] NIH-UC Expert Panel for Corticosteroids as Adjunctive Therapy for Pneumocystis Pneumonia: Consensus statement for use of corticosteroids as adjunctive therapy for pneumocystis pneumonia in AIDS. N Engl J Med 1990;323:1451–7.

[21] Markowitz N, Hansen NI, Hopewell PC, et al. Incidence of tuberculosis in the United States among HIV-infected persons: the pulmonary complications of HIV infection study group. Ann Intern Med 1997;126:123–32.

[22] Perlman DC, El-Sadr WM, Nelson ET, et al. Variation of chest radiographic patterns in pulmonary tuberculosis by degree of human immunodeficiency virus-related immunosuppression. Clin Infect Dis 1997;25:242–6.

[23] Centers for Disease Control and Prevention. Prevention and treatment of tuberculosis in patients infected with human immunodeficiency virus: principles of therapy and revised recommendations. MMWR Morb Mortal Wkly Rep 1998;47:1–58.

[24] Blumberg HM, Leonard MK Jr, Jasmer RM. Update on the treatment of tuberculosis and latent tuberculosis infection. JAMA 2005;293:2776–84.

[25] Drugs for tuberculosis. The Medical Letter 2007;5:19.

[26] Rizzi EB, Schinina V, Bellussi A, et al. Pulmonary mycosis in AIDS. Eur J Radiol 2001;37:42–6.

[27] Milei J, Grana D, Alonso GF, et al. Cardiac involvement in acquired immunodeficiency syndrome: a review to push action. Clin Cardiol 1998;21:465–72.

[28] Chu WW, Sosman JM, Stein JH. Clinical cardiac manifestations of HIV infection: a review of current literature. WMJ 2002;101:39–45.

[29] Barbaro G, Fisher SD, Giancaspro G, et al. HIV-associated cardiovascular complications: a new challenge for emergency physicians. Am J Emerg Med 2001;19:566–74.

[30] Bonacini M. Medical management of benign oesophageal disease in patients with human immunodeficiency virus infection. Dig Liver Dis 2001;33:294–300.

[31] Hunter PR, Nichols G. Epidemiology and clinical features of *Cryptosporidium* infections in immunocompromised patients. Clin Microbiol Rev 2002;15:145–54.

[32] Levin ML, Palella F, Shah S, et al. HIV-associated nephropathy occurring before HIV antibody seroconversion. Am J Kidney Dis 2001;37:E39.

[33] Golden MR, Marra CM, Holmes KK. Update of syphilis: resurgence of an old problem. JAMA 2003;290:1510–4.

[34] Fleming DT, Wasserheit JN. From epidemiological synergy to public health policy and practice: the contribution of other sexually transmitted diseases to sexual transmission of HIV infection. Sex Transm Infect 1999;75:3–17.

[35] Silva A, Glick NR, Lyss SB, et al. Implementing an HIV and sexually transmitted disease screening program in an emergency department. Ann Emerg Med 2007;49:564–72.

[36] Nasti G, Errante D, Santarossa S, et al. A risk and benefit assessment of treatment for AIDS-related Kaposi's sarcoma. Drug Saf 1999;20:403–25.

[37] Treisman G, Fishman M, Lyketsos C, et al. Evaluation and treatment of psychiatric disorders associated with HIV infection. Res Publ Assoc Res Nerv Ment Dis 1994;72:239–50.

[38] Moses A, Nelson J, Bagby GC. The influence of human immunodeficiency virus-I on hematopoiesis. Blood 1998;91:1479–95.

[39] Church JA. Pediatric HIV in the emergency department. Clin Ped Emerg Med 2007;8: 117–22.

[40] Palella FJ, Delaney KM, Moorman AC, et al. Declining morbidity and mortality among patients with advanced human immunodeficiency virus infection. N Engl J Med 1998;338: 853–60.

[41] Department of Health and Human Services, Panel on Clinical Practices for Treatment of HIV Infection. Guidelines for the use of antiretroviral agents in HIV-infected adults and adolescents. Available at: www.hivatis.org. Accessed February 8, 2008.

[42] Drugs for HIV infection. Med Lett 2006;4:67–76.

[43] Carpenter CC, Cooper DA, Fischl MA, et al. Antiretroviral therapy in adults: updated recommendations of the International AIDS Society–USA Panel. JAMA 2000;283:381.

[44] Warren KJ, Boxwell DE, Kim NY, et al. Nevirapine-associated Stevens-Johnson syndrome. Lancet 1998;351:567.

[45] Hovanessian HC. New developments in the treatment of HIV disease: an overview. Ann Emerg Med 1999;33:546–55.

[46] A once-daily combination tablet (Atripla) for HIV. Med Lett Drugs Ther 2006;48:78–9.

[47] Two once-daily fixed-dose NRTI combinations for HIV. Med Lett Drugs Ther 2005;47: 19–20.

[48] US Department of Health and Human Services. Recommended HIV treatment regimens. Available at: http://www.aidsinfo.nih.gov/ContentFiles/AboutHIVTreatmentGuidelines_FS_en.pdf. Accessed February 8, 2008.

[49] Ippolito G, Puro V, Heptonstall J, et al. Occupational human immunodeficiency virus infection in health care workers: worldwide cases through September 1997. Clin Infect Dis 1999;28:365–83.

[50] Updated US Public Health Service guidelines for the management of occupational exposures to HBV, HCV and HIV and recommendations for postexposure prophylaxis. MMWR Morb Mortal Wkly Rep 2001;50(RR–1):1–52.

[51] Phillips KA, Lowe RA, Kahn JG, et al. The cost-effectiveness of HIV testing of physicians and dentists in the United States. JAMA 1994;271:851–8.

[52] Gerberding JL. Occupational exposure to HIV in health care settings. N Engl J Med 2003; 343:826–33.

[53] Moran GJ. Emergency department management of blood and body fluid exposures. Ann Emerg Med 2000;35:47–62.

[54] Centers for Disease Control. Updated U.S. Public Health Service guidelines for the management of occupational exposures to HBV, HCV, and HIV and recommendations for postexposure prophylaxis. Available at: http://www.cdc.gov/mmwr/preview/mmwrhtml/rr5011a1.htm. Accessed February 8, 2008.

[55] Merchant RC. Nonoccupational HIV postexposure prophylaxis: a new role for the emergency department. Ann Emerg Med 2000;36:366–75.
[56] McCausland JB, Linden JA, Degutis LC, et al. Nonoccupational postexposure HIV prevention: emergency physicians' current practices, attitudes, and beliefs. Ann Emerg Med 2003;42:651–6.
[57] Katz MH, Gerberding JL. The care of persons with recent sexual exposure to HIV. Ann Intern Med 1998;128:306–12.

ELSEVIER
SAUNDERS

Emerg Med Clin N Am
26 (2008) 389–411

EMERGENCY
MEDICINE
CLINICS OF
NORTH AMERICA

Pneumonia in the Emergency Department

Joseph F. Plouffe, MD[a],*, Daniel R. Martin, MD[b]

[a]5205 Canterbury Drive, Sarasota, FL 34243, USA
[b]Department of Emergency Medicine, The Ohio State University Medical Center,
410 West 10th Avenue, Columbus, OH 43210, USA

Pneumonia is an important cause of morbidity and mortality in adults, with more than 5 million cases occurring annually in United States. Guidelines for the diagnosis and treatment of community-acquired pneumonia (CAP) have evolved since initial meetings in Halifax, Nova Scotia in 1991 [1]. Recent consensus guidelines for CAP have been published by a committee consisting of members from the Infectious Diseases Society of America (IDSA), American Thoracic Society (ATS), and Centers for Disease Control and Prevention (CDC) and are referred to as the 2007 CAP guidelines [2]. Guidelines for health care–associated pneumonia (HCAP) reflecting broader etiologies, including resistant gram-negative bacilli and *Staphylococcus aureus*, have been published by the ATS and IDSA [3]. This article draws extensively from these guidelines and their cited references. Our references emphasize more recent publications. The reader is referred to published guidelines for in-depth discussions and older references.

Common bacterial etiologies of CAP (Fig. 1) include *Streptococcus pneumoniae*, *Mycoplasma pneumoniae*, *Chlamydophila pneumoniae*, *Haemophilus influenzae*, *Legionella pneumophila*, anaerobes associated with aspiration, *S aureus*, and gram-negative bacilli. Viral causes of CAP include influenza, parainfluenza, respiratory syncytial virus, metapneumonia virus, Hanta virus, coronavirus, varicella, and rubeola. *S pneumoniae* is the most commonly diagnosed etiology of CAP among patients treated in the hospital. *M pneumoniae*, *C pneumoniae*, and viruses are more common in patients treated at home. *S pneumoniae* is more common than *M pneumoniae* and *C pneumoniae* among patients who have moderate disease. *S pneumoniae*

---

* Corresponding author.
E-mail address: jsplouf@aol.com (J.F. Plouffe).

0733-8627/08/$ - see front matter © 2008 Elsevier Inc. All rights reserved.
doi:10.1016/j.emc.2008.02.005
emed.theclinics.com

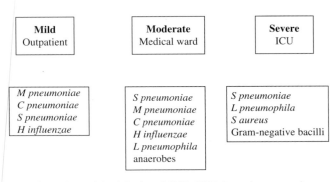

Fig. 1. Bacterial etiologies of CAP. ICU, intensive care unit.

and *L pneumophila* are more common in patients who have severe disease and are treated in the intensive care unit (ICU).

More recently, *S pneumoniae* has become more resistant to penicillin and the macrolides. A small proportion of cases are also resistant to fluoroquinolones. Recent antimicrobial use (within 3 months) is associated with resistance to the same class of antibiotics [4]. The 2007 guidelines emphasize the importance of recent prior antibiotic therapy and prescribing a different class of antimicrobial therapy. There is also evidence that resistance to penicillin and cephalosporins may be decreasing or stabilizing, whereas the resistance to erythromycin is increasing. Doern and colleagues [5], using data from 44 US centers, demonstrated a stable rate of penicillin resistance of 34.2%, with 15.7% intermediate resistance and 18.5% high resistance. Macrolide resistance had increased, although most was efflux pump mediated and considered to be low-level resistance. Nevertheless, the mean macrolide resistance of pneumococci was 27.2% in a recent meta-analysis [6]. Despite this relatively high rate, it is widely believed that this is likely attributable to the efflux pump mechanism, which is more a laboratory phenomenon, because significant failure rates with the newer macrolides have not been reported. Fluoroquinolone resistance was less than 1%. The most active β-lactam was ceftriaxone, with a resistance rate of 6.9%. Although prior antibiotic use of macrolides, penicillins, cephalosporins, and sulfonamides increased the likelihood of future pneumococcal antibiotic resistance to all these agents, this was not the case for fluoroquinolones, wherein pneumococci resistant to other antibiotics remained susceptible to fluoroquinolones [7]. The fluoroquinolone clinical failures that have been reported mainly have been with ciprofloxacin and levofloxacin. Ciprofloxacin is not considered an antipneumococcal fluoroquinolone, and levofloxacin failures occurred mainly at lower dose ranges [8]. The 2007 CAP guidelines caution that inappropriate overuse of fluoroquinolones (ie, acute bronchitis) hastens the development of resistance.

More recent data suggest that empiric coverage in all levels of CAP severity should include atypical organisms, such as *M pneumoniae*, *C pneumoniae*, and *L pneumophila*, although some reports [9,10] that analyzed several studies by meta-analysis or review of published studies reported no difference in outcomes in hospitalized patients treated with atypical coverage versus β-lactams. These studies used antibiotics that included mainly monotherapy (macrolides or quinolones) in the treatment regimens for atypical organisms rather than a treatment regimen that included β-lactams in addition to atypical coverage, however. A recent report from Arnold and colleagues [11] evaluated the effects of treating CAP in four different worldwide regions with a β-lactam alone versus therapy, including atypical coverage, and reported significant benefits in time to clinical stability, decreased length of stay, decreased total mortality, and decreased CAP-related mortality when atypicals were treated.

One unanticipated result of previous guidelines was with pay-for-performance measure PN-5b, which recommended that antibiotics for patients who have CAP be administered within 4 hours of emergency department (ED) triage. Patients with respiratory symptoms who did not have pneumonia were inappropriately receiving antibiotics. In fact, one study [12] reported that 28.5% of patients with an admission diagnosis of CAP received antibiotics for CAP without radiographic abnormalities and this represented an increased from previous data (20.6%). In this study, the final diagnosis of CAP decreased to 58.9%. Data were publicly available. Local media compared hospitals regarding their success in treating CAP quickly.

Pines and colleagues [13] performed a survey of 90 academic ED directors or chairpersons, which revealed that 69% did not believe receiving antibiotics within the 4-hour time window would improve patient care. Most EDs instituted policies to improve timing of antibiotic therapy for patients suspected of having pneumonia, 46 (51%) automated chest radiograph (CXR) ordering at triage, 37 (41%) prioritized patients suspected of having pneumonia, and 33 (37%) administered antibiotics before obtaining CXR results. Despite these efforts, the increasing volumes in US EDs and resulting overcrowding made achieving 4-hour quality standards much less likely [14,15]. Another source of barriers to administer appropriate antibiotics rapidly is the atypical presentation of many patients who have CAP. One study found that altered mental status, absence of fever, absence of hypoxia, and elderly age were significant predictors of antibiotic delays, but it was not clear that such delays contributed to mortality [16]. Pines and colleagues [17] found that less severe illness and nonclassic presentation were associated with antibiotic delays. In another study, Metersky and colleagues [18] found that 22% of their cohort of admitted Medicare patients who had CAP presented in a manner that was atypical enough to cause delays in antibiotic administration. Fee and Weber [19] found that many of the "outliers" who were given their antibiotics after 4 hours did not have a diagnosis of ED CAP and many did not have an abnormal chest radiograph.

The two articles most often quoted regarding the benefit of early antibiotic therapy were by Meehan and colleagues [20] and Houck and colleagues [21], and as has been pointed out by others, these studies have numerous limitations [22]. For example, the sample used was taken from the National Pneumonia Project from the Centers for Medicare and Medicaid Services (CMS) and included patients 65 years of age and older but excluded many patients who have immune-compromising conditions. Moreover, although it is assumed that these patients were treated in both studies by emergency medicine physicians in an ED before hospital admission, these details are never described anywhere in either paper; in fact, the term *emergency department* is not even used in the publications. Several recent editorials and opinion papers [23,24] have criticized this 4-hour time recommendation. The CMS is in the process of changing the 4-hour window (PN-5b) to a 6-hour window (PN-5c) for reporting purposes. The 2007 CAP guidelines have changed the focus from an absolute time frame to recommending that patients receive the initial antibiotic dose during their time in the ED before being admitted to the hospital. Hospitals were also urged to monitor for inappropriate antimicrobial treatment of patients who do not have CAP [2].

Patients come to the ED based on the severity of their symptoms. The ED physician faces a series of critical decisions. Initially, one must decide if the patient has pneumonia and, if so, where and how the patient should be treated. National guidelines suggest that local pneumonia protocols be established at each hospital. Patients treated at hospitals that follow CAP guidelines have been shown to have improved outcomes. Use of local protocols should facilitate improved patient care and documentation for reimbursement. Pham and colleagues [25] reported data on ED treatment of acute myocardial infarction (AMI) and pneumonia from the National Hospital Ambulatory Medical Care Survey involving 544 EDs from 1998 through 2004. Recommended antibiotics were administered to 69% of patients who had pneumonia, and pulse oximetry was measured in 46% of patients who had pneumonia. There were more than 2.7 million opportunities to improve care and 22,000 excess deaths per year associated with current treatment of AMI and pneumonia. These data suggest that we can continue to improve. ED physicians can be valuable team members in the development of local pneumonia protocols.

Local hospital pneumonia protocols

Each hospital should have its own protocol that reflects the local environment, resources, and patient population. Some of the factors to be considered in developing or redefining a local pneumonia protocol are listed here. Obviously, some cost is going to be expended. Hospital administrators need to be convinced that the pneumonia protocol is valuable. Certainly, adverse publicity can be avoided with good adherence. Local pneumonia protocols could be cost-saving, because fewer health care dollars would be spent by identifying patients who have mild disease and could be treated at home. Information from 2007 guidelines on site of care should provide important criteria [26,27]. The cost differential is hundreds of dollars for outpatient treatment compared with thousands of dollars for an admission. Adherence to protocols also has resulted in shorter hospitalization stays with cost savings.

Factors to be included in local guidelines

Define local epidemiologic factors that may influence care
  Proportion of antimicrobial resistance in *S pneumoniae*
  Presence of outbreaks in community: influenza, methicillin-resistant *Staphylococcus aureus* (MRSA)
Type of patient population
Isolation procedures in the ED
Notification of local health authorities
Triage
  Identify patients with respiratory symptoms
  Rapid identification of patients with vital sign abnormalities
  Define patients who should have pulse oximetry
  Facilitate obtaining CXR and appropriate laboratory studies
Historical information (checklist may be a useful aid for documentation and completeness, especially to identify unusual circumstances)
Differential diagnosis
Factors that may influence the site and type of initial care
Immunization status: documentation
Physical examination
  Mental status, vital signs, and oxygenation status are critical in profiling disease severity (Box 1)
  Findings important in the differential diagnosis (Box 2)
Radiology: CXR and other imaging studies
Laboratory studies: results should be available promptly. It is important to note that most patients who have CAP come to ED outside of office hours. Adequate staffing can facilitate timely and appropriate treatment of patients.
Classification of pneumonia type (CAP versus HCAP)

Box 1. CURB65

Confusion: recent disorientation to person, place, or time
Uremia: blood urea nitrogen greater than 20 mg/dL (17 mmol/L)
Respiratory rate: 30 breaths per minute or greater
Blood pressure: systolic <90 mm Hg, or diastolic 60 mm Hg or less
Age 65 years or older

If the patient was transported to the ED by emergency medical technicians (EMTs), initial vital signs obtained by EMTs should be used to profile the patient. One point for each abnormal variable (0–5 points) should be assigned.

Box 2. Nonpneumonic illnesses masquerading as pneumonia

Acute bronchitis: clear CXR

Chronic obstructive pulmonary disease (COPD) with
   exacerbation: change in dyspnea, sputum volume, or
   purulence

Asthma: prior episodes, wheezing

Pleuritis: pleuritic chest pain

Myocardial infarction: coronary artery disease, risk factors

Congestive heart failure (CHF): prior myocardial infarction,
   orthopnea, peripheral edema

Pulmonary emboli: leg pain, venous thrombosis, prior emboli,
   malignancy, recent prolonged plane or car travel

Lung cancer: weight loss, hemoptysis, smoker

Ruptured esophagus: protracted vomiting, severe chest pain

Profile CAP severity and site of care
Prescribe initial empiric therapy

Adequate follow-up for patients sent home

ED physicians and hospital administrators can address several of these issues and incorporate potential solutions in local pneumonia protocols (ie, provide oral antimicrobial therapy, set up ED holding area for initial observation, make follow-up telephone calls, arrange for ED follow-up visit for patients without a primary care physician).

Regardless of whether all these factors can be implemented into a local protocol for treatment of patients who have CAP, collection of subsequent quality improvement (QI) data is key to determine the successful adherence to these protocols.

Monitored data

National performance indicators
   1. Initial antimicrobial therapy is consistent with 2007 CAP guidelines.
   2. Initial antimicrobial therapy for hospitalized patients should be given in the ED.
   3. Mortality data should be stratified by site of care in the hospital.
   4. Is immunization for influenza or pneumococci recommended for the patient? Is the patient's immunization status up to date?
Additional data that may assist hospitals in improving care and documenting protocol success
   Admitted or discharged?

Adequacy of follow-up for those treated at home?

Admitted to the ward or intensive care unit (ICU) and mortality rate for each?

Blood cultures in ICU admissions?

Documentation of antismoking advice?

Number of patients admitted to the ward and then transferred to the ICU (mortality)?

Length of stay?

Readmission rate?

Time back to work or prepneumonia activity?

Costs?

Protocol adherence

It seems logical that once a local protocol is put together, physicians should abide by the recommendations. Recent data from Australia showed minimal compliance with national recommendations, however [28]. Documentation of the pneumonia severity index (PSI) was only 5%. Concordance with antibiotic recommendations was less than 20%. Educational efforts are a critical part of protocol implementation and should be underway to improve acceptance and compliance. These efforts must include a defined educational campaign and a mechanism for auditing and providing feedback to ED physicians and ED QI committees.

Decisions to be made in the emergency department

1. Does the patient have pneumonia? (Fig. 2)
2. CAP versus HCAP? (Fig. 3)
3. How severe is the pneumonia, and where should the patient be treated? (Fig. 4)
4. What studies should be obtained in the ED?
5. Determine empiric antimicrobial therapy (Figs. 5–7)
6. Do unusual circumstances exist?
7. What are the new areas of diagnosis and treatment in the ED?

Available data to assist with decisions

National guidelines

Local guidelines

History and physical examination

Radiologic studies

Laboratory studies

Microbiologic studies

Consultation for unusual circumstances

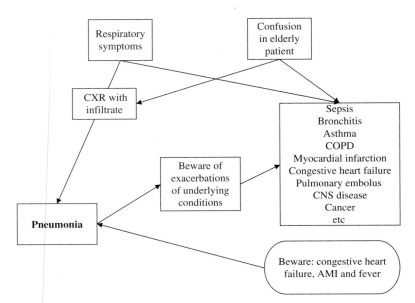

Fig. 2. Does patient have pneumonia, an alternative diagnosis, or perhaps both? CNS, central nervous system.

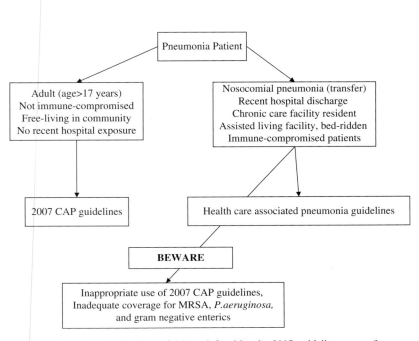

Fig. 3. Does patient have CAP as defined by the 2007 guidelines or not?

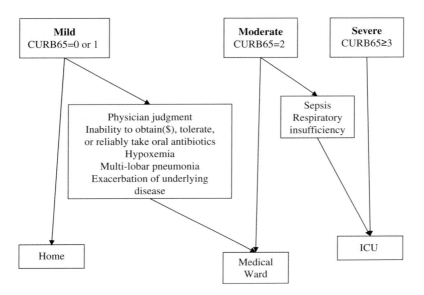

Fig. 4. Profile of disease severity.

Does the patient have pneumonia?

The patient who has pneumonia usually presents to ED with the recent onset of some respiratory symptoms that may include fever, acute cough (with or without sputum production), dyspnea, tachypnea, or chest pain.

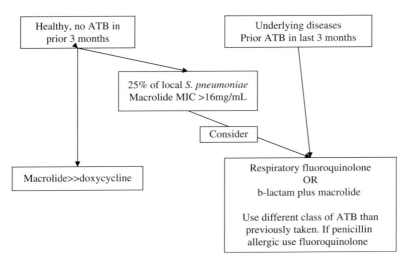

Fig. 5. Therapy for a patient who has CAP to be treated as an outpatient. ATB, antibiotics; MIC, minimum inhibitory concentration.

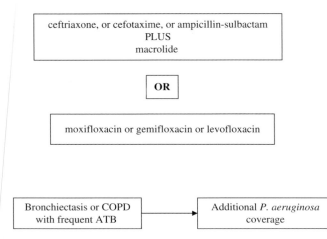

Fig. 6. Empiric therapy for patients who have CAP on the general ward. ATB, antibiotics.

Unfortunately, most patients do not have all the classic symptoms. In elderly patients, the presenting symptoms may not even point directly to the respiratory system (ie, decreased mentation, nonspecific aches and pains).

Symptoms may be associated with severe vital sign abnormalities. Immediate action may be required, including treatment of sepsis and respiratory failure.

As many as 30% of patients may have been pretreated with antimicrobial agents (personal physician, prior ED visit, or self-prescribed). Symptoms may not have resolved, or had a chance to resolve, or may have progressed. Infrequently, side effects from the antimicrobial agents bring the patient to the ED.

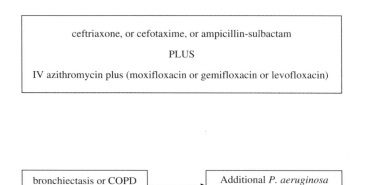

Fig. 7. Empiric therapy for patients in the ICU who have CAP. ATB, antibiotics.

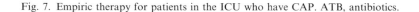

The presenting respiratory symptoms may be caused by a nonpneumonic illness. The ED physician should identify the patient with a realistic possibility of pneumonia and differentiate patients presenting with other illnesses and similar symptoms (see Fig. 2). Information obtained from the history and physical examination should be helpful in making alternative diagnoses more or less likely. The presence of underlying diseases and medication history may be useful in defining the type of pneumonia and profiling its severity. Metlay and colleagues [29] reported that the absence of any vital sign abnormality or any abnormalities on chest auscultation can substantially reduce the likelihood of CAP. Several studies, including an emergency medicine evidenced-based review [30], make the point that there is no one historical finding or physical examination finding or combination of findings that can accurately rule in or rule out the diagnosis of pneumonia. Nevertheless, it is still recommended by these authors that history and physical examination findings can help to contribute to the diagnosis of pneumonia; thus, the concept of performing a complete history and physical examination findings continue to be an integral part of evaluating these patients. Moreover, pertinent history and examination findings can help the emergency physician to determine if certain organisms are more likely causative agents and whether antimicrobial resistance is likely.

The indications for a CXR in suspected CAP have been widely debated. An early report by Heckerling and colleagues [31] determined that certain findings, such as fever, tachycardia, decreased breath sounds, and absence of asthma were predictors of finding CAP on CXR. Subsequent studies suggest that no one symptom, sign or examination finding is statistically powerful enough to rule in or rule out the diagnosis of pneumonia on CXR. The absence of any vital sign abnormality, coupled with a normal examination, may nearly excluded the diagnosis, with only a 5% miss rate, as reported recently by O'Brien and colleagues [32]. Despite the lack of predictors to rule in the diagnosis, several vital sign abnormalities (hypoxia, fever, tachycardia, or tachypnea) make the diagnosis of pneumonia more likely [33]. Most consensus recommendations state that a CXR should be obtained in patients older than the age of 40 years and in patients with abnormal vital signs or physical examination findings or the presence of significant comorbidities.

CXR demonstrating an acute infiltrate is part of the definition of CAP in the 2007 guidelines. Unfortunately, the CXR rarely suggests a specific etiology. Multilobar infiltrates and cavity infiltrates are associated with poor outcomes. The presence of a pleural effusion may suggest empyema. The presence of hyperinflated airways or flattened diaphragms may suggest COPD, with the need for arterial blood gases and more cautious assessment. In patients with fever and a CXR interpreted as congestive heart failure (CHF), coexisting pneumonia should be considered.

Another limitation of the CXR is that despite the fact that it is considered the "gold standard" by many, it also has several limitations and does not have 100% sensitivity or 100% specificity. In one study, one third of admitted patients were found to have a normal CXR on admission, and these patients had similar rates of positive blood and sputum cultures [34]. Although the CXR is still considered the standard of care for diagnosing CAP, high-resolution CT scanning may be more sensitive. In a frequently cited study [35], chest radiography missed 31% of cases of possible pneumonia (8 of 26 cases) that were subsequently diagnosed on high-resolution CT. Diagnosis by CT is being made even more commonly, given the increasing numbers of CT scans done to rule out common causes of chest pain, such as CT pulmonary embolus studies to rule out pulmonary embolus and CT aneurysm studies to rule out aortic dissection. The precise role of CT scanning to rule in or rule out CAP remains to be determined, however, and studies connecting the CT diagnosis with some microbiologic diagnoses are still lacking.

Is the pneumonia community-acquired pneumonia or health care–associated pneumonia?

Most patients who have pneumonia and are seen in the ED have CAP, and the approach to these patients can be as recommended in 2007 CAP guidelines (see Fig. 3). Previously, many ED studies of pneumonia lumped all pneumonia cases together. The ED physician must be alert to the occasional patient who has pneumonia who has HCAP or reasons cited here that exclude them from the 2007 CAP guidelines.

Children aged 17 years or younger are not covered by the recent CAP guidelines.

Patients exposed to an environment that has been altered by selective pressure of antimicrobial agents, such as those recently hospitalized (within 3 months), those residing in chronic care facilities, and those nonambulatory residents of nursing homes or assisted living facilities, should be considered to have HCAP. These patients have an expanded spectrum of etiologic agents that would be better addressed using the HCAP guidelines [3] with broader spectrum therapy. Appropriate consultation in this small group of patients is suggested. Ambulatory residents of assisted living facilities would be expected to have etiologies similar to those patients who have CAP.

Patients whose immune systems are compromised may have pneumonia caused by typical community organisms. A wide variety of unusual organisms may cause the pneumonia, however. The 2007 CAP guidelines exclude transplant recipients, lymphatic malignancies, neutropenic patients, patients receiving chemotherapy or high-dose steroids for at least a month, and HIV-infected patients with CD4 counts less than 350 cells/mm^3 [2]. Appropriate consultation should assist in prescribing initial therapy in these patients because they generally require broader spectrum coverage.

There are minimal data on the proportions of patients presenting to the ED with pneumonia who have CAP versus HCAP. It has been the authors' experience that most patients presenting to ED with pneumonia have CAP. A recent study [36] from Barnes Hospital in St. Louis of 639 patients admitted between 2001 and 2003 who had culture-positive pneumonia reported twice as many HCAP admissions as CAP admissions. *S aureus* (MRSA and methicillin-sensitive *Staphylococcus aureus* [MSSA]), *S pneumoniae*, *P aeruginosa*, and *H influenzae* were the most common pathogens identified overall. Patients who had HCAP frequently received inadequate empiric therapy (28.3%) and had a higher mortality rate (24.6%) than did patients who had CAP (inappropriate therapy of 13.0%, mortality rate of 9.1%). This series of patients is a different population from usually seen in EDs because it includes direct admissions from those caring for immune-compromised patients in a large medical center. The study also only addresses culture-positive patients. The data presented emphasize the importance in obtaining thorough historical information to distinguish accurately between patients who have CAP and HCAP, however.

Many of the patients admitted who have CAP are older and have associated chronic diseases. The stress of hypoxemia and or sepsis may worsen many of these conditions. Musher and colleagues[37] reported on 170 patients who had pneumococcal pneumonia, of whom 33 (19.4%) had concomitant severe acute cardiac conditions; CHF (new or worsening), arrhythmias, or AMI. Mortality was significantly higher in patients who had associated acute cardiac events. Lichtman and colleagues [38] reviewed 3904 cases of AMI and found 267 (6.8%) patients who also had an acute, severe, noncardiac condition in the initial 24 hours. Pneumonia was the most common coexisting illness. The adjusted mortality rate was fivefold greater for patients who had AMI and an additional acute severe illness. ED physicians must be vigilant for patients who have more than one acute disease.

How severe is the pneumonia, and where should the patient be treated?

Previous recommendations for deciding on the site and type of care were based, in part, on the PSI [26]. The PSI was made up of 20 variables and was somewhat cumbersome to use in many EDs. The 2007 guidelines favor the CURB65 (see Box 1) designed by the British Thoracic Society [27]. Only 5 variables are required: newly developed confusion (C), uremia (U), increased respiratory rate (R), decreased blood pressure (B) and age older than 65 years. Niederman [39] suggested that the two instruments should be complementary, because each has its limitations. Although the PSI has been used to determine which patients have a low mortality risk, it can occasionally underestimate CAP severity, especially in younger patients who do not have comorbid illnesses. In one study comparing both instruments in patients in the ED [40], both successfully predicted which patients had a low risk for mortality. The CURB65 had a better gradation of severe disease, however, with those patients having scores from 2 to 5 having a progressively greater mortality rate compared with the PSI, which has only two categories of severe illness (IV and V). Interestingly, both tools were designed to predict mortality and not to determine the optimal site of care. Renaud and colleagues [41] found that the routine use of the PSI increased the percentage of patients in PSI classes I and II who were treated as outpatients (42.8%) compared with an ED in which the PSI was not routinely used (23.9%). The increased outpatient treatment was not associated with any compromise in patient safety. The accompanying editorial by Marrie [42] emphasized the need for prospective trials of patients discharged from the ED and managed on an ambulatory basis.

The most common recommendations have been that patients with a PSI class of I or II or a CURB65 score of 0 or 1 generally be considered "low risk" and may be considered for outpatient treatment (see Fig. 4). Patients who have mild pneumonia have low mortality rates (0.7%–2.1%) and prefer to be treated at home. Physician judgment can and should override site of care suggestion from low PSI or CURB65 scores in certain circumstances (see Fig. 4) [43,44]. Does the patient appear sicker than a "mild pneumonia"? Perhaps an underlying disease, such as CHF, coronary artery disease, diabetes, or COPD, has been exacerbated. Perhaps the patient is hypoxemic and requires oxygen supplementation even though the respiratory rate is less than 30 breaths per minute. Perhaps the pneumonia is more severe but has not yet been associated with systemic dysfunction (ie, multilobar infiltrates, cavitary disease). The patient must be able to fill a potentially expensive prescription in a timely fashion and tolerate and reliably take the antimicrobial therapy. Is there adequate supervision available for the patient over the subsequent 24 to 48 hours, and can adequate medical follow-up be arranged?

ED physicians and hospital administrators can address several of these issues and incorporate potential solutions in local pneumonia protocols (ie, provide oral antimicrobial therapy or the initial doses until a prescription can be filled, set up an ED holding area for initial observation, make follow-up telephone calls, arrange for ED follow-up visit for patients without a primary care physician). The cost of treating a patient who has pneumonia at home is hundreds of dollars versus thousands of dollars for treating patients in the hospital. Innovative partnerships with nursing home physicians may prevent hospitalizations for some patients better treated at the nursing home or for patients who have indicated a preference not to be hospitalized [45].

Patients who have mild pneumonia (CURB65 = 0 or 1) with confounding problems, as listed previously, may require admission to the general medical ward.

Most patients (90%) admitted to the hospital have moderate disease (CURB65 = 2) and are admitted to the general medical ward. The mortality rate for this group is 9.2%. There is an increased mortality rate among patients initially admitted to medical ward and then later transferred to the ICU. The reason for more intensive care is usually progressive respiratory failure. It has been difficult to predict this heterogeneous population that develops clinical deterioration after admission [46]. The 2007 guidelines suggest cautious assessment of patients who have hypothermia, multilobar infiltrates, leukopenia, and thrombocytopenia. Recent data suggest that patients who have COPD and CAP have higher mortality rates and more frequently require mechanical ventilation [47,48].

Approximately 10% of admitted patients go directly to the ICU, with 80% of these patients requiring ventilatory support [46]. Patients in septic shock or with respiratory insufficiency are admitted directly to the ICU. Patients who have severe disease (CURB65 = 3, 4, or 5) usually are admitted to the ICU. Mortality is high in this population. Recent data from Spain [49] in patients who had CAP and were admitted to the ICU reported that a delay in the ED of longer than 1 hour in obtaining pulse oximetry resulted in a delay in initial antibiotic therapy. An ED delay in obtaining pulse oximetry of longer than 3 hours was associated independently with a twofold increase in mortality.

What studies should be obtained in the emergency department?

With regard to laboratory data, pulse oximetry should be part of the initial vital signs evaluation in all patients with a possible diagnosis of pneumonia.

For the patient who has mild disease who is to be treated at home, minimal or no additional laboratory data are needed.

In the sicker patient who is to be admitted, laboratory studies should include blood urea nitrogen (BUN; CURB65), complete blood cell count (CBC), differential, platelet count, and basic admission tests. In patients who have COPD, pulse oximetry is suboptimal. Arterial blood gases are necessary to define the carbon dioxide content. Urine antigen assays should be obtained for *Legionella* and pneumococci in sicker patients. These assays can be performed in 15 minutes, and results should be available to ED physicians in the same time frame as CBC results. In general the more severe the pneumonia, the more aggressive the diagnostic studies should be.

With regard to blood cultures, there has been debate about the cost-effectiveness of blood and sputum cultures in patients who have CAP [50]. Certainly, the low mortality rate in patients treated at home does not justify a search for an etiologic agent. The criticism of routinely obtaining blood cultures is that studies show that they rarely change therapy. A recent emergency medicine study reported that blood cultures altered therapy in only 3.6% of patients and that most of these were changes to narrow therapy, with only 1.0% of patients having their antibiotics broadened [51]. The accompanying editorial by Moran and Abrahamian [52] rationalized that blood cultures still make sense for patients in the ICU because they are more likely to be bacteremic and they are more at risk should empiric therapy be inappropriate. The editorial by Walls and Resnick [23] in the same issue criticized the JCAHO and CMS for adopting the original policy to require blood cultures for all admitted patients who have CAP, because the weight of evidence clearly does not support this. The 2007 guidelines recommend obtaining blood and respiratory cultures in all patients admitted to the ICU. They also suggest obtaining blood cultures in a subset of patients admitted to the ward who have comorbid conditions associated with potentially higher bacteremic rates. Blood cultures should be obtained before empiric antimicrobial therapy. If patients were pretreated with antibiotics, blood cultures still should be obtained in appropriate patients, because resistant organisms may be present. In patients who have bacteremia, antimicrobial susceptibility can guide continued therapy and the appropriate switch to oral agents.

The value of microbiologic examination of sputum has always been debated. There is no value in examining saliva. If the patient is producing purulent sputum, however, important data can be obtained. MRSA is becoming a common pathogen in skin infections among community residents. Unfortunately, it is likely that as MRSA colonizes more community residents, it is going to become a more common cause of CAP. MRSA pneumonia has already been seen in children who have influenza. A Gram stain of an appropriate sputum specimen can be diagnostic for pneumonia caused by *S aureus*.

A sputum Gram stain and culture can be helpful in the patient with COPD who also has CAP. These patients have frequently been exposed to multiple courses of antibiotics and might have resistant pathogens. Recent data suggest that patients who have COPD and CAP are sicker and have a higher mortality rate than patients who do not have COPD [47,48].

Determining empiric antimicrobial therapy

Prior exposure to antibiotics or to an antibiotic-pressured environment can assist in deciding whether empiric therapy need cover antibiotic resistant *S pneumoniae*. Did the patient take any antibiotics in past 3 months? What kind of antibiotics? Has there been a recent hospitalization, prolonged exposure to medical outpatient clinics, or exposure to day care or preschool (direct or indirectly)? Many patients claim allergies to various antimicrobial agents. It is important to define the patient's definition of allergic symptoms (eg, anaphylaxis, hives, rash, upset stomach, diarrhea). In patients who state that they are allergic to penicillin, it is important to ask if they have been treated with cephalosporin antibiotics without allergic symptoms.

Recognition of epidemiologic clues may assist the ED physician in ordering empiric therapy, appropriate isolation procedures, and consultations. The epidemiologic information may be specific to the individual patient, such as exposure to the health care system, recent hospitalization, or residence in a chronic or extended care facility. The patient may have had a known exposure to a sick individual who had tuberculosis, chicken pox, or measles. A history of alcohol abuse, drug abuse, or neurologic disorders may suggest an increased likelihood of aspiration pneumonia.

Travel history should be documented in all patients (variance from local pneumonia protocol). The patient may have visited other communities with higher rates of resistant pneumococci. The patient may have been to a foreign country with an outbreak of viral hemorrhagic fever, severe acute respiratory syndrome (SARS), or avian influenza. A recent cruise, whirlpool spa exposure, or travel away from home in the past 2 weeks may be associated with Legionnaire's disease.

If animal or bird exposure has occurred, consider the following associations:

Rabbit hunting: tularemia
Psittacine birds: psittacosis
Cattle, pregnant cats: Q fever
Cave exploring, bat exposure: histoplasmosis

Similarly, the type of employment should be documented (ie, day care, preschool, chronic care, extended care facility, laboratory worker, pet store employee). Importantly, is the patient in residence at a chronic care or an assisted living facility (ambulatory)?

Physical examination may suggest particular diagnoses or important coexisting illnesses, including mental status changes, such as a recent change in the ability to recognize persons, place, and time, and patients who have neurologic disorders and those with drug or alcohol abuse may have an increased incidence of aspiration pneumonia. Intravenous drug abuse may be associated with undiagnosed HIV infection.

Presence of nuchal rigidity: meningitis may be also present.
Red, swollen, tender joint: septic arthritis may be present.
Rash: varicella, rubeola, hemorrhagic fever, or stigmata of intravenous drug or alcohol abuse may be present.

The lung examination and auscultatory findings may indicate consolidation; dullness to percussion; or diminished breath sounds, which may also suggest pleural effusion (may suggest obtaining a lateral decubitus film). Signs of COPD are useful in categorization of the patient and suggest the need for measurement of arterial blood gases.

Cardiac examination may reveal pericarditis or signs of CHF. Abdominal examination may assist in the diagnosis of findings consistent with cirrhosis, such as ascites, small liver, or jaundice. Extremity examination may reveal swelling, calf tenderness, needle tracts, or diminished pulses.

Fig. 5 summarizes outpatient empiric treatment recommendations that are designed to treat atypical pathogens, S pneumoniae, and H influenzae. For uncomplicated CAP, a newer macrolide or less optimally doxycycline is usually recommended. If there are problems with local macrolide resistance for S pneumoniae or recent use of antibiotics, a respiratory fluoroquinolone or combination oral therapy is recommended. Although not well studied, it seems logical that patients who have mild CAP and are to be treated at home should receive their first dose of oral antibiotics in the ED unless the prescription can be filled immediately.

With regard to macrolides, azithromycin and clarithromycin are better tolerated than erythromycin. Azithromycin has better activity against *H influenzae*. Doxycycline as a macrolide alternative is a less expensive, although there are few data in comparison trials.

With regard to respiratory fluoroquinolones, moxifloxacin, gemifloxacin, and levofloxacin have good activity against atypical pathogens, *S pneumoniae*, and *H influenzae*.

With regard to oral β-lactams to be used with macrolides for outpatient therapy, high-dose amoxicillin, 1 g, administered three times daily or amoxicillin-sulbactam, 2 g, administered twice daily is preferred in the 2007 guidelines because of their activity against *S pneumoniae*. Less preferred alternatives include cefpodoxime, cefuroxime, or parenteral ceftriaxone.

In patients admitted to the general medical ward with moderate pneumonia, parenteral antimicrobial therapy is generally recommended (see Fig. 6). Empiric therapy is designed to cover *S pneumoniae*, *H influenzae*, and the atypical pathogens, including *Legionella* spp. The two major choices would be combination therapy with a β-lactam and a macrolide or monotherapy with a fluoroquinolone. Both of these regimens are suboptimal for pneumonia caused by MRSA, some gram-negative enterics, and *P aeruginosa*. Care must be taken to search for clues for unusual circumstances that would make these organisms more likely possible etiologic agents. For patients who have bronchiectasis or COPD with frequent antibiotic courses, obtain consultation for additional *P aeruginosa* coverage.

The β-lactams (parenteral) recommended for inpatients include ceftriaxone, cefotaxime, and ampicillin-sulbactam because of their activity against *S pneumoniae*.

Patients admitted to the ICU who have severe pneumonia should receive the broadest empiric therapy (see Fig. 7) because they are in imminent danger of respiratory failure and death. All patients should receive combination therapy with a β-lactam plus intravenous azithromycin or intravenous fluoroquinolone. As with patients admitted to the general medical ward, if the patient has bronchiectasis or COPD associated with frequent antibiotic therapy, additional *P aeruginosa* therapy should be added.

Do unusual circumstances exist?

Historical information associated with travel, an unusual living environment, unusual exposures, or work or leisure activities should prompt additional questions and perhaps consultation. Local pneumonia protocols need to be updated if organisms, such as MRSA, become a community problem.

Penicillin allergy may be claimed by 20% to 30% of patients who have pneumonia. Carefully define what the patient means by penicillin allergy. Has the patient taken cephalosporins without difficulty? If not a type 1 hypersensitivity, cephalosporins may be used for inpatients. For outpatients, if macrolides are not an option, use a respiratory fluoroquinolone. Similarly, for patients admitted to a medical ward in which macrolides are not an option, use fluoroquinolones rather than combination therapy. In patients admitted to the ICU, the 2007 guidelines recommend using a respiratory fluoroquinolone and aztreonam. Local pneumonia guidelines need to address this issue, because many pharmacies may not stock aztreonam. Appropriate consultation may be helpful in these patients.

If an outbreak of influenza is occurring in the community, patients suspected of having influenza should be placed on respiratory isolation in the ED. If the results of rapid antigen testing for influenza are positive, antiviral therapy should be prescribed. The most common cause of bacterial pneumonia in patients who have influenza is *S pneumoniae*. Other organisms to consider include *S aureus* (MSSA or MRSA), *H influenzae*, and *Neisseria meningitidis* (with concomitant meningitis). A Gram stain and culture of purulent sputum may assist with the diagnosis of staphylococcal pneumonia. Blood cultures should be obtained in these patients.

What are the new areas of diagnosis and treatment in the emergency department?

Rapid diagnosis of pathogens to aid in the choice of initial antibiotics
Unfortunately, most of the antimicrobial therapy in the ED is empiric, because we have few rapid diagnostic assays to identify etiologic agents. Rapid assays for detection of *S pneumoniae* antigens in urine, *L pneumophila* serogroup 1 antigens in urine, and throat swabs for influenza A and B antigens are available. Pneumococcal urinary antigen detection is highly specific in the adult population with pneumococcal pneumonia [53,54] Rarely, recent (within days) administration of a pneumococcal vaccine may be associated with a false-positive result on a pneumococcal urinary antigen assay [55]. A negative pneumococcal urinary antigen result does not exclude bacteremic pneumococcal pneumonia.

A positive *Legionella* urinary antigen assay result is highly specific for pneumonia caused by *L pneumophila* serogroup 1 [56]. A negative urinary antigen result for *Legionella* can be seen in mild *L pneumophila* serogroup 1 disease or in pneumonia caused by other serogroups or species of *Legionella* [57]. In the United States, most cases of Legionnaire's disease are caused by *L pneumophila* serogroup 1 [58].

Influenza antigen detection is useful early in an influenza community outbreak. There are 15 rapid antigen detection kits approved by US Food and Drug Administration (FDA) [59]. The sensitivity is approximately 75%. Influenza antigen detection can also be useful in immune-compromised patients who have pneumonia, because antigen detection is associated with influenza replication. Antiviral therapy should be administered, and a search for a secondary bacterial pneumonia should be initiated.

Polymerase chain reaction (PCR) assays for a wide array of respiratory pathogens have been reported in the literature; however, to date, they have not been clinically available to ED physicians. Costs and logistical problems should be solved in the future, however.

Rapid antigen detection of MRSA is being developed and would be a useful addition [60,61]. Current empiric regimens do not cover for MRSA. Currently, the sputum Gram stain is the most rapid diagnostic test for staphylococcal pneumonia.

Using serum markers to predict poor outcomes and adjunctive therapy

Inflammatory markers are elevated in patients who have CAP [39]. C-reactive protein and procalcitonin are more elevated initially in those with poorer outcomes [62]. These markers may useful in evaluating immune-modulating therapy with such agents as activated protein C [63] or steroids [64–66]. Research continues into the possible role of adjunctive immune-modulating therapy in patients who have severe CAP. A review by Gorman and colleagues [67] states that with current data, corticosteroids cannot be recommended for adjunctive treatment of severe CAP.

Summary

Pneumonia is a common disease seen in the ED. More structured approaches to patients who have pneumonia have evolved. Recent 2007 CAP guidelines from the ATS, IDSA, and CDC are summarized. The importance and outline for a local CAP protocol are discussed. An approach to the patient who has pneumonia is presented, including the differential diagnosis, CAP or non-CAP disease, severity of pneumonia, site of care, initial therapy, and unusual circumstances.

References

[1] Marrie TJ. The halo effect of adherence to guidelines extends to patients with severe community-acquired pneumonia requiring admission to an intensive care unit. Clin Infect Dis 2005;41:1717–9.
[2] Mandell LA, Wunderink RG, Anzueto A, et al. Infectious Diseases Society of America/ American Thoracic Society consensus guidelines on the management of community-acquired pneumonia in adults. Clin Infect Dis 2007;44:S27–72.
[3] Guidelines for the management of adults with hospital-acquired, ventilator-associated, and healthcare-associated pneumonia. Am J Respir Crit Care Med 2005;171:388–416.
[4] Vanderkooi OG, Low DE, Green K, et al. Predicting antimicrobial resistance in invasive pneumococcal infections. Clin Infect Dis 2005;40:1288–97.
[5] Doern GV, Richter SS, Miller A, et al. Antimicrobial resistance among *Streptococcus pneumoniae* in the United States: have we begun to turn the corner on resistance to certain antimicrobial classes? Clin Infect Dis 2005;41:139–48.
[6] Halpern MT, Schmier JK, Snyder LM, et al. Meta-analysis of bacterial resistance to macrolides. J Antimicrob Chemother 2005;55:748–57.
[7] Neuman MI, Kelley M, Harper MB, et al. Factors associated with antimicrobial resistance and mortality in pneumococcal bacteremia. J Emerg Med 2007;32:349–57.
[8] Fuller JD. A review of Streptococcus pneumoniae infection treatment failures associated with fluoroquinolone resistance. Clin Infect Dis 2005;41:118–21.

[9] Shefet D, Robenshtok E, Paul M, et al. Empirical atypical coverage for inpatients with community-acquired pneumonia: systemic review of randomized controlled trials. Arch Intern Med 2005;165:1992–2000.

[10] Mills GD, Oehley MR, Arrol B. Effectiveness of beta lactam antibiotics compared with antibiotics active against atypical pathogens in non-severe community acquired pneumonia: meta-analysis. BMJ 2005;330:456.

[11] Arnold FW, Summersgill JT, Lajoie AS, et al. A worldwide perspective of atypical pathogens in community acquired pneumonia. Am J Respir Crit Care Med 2007;175:1086–93.

[12] Kanwar M, Brar N, Khatib R, et al. Misdiagnosis of community-acquired pneumonia and inappropriate utilization of antibiotics: side effects of the 4-h antibiotic administration rule. Chest 2007;131:1865–9.

[13] Pines JM, Hollander JE, Lee H, et al. Emergency department operational changes in response to pay-for-performance and antibiotic timing in pneumonia. Acad Emerg Med 2007;14:545–8.

[14] Fee C, Weber EJ, Maak CA, et al. Effect of emergency department crowding on time to antibiotics in patients admitted with community-acquired pneumonia. Ann Emerg Med 2007;50:501–9.

[15] Pines JM, Localio AR, Hollander JE, et al. The impact of emergency department crowding measures on time to antibiotics for patients with community-acquired pneumonia. Ann Emerg Med 2007;50:510–6.

[16] Waterer GW, Kessler LA, Wunderink RG. Delayed administration of antibiotics and atypical presentation in community-acquired pneumonia. Chest 2006;130:11–5.

[17] Pines JM, Morton MJ, Datner EM, et al. Systemic delays in antibiotic administration in the emergency department for adult patients admitted with pneumonia. Acad Emerg Med 2006; 13:939–45.

[18] Metersky ML, Sweeney TA, Getzow MB, et al. Antibiotic timing and diagnostic uncertainty in Medicare patients with pneumonia: is it reasonable to expect all patients to receive antibiotics within 4 hours? Chest 2006;130:16–21.

[19] Fee C, Weber EJ. Identification of 90% of patients ultimately diagnosed with CAP within four hours of emergency department arrival may not be feasible. Ann Emerg Med 2007; 49:553–9.

[20] Meehan TP, Fine MJ, Krumholz HM, et al. Quality of care, process, and outcomes in elderly patients with pneumonia. JAMA 1997;278:2080–4.

[21] Houck PM, Bratzler DW, Nsa W, et al. Timing of antibiotic administration and outcomes for Medicare patients hospitalized with community-acquired pneumonia. Arch Intern Med 2004;164:637–44.

[22] Pines JM. Profiles in patient safety: antibiotic timing in pneumonia and pay-for performance. Acad Emerg Med 2006;13:787–90.

[23] Walls RM, Resnick J. The Joint Commission on Accreditation of Healthcare Organization and Center for Medicare and Medicaid Services CAP initiative: what went wrong? Ann Emerg Med 2005;46:409–11.

[24] Rothman RE, Quianzon CC, Kelen GD. Narrowing in on JCAHO recommendations for community-acquired pneumonia. Acad Emerg Med 2006;13:983–5.

[25] Pham JC, Kelen GD, Pronovost PJ. National study on the quality of emergency department care in the treatment of acute myocardial infarction and pneumonia. Acad Emerg Med 2007; 14:856–63.

[26] Fine MJ, Auble TE, Yealy DM, et al. A prediction rule to identify low-risk patients with community-acquired pneumonia. N Engl J Med 1997;336:243–50.

[27] Lim WS, van der Eerden MM, Laing R, et al. Defining community acquired pneumonia severity on presentation to hospital: an international derivation and validation study. Thorax 2003;58:377–82.

[28] Maxwell DJ, McIntosh KA, Pulver LK, et al. Empiric management of community-acquired pneumonia in Australian emergency departments. Med J Aust 2005;183:520–4.

[29] Metlay JP, Kapoor WN, Fine MJ. Does this patient have CAP? Diagnosing pneumonia by history of a physical examination. JAMA 1997;278:1440–5.

[30] Rosh AJ, Newman DH. Diagnosing pneumonia by medical history and physical examination. Ann Emerg Med 2005;46:465–7.

[31] Heckerling PS, Tape TG, Wigton RS, et al. Clinical prediction rule for pulmonary infiltrates. Ann Intern Med 1990;113:664–70.

[32] O'Brien WT Sr., Rohweder DA, Lattin GE Jr, et al. Clinical indicators of radiographic findings in patients with suspected community acquired pneumonia: who needs a chest x-ray? J Am Coll Radiol 2006;3:703–6.

[33] Nolt BR, Gonzales R, Maselli J, et al. Vital-sign abnormalities as predictors of pneumonia in adults with acute cough illness. Am J Emerg Med 2007;25:631–6.

[34] Basi SK, Marrie TJ, Huang JQ, et al. Patients admitted to the hospital with suspected pneumonia and normal chest radiographs: epidemiology, microbiology and outcomes. Am J Med 2004;117:305–11.

[35] Syrjälä H, Broas M, Suramo I, et al. High-resolution computerized tomography for the diagnosis of community acquired pneumonia. Clin Infect Dis 1998;27:358–63.

[36] Micek ST, Kollef KE, Reichley RM, et al. Health care-associated pneumonia and community-acquired pneumonia: a single-center experience. Antimicrob Agents Chemother 2007; 51:3568–73.

[37] Musher DM, Rueda AM, Kaka AS, et al. The association between pneumococcal pneumonia and acute cardiac events. Clin Infect Dis 2007;45:158–65.

[38] Lichtman JH, Spertus JA, Reid KJ, et al. Acute noncardiac conditions and in-hospital mortality in patients with acute myocardial infarction. Circulation 2007;116:1925–30.

[39] Niederman MS. Recent advances in community acquired pneumonia: inpatient and outpatient. Chest 2007;131:1205–15.

[40] Aujesky D, Auble TE, Yealy DM, et al. Prospective comparison of three validated prediction rules for prognosis in community acquired pneumonia. Am J Med 2005;118:384–92.

[41] Renaud B, Coma E, Labarere J, et al. Routine use of the PSI for guiding the site-of-treatment decision of patients with pneumonia in the emergency department: a multicenter, prospective observational controlled cohort study. Clin Infect Dis 2007;44:41–9.

[42] Marrie TJ. The PSI score: time to move to a prospective study of patients with community acquired pneumonia who are discharged from emergency departments to be managed on an ambulatory basis. Clin Infect Dis 2007;44:50–2.

[43] Marrie TJ, Huang JQ. Low-risk patients admitted with community-acquired pneumonia. Am J Med 2005;118:1357–63.

[44] Labarere J, Stone RA, Obrosky DS, et al. Comparison of outcomes for low-risk outpatients and inpatients with pneumonia: a propensity-adjusted analysis. Chest 2007;131:480–8.

[45] Loeb M, Carusone SC, Goeree R, et al. Effect of a clinical pathway to reduce hospitalizations in nursing home residents with pneumonia. JAMA 2006;295:2503–10.

[46] Marrie TJ, Shariatzadeh MR. Community-acquired pneumonia requiring admission to an intensive care unit: a descriptive study. Medicine 2007;86:103–11.

[47] Restrepo MI, Mortensen EM, Pugh JA, et al. COPD is associated with increased mortality in patients with community-acquired pneumonia. Eur Respir J 2006;28:346–51.

[48] Rello J, Rodriguez A, Torres A, et al. Implications of COPD in patients admitted to the intensive care unit by community-acquired pneumonia. Eur Respir J 2006;27:1210–6.

[49] Blot SI, Rodriguez A, Solé-Violán J, et al. Effects of delayed oxygenation assessment on time to antibiotic delivery and mortality in patients with severe community-acquired pneumonia. Crit Care Med 2007;35:2509–14.

[50] File TM Jr, Gross PA. Performance measurement in community-acquired pneumonia: consequences intended and unintended. Clin Infect Dis 2007;44:942–4.

[51] Kennedy M, Bates DW, Wright SB, et al. Do emergency department blood cultures change practice in patients with pneumonia? Ann Emerg Med 2005;46:393–400.

[52] Moran GJ, Abrahamian FM. Blood cultures for community-acquired pneumonia: can we hit the target without a shotgun? Ann Emerg Med 2005;46:407–8.
[53] Boulware DR, Daley CL, Merrifield C, et al. Rapid diagnosis of pneumococcal pneumonia among HIV-infected adults with urine antigen detection. J Infect 2007;55:300–9.
[54] Briones ML, Blanquer J, Ferrando D, et al. Assessment of analysis of urinary pneumococcal antigen by immunochromatography for etiologic diagnosis of community-acquired pneumonia in adults. Clin Vaccine Immunol 2006;13:1092–7.
[55] Priner M, Cornillon C, Forestier D, et al. Might *Streptococcus pneumoniae* urinary antigen test be positive because of pneumococcal vaccine? J Am Geriatr Soc 2008;56:170–1.
[56] Plouffe JF, File TM Jr, Breiman RF, et al. Reevaluation of the definition of Legionnaires' disease: use of the urinary antigen assay. Community Based Pneumonia Incidence Study Group. Clin Infect Dis 1995;20:1286–91.
[57] Blázquez RM, Espinosa FJ, Martínez-Toldos CM, et al. Sensitivity of urinary antigen test in relation to clinical severity in a large outbreak of Legionella pneumonia in Spain. Eur J Clin Microbiol Infect Dis 2005;24:488–91.
[58] Yu VL, Plouffe JF, Pastoris MC, et al. Distribution of Legionella species and serogroups isolated by culture in patients with sporadic community-acquired legionellosis: an international collaborative survey. J Infect Dis 2002;186:127–8.
[59] Centers for Disease Control and Prevention (CDC). Influenza-testing and antiviral-agent prescribing practices—Connecticut, Minnesota, New Mexico, and New York, 2006–07 influenza season. MMWR Morb Mortal Wkly Rep 2008;57:61–5.
[60] Francois P, Scherl A, Hochstrasser D, et al. Proteomic approach to investigate MRSA. Methods Mol Biol 2007;391:179–99.
[61] Hardy KJ, Szczepura A, Davies R, et al. A study of the efficacy and cost-effectiveness of MRSA screening and monitoring on surgical wards using a new, rapid molecular test (EMMS). BMC Health Serv Res 2007;7:160.
[62] Menéndez R, Cavalcanti M, Reyes S, et al. Markers of treatment failure in hospitalized community-acquired pneumonia. Thorax 2008 Feb 1 [Epub ahead of print].
[63] Laterre PF, Garber G, Levy H, et al. Severe community-acquired pneumonia as a cause of severe sepsis: data from the PROWESS study. Crit Care Med 2005;33:952–61.
[64] Confalonieri M, Urbino R, Potena A, et al. Hydrocortisone infusion for severe community-acquired pneumonia: a preliminary randomized study. Am J Respir Crit Care Med 2005;171:242–8.
[65] Mikami K, Suzuki M, Kitagawa H, et al. Efficacy of corticosteroids in the treatment of community-acquired pneumonia requiring hospitalization. Lung 2007;185:249–55.
[66] Garcia-Vidal C, Calbo E, Pascual V, et al. Effects of systemic steroids in patients with severe community-acquired pneumonia. Eur Respir J 2007;30:951–6.
[67] Gorman SK, Slavik RS, Marin J. Corticosteroid treatment of severe community-acquired pneumonia. Ann Pharmacother 2007;41:1233–7.

ELSEVIER
SAUNDERS

Emerg Med Clin N Am
26 (2008) 413–430

EMERGENCY
MEDICINE
CLINICS OF
NORTH AMERICA

Urinary Tract Infections: Diagnosis and Management in the Emergency Department

Donald L. Norris II, MD[a,*],
Jeremy D. Young, MD, MPH[b]

[a]Department of Emergency Medicine, The Ohio State University Medical Center,
146 Means Hall, 1654 Upham Drive, Columbus, OH 43210, USA
[b]Division of Infectious Diseases, Department of Internal Medicine, The Ohio State University
Medical Center, N-1101 Doan Hall, 410 West 10th Avenue, Columbus, OH 43210, USA

Urinary tract infections (UTIs) are among the most common infectious diseases encountered by emergency physicians in the United States. Therefore, it is important to review and update the evidence-based guidelines for evaluation and treatment of cystitis and pyelonephritis in the emergency department. This is particularly important in light of increasing antibiotic resistance among the typical UTI pathogens and the increase in complicated hosts in the community, such as those with anatomic and immunologic abnormalities from solid organ transplantation.

It is estimated that between 7 and 8 million outpatient visits and more than 1 million hospitalizations occur each year because of UTIs [1]. Women are five times more likely than men to be hospitalized with pyelonephritis, but they have a lower mortality rate (7.3 versus 16.5 deaths per 1000 cases) [2], likely because of the complicated nature of UTIs in men. The most common bacterium associated with UTIs remains *Escherichia coli*, but other aerobic gram-negative bacteria and gram-positive bacteria, such as *Staphylococcus saprophyticus* and enterococci, are frequently isolated [2]. Enterococcal cystitis and pyelonephritis are particularly common in older men with urinary tract obstruction, such as from prostatic hypertrophy or cancer.

The diagnostic workup of UTIs has changed little in the past few decades; however, the management has become much more complex. With the emergence of *E coli* resistant to ampicillin, trimethoprim-sulfamethoxazole (TMP-SMX), and the fluoroquinolones, the choice of empiric antibiotic

---

* Corresponding author.
E-mail address: donald.norris@osumc.edu (D.L. Norris).

doi:10.1016/j.emc.2008.02.003

therapy has become more challenging. The goals of this article are to summarize the pathophysiology, epidemiology, diagnosis, and treatment of uncomplicated and complicated UTIs in the emergency department; discuss the practical implications of emerging antibiotic resistance; and summarize the data supporting the use of fluoroquinolones as the current antibiotic class of choice for empiric treatment of uncomplicated UTIs. The authors also address the treatment of asymptomatic bacteriuria and antibiotic use in the pregnant patient.

Definitions

To discuss infection of the urinary tract, it is necessary to begin by defining the various diagnostic categories of UTI *Urinary tract infection* is a general term used to describe an inflammatory response of any of the cells lining the urinary tract to micro-organisms [3]. This may involve the upper tract (ureters and kidneys), lower tract (bladder), or both.

Cystitis is an inflammatory response of the bladder to micro-organisms without involvement of the upper tract. Symptoms commonly include dysuria, frequency, urgency, hematuria, and suprapubic pain [3].

Pyelonephritis refers to an infection of the upper structures of the urinary tract, specifically the ureters, renal pelvis, and renal parenchyma. Pyelonephritis is often separated into acute versus chronic infection, which has significant implications regarding treatment. The term *chronic pyelonephritis* typically refers to recurrent upper tract infections, which are often the result of an underlying anatomic abnormality, such as neurogenic bladder with vesicoureteral reflux. Common complaints of patients who have pyelonephritis include fever, chills, and flank or low back pain [3]. The Infectious Diseases Society of America (IDSA) guidelines suggest that a urine culture growing at least 10,000 colony-forming units (CFUs) per cubic millimeter of bacteria should be used as a criterion to support this diagnosis [2]. As addressed elsewhere in this article, however, it is important to note that some patients who have pyelonephritis do have lower colony counts.

Uncomplicated UTI is one in which the structure and function of the genitourinary tract are normal. Essentially, this occurs in young, healthy, nonpregnant women with normal urinary tract anatomy [3].

Complicated UTI is associated with an underlying structural or functional problem with the genitourinary tract, obstruction, immune dysfunction, recent urinary tract instrumentation, health care–associated infection, male gender, or pregnancy. Some examples of patients who would fall into this category would be those who have renal stones, neurogenic bladder, an indwelling urinary catheter, diabetes, a fistula to the urinary tract, or polycystic kidney disease; recently hospitalized patients; patients with renal or other solid organ transplantation; patients who are immunocompromised for other reasons; and older patients. For all practical purposes, any patient other than a young, healthy, nonpregnant woman from the community is considered complicated. The distinction between complicated and uncomplicated UTIs is vital because it has implications regarding the clinical evaluation, choice of empiric antibiotic therapy, consideration of surgical interventions (eg, to relieve obstruction), and length of antibiotic therapy.

Pathophysiology

The ascending route is the most common way in which UTIs are initiated. Bacteria enter the urinary tract through the urethra and ascend to the bladder, and possibly the collecting system. This occurs more frequently in women because of a shorter distance from the urethra to the bladder and the close proximity to the vagina and perirectal area, both of which contain a high concentration of potentially pathogenic bacteria. UTIs are less common in men because of the increased distance of the urethral meatus from the bladder. Men do occasionally develop infections of the urinary tract, but they are more commonly seen in those with prostatic hypertrophy, renal stones, bladder catheterization, recent cystoscopy, and immunocompromise. Because of these associations, all UTIs in men should be considered complicated. The main host defense against bacterial infection is the flow of sterile urine through the urethra. This decreases the bacterial load, thus decreasing the likelihood of a bacterial infection occurring [4].

Epidemiology and microbiology

The common risk factors for the development of cystitis and pyelonephritis have been well studied. In women, recent sexual intercourse, use of a spermicide or diaphragm, and history of previous UTI all place the patient at increased risk [1]. The classic teachings involving increased water intake, direction of wiping, cranberry juice, and voiding promptly after intercourse have not been supported in the data [5]. Risk factors for the development of UTI in healthy men include insertive anal intercourse, lack of circumcision, and a sexual partner with the same uropathogen. Such conditions as recent instrumentation of the genital tract, presence of a renal stone, and prostatic hypertrophy also increase the risk for UTI in men [4].

The uropathogens responsible for UTI have changed little through the decades. *E coli* is still responsible for 75% to 95% of uncomplicated cases. *S saprophyticus* is isolated in 5% to 15% of UTIs, and enterococci, *Klebsiella*, and *Proteus mirabilis* make up the remaining 5% to 10% [6]. *Enterococcus* tends to be a urinary tract pathogen in older men with abnormalities of the prostate gland [7]. In general, the uropathogens leading to uncomplicated cystitis are much the same as those causing acute uncomplicated pyelonephritis. These pathogens are relatively adept at ascending, colonizing, and causing infection in the urinary tract.

The virulence of the pathogen is less important than the host in considering the infection "complicated." Structural abnormalities, including prostatic hypertrophy or neurogenic bladder; an immunocompromised state, such as HIV; or metabolic changes, such as those that occur in the diabetic host, may allow bacteria that would not normally cause infection to cause a UTI in these patients [8]. Although susceptible *E coli* remains the dominant pathogen in complicated UTIs, these patients are at risk for infection with antibiotic-resistant organisms, including fluoroquinolone-resistant *E coli*; *Pseudomonas aeruginosa*; vancomycin-resistant *Enterococcus* (VRE); and extended-spectrum β-lactamase (ESBL)–producing *E coli*, *Klebsiella*, or *Proteus*. As addressed elsewhere in this article, this should be considered when choosing empiric therapy for patients who have complicated UTI.

Clinical presentation

Cystitis

Cystitis is most commonly seen in women of reproductive age. Patients who have cystitis often present with localized signs and symptoms, such as dysuria, frequency, urgency, hematuria, and suprapubic pain. These patients are typically not systemically ill in that they tend to lack fevers, chills, nausea, or vomiting. It is important to consider the diagnosis of vaginitis (trichomoniasis or candidiasis) or urethritis (*Neisseria gonorrhoeae* or *Chlamydophila trachomatis*) when evaluating female patients who have urinary tract complaints. Historical findings that are consistent with vaginitis or urethritis include vaginal discharge or bleeding, absence of frequency or urgency, dyspareunia, and lack of bacteria on urinalysis. If symptoms are consistent with vaginitis or urethritis, a pelvic examination with a DNA probe for gonococcus and chlamydia, potassium hydroxide (KOH) preparation with a whiff test, and wet preparation are indicated [9].

As stated previously, men do present with cystitis, but it is usually seen after the age of 50 years. Often, cystitis in men is related to abnormalities of the prostate (80%), specifically prostatic hypertrophy, or instrumentation of the urinary tract (Foley catheterization or cystoscopy). It is important to consider prostatitis in the differential diagnosis, which can be present concurrently with cystitis. A digital rectal examination and urine culture is indicated in all men who present with signs or symptoms of cystitis [9]. Consideration should be given to radiographic imaging to evaluate the urinary tract in male patients who present with pyelonephritis. A noncontrast CT scan of the abdomen and pelvis is typically the study of choice.

Pyelonephritis

The distinction between cystitis and pyelonephritis is important because antibiotic choice and length of treatment are different. Patients who have pyelonephritis may be relatively well appearing or may be quite ill, presenting with sepsis. They most commonly complain of flank pain, abdominal pain, fevers, and chills. Nausea and vomiting also occur frequently. Often, symptoms of cystitis are present as well, but it is possible to have pyelonephritis without having the concurrent symptoms of cystitis. It is important to note that in elderly patients, signs or symptoms not referable to the urinary tract often predominate, including acute delirium. In the elderly, up to 20% of those with pyelonephritis present with predominantly respiratory or gastrointestinal symptoms. It is also essential for the clinician to consider that fever is absent in up to 33% of elderly patients who have pyelonephritis [2].

Diagnostic evaluation

Before discussing the various diagnostic modalities available to the emergency physician to assist with the diagnosis of UTIs, let us first discuss the practice of treating based on patient history alone. In a study done by Bent and colleagues [10] in 2002, the likelihood ratios of various signs and symptoms of UTI were evaluated. Using these data, the combination of dysuria and frequency without vaginal discharge or irritation had a likelihood ratio of 24.6. Patients who had recurrent UTI and made a self-diagnosis had a likelihood ratio of 4.0. This study seems to support the practice of treating uncomplicated cystitis in female patients based on history alone. Further diagnostic evaluation, including urinalysis and urine culture, should be performed in all patients who present with pyelonephritis or any complicated UTI, including complicated cystitis.

Urine dipstick

This is often the first diagnostic test performed on a patient with urinary complaints. On a clean-catch urine specimen, leukocyte esterase (LE) is an enzyme released from white blood cells (WBCs). Nitrites, which are converted from urinary nitrates in the presence of certain bacteria or blood, may suggest the presence of a UTI. Taken alone, nitrite sensitivity on dipstick urinalysis (UA) is 81%, whereas LE sensitivity is 77%. If both are present, the sensitivity increases to 94%. It is important to note that nitrites are only present when infections are caused by the *Enterobacteriaceae* (eg, *E coli*), which convert urinary nitrate to nitrite. The absence of nitrites on a urine dipstick certainly does not exclude the presence of other common pathogens, including *S saprophyticus* and the enterococci. Nitrites are more specific for the diagnosis of UTI than LE (87% versus 54%) [11]. This makes scientific sense considering the noninfectious conditions that can lead to pyuria, such as interstitial nephritis and pyelonephritis. In 2001, Lammers and colleagues [12] found that if the urine dipstick definition of UTI was a positive LE and nitrite, the overtreatment rate for UTI was 47% and the undertreatment rate was 13%. This illustrates the inability of dipstick UA to predict UTI accurately.

It is important to note that there are situations in which the urine nitrite may be falsely negative. Any of the following can cause nitrite to be falsely negative:

- Inadequate dietary nitrates can reduce substrates.
- Vitamin C can prevent the proper chemical reaction to cause dipstick positivity.
- An old dipstick exposed to air may not properly undergo color change.
- Unusually high urine urobilinogen or low urine pH (<6.0)
- Urinary frequency may not allow enough time for conversion from nitrate to nitrite.

Urine microscopy

Sending the urine to the laboratory for formal microscopic analysis is another tool available to the emergency physician to assist with the diagnosis of UTI. Classically, the presence of more than five leukocytes (WBCs) per high-power field (hpf), more than five red blood cells (RBCs) per hpf, or more than 2+ bacteria is consistent with a diagnosis of UTI. In the study by Lammers and colleagues [12] discussed previously, it was discovered that by using a cutoff of more than three WBCs per hpf and more than five RBCs per hpf on the urinalysis, the overtreatment rate was 44% and the undertreatment rate was 11% [12]. When comparing these findings with their findings regarding the urine dipstick, it is clear that the under-treatment and overtreatment rates are nearly the same. Given the increased cost and time involved in performing a formal microscopic analysis, the urine dipstick is the screening test of choice in most scenarios to make the diagnosis of UTI.

Urine gram stain

Although not available to many emergency physicians, the urine Gram stain is a sensitive and specific test. In a study done by Wiwanitkit and colleagues [13] in 2005, the sensitivity of the urine Gram stain was found to be 96.2%, with a specificity of 93.0%. These data were compared with the sensitivity and specificity of urine microscopy, which were 65.4% and 74.4%, respectively. The problem with this test is its lack of availability in many emergency departments and the increased time it may take to get the results. If available, however, the urine Gram stain can be quite enlightening to the clinician.

Urine culture

Clearly, not every patient needs a urine culture in the workup of UTI. In young women with uncomplicated cystitis, it is not generally indicated to perform a urine culture. In these patients, the pathogens are fairly predictable and most of these are susceptible to standard antibiotics used for

UTI. Therefore, the workup of uncomplicated cystitis is more algorithmic, and the therapy is entirely empiric, with a high rate of success using this approach.

Nevertheless, it is standard of care to culture the urine of all patients who have pyelonephritis, those who are pregnant, immunocompromised individuals, the elderly ($\geq$65 years of age), those who have recurrent UTIs, male patients, or any other patient with the diagnosis of complicated infection. Urine cultures should be collected before the administration of antibiotics to maximize the diagnostic yield and avoid false-negative results. The traditional standard, based on prospective studies, is that 10^5 or more CFUs of a uropathogen per milliliter of midstream clean-catch urine is indicative of significant bacteriuria [14]. Although 80% to 95% of episodes of uncomplicated pyelonephritis are associated with such colony counts, a significant proportion of patients may present with counts as low as 10^2 CFUs/mL, which may be significant in the setting of fever, flank pain, costovertebral angle (CVA) tenderness, and pyuria and in catheterized patients [15,16].

Alternative diagnoses and workup

A wide differential diagnosis needs to be considered in a patient who presents with signs and symptoms of pyelonephritis, which are relatively nonspecific. Fever, chills, nausea and vomiting, flank pain, or CVA tenderness can be seen in a variety of disorders, including cholecystitis, appendicitis, pancreatitis, perforated viscus, tubo-ovarian abscess, ectopic pregnancy, nephrolithiasis, and lower lobe pneumonia. The emergency physician should be particularly aware of the potential for an alternative diagnosis in a patient with urine dipstick or microscopy findings that are not consistent with infection of the urinary tract. Further diagnostic workup, such as pregnancy testing, pelvic examination, abdominal imaging (ultrasound or CT), and chest radiography, should be considered on a case-by-case basis. The specifics of the appropriate clinical approach to these other disorders are beyond the scope of this review.

In patients in whom vaginitis or urethritis is suspected, a cervical, vaginal, or urethral swab is indicated. Patients should be worked up for the most common causes of vaginitis, including trichomoniasis, candidiasis, and bacterial vaginosis. The patient should also be evaluated for the presence of sexually transmitted infections if urethritis or cervicitis is present. This should include a Gram stain of urethral discharge and a DNA probe or nucleic acid amplification test (NAAT) of a cervical specimen of the urine to evaluate for gonorrhea and chlamydia. It is also important to consider helical CT in a patient in whom a renal stone is suspected. Other studies may include blood chemistry to evaluate creatinine and a urine pregnancy test.

If the patient is to be admitted to the hospital, the authors recommend that a complete blood cell count (CBC), chemistries, and blood cultures be performed in all such patients. Blood cultures should be considered a high priority in the following situations: the patient has signs of sepsis, if the diagnosis of pyelonephritis is not clear, if a urine culture cannot be obtained, or in the case of endocarditis in which there is a possible hematogenous origin of pyelonephritis with seeding of the kidneys [17].

Antibiotic resistance

Since the guidelines for the treatment of UTIs were published by the IDSA in 1999, much new consideration has been given to empiric antibiotic choices in patients who have UTI [18]. Of particular interest is the fact that resistance to TMP-SMX and fluoroquinolones has been increasing. Before 1990, E coli resistance to TMP-SMX was between 0% and 5%. This increased to between 7% and 18% by the mid-1990s. In 2001, it was found to be 16% [19]. There seems to be geographic variability to TMP-SMX resistance. It ranges from a low of 10% in the northeastern United States to a high of 22% in the southwestern United States [20]. The wide geographic range in the prevalence of antibiotic resistance is striking, and knowledge of general uropathogen resistance patterns, particularly local trends, is essential for the emergency physician.

Resistance patterns to the fluoroquinolones have been changing as well. Presently, in the United States, approximately 3% of E coli strains are resistant [21], but the prevalence varies by geography. A 2002 study examined a 10-year trend in E coli resistance to fluoroquinolones in England and Wales. The study investigators found an increase from 0.8% in 1990 to 3.7% in 1999 [22]. There does seem to be a difference in susceptibility between different age groups as well. Women older than the age of 50 years were found to have an increased prevalence of resistance to fluoroquinolones [20]. It is thought that this is attributable not only to increasing resistance patterns but to the higher prevalence of enterococci in this age group.

An important aspect of antibiotic resistance to address is the use of hospital antibiograms when making treatment decisions regarding uncomplicated UTIs. Although antibiotic resistance is growing, and the concern for fluoroquinolone resistance in E coli is justified, many clinicians are now avoiding the use of standard antibiotic therapy, such as TMP-SMX and ciprofloxacin, for uncomplicated infection, based on hospital antibiograms. Nevertheless, it is vital to note the inherent selection bias in these data. Most young, healthy, nonpregnant women with UTI do not have urine collected for culture because it is not clinically indicated. Therefore, hospital antibiograms tend to reflect the spectrum of pathogens in hospitalized patients or in those who have complicated UTI. These patients are at higher risk for infection with antibiotic-resistant organisms, giving an overestimation of overall antibiotic resistance in the community. As a result of this bias, most hospitals and clinics do not have accurate susceptibility data for the pathogens that cause uncomplicated UTI. Although antibiograms can provide some insight into local resistance patterns, and should not be discounted, the empiric treatment of uncomplicated UTI should not be based on hospital antibiograms alone. Even large studies, such as those published by the North American Urinary Tract Infection Collaborative Alliance (NAUTICA) [23,24], include a significant proportion of men and others with complicated infections and rely on clinicians to collect isolates when deemed necessary, thus sharing the biases of antibiogram data.

Although clinicians are often tempted and encouraged to use an algorithmic approach in the treatment of UTI, risk factors for individual patients must be taken into account when choosing empiric therapy. Small studies suggest, logically, that patients who have had significant previous exposure to fluoroquinolones, particularly for recurrent UTI, are at increased risk for fluoroquinolone resistance [25]. One prospective evaluation found fluoroquinolone-resistant *E coli* in a rectal culture of one patient after a short course of ciprofloxacin for uncomplicated cystitis [26]. Therefore, it stands to reason that patients who have complicated, recurrent, or health care–associated UTI, or those with substantial previous fluoroquinolone exposure, are potentially poor candidates for empiric ciprofloxacin therapy. In areas in which fluoroquinolone resistance remains low, this class of drugs may be used as first-line therapy in uncomplicated cystitis and pyelonephritis.

Another concept that has gained more attention recently is that of cross-resistance. Data suggest that if the *E coli* strain isolated from the urine is resistant to TMP-SMX, there is an increased likelihood of it being resistant to other commonly prescribed antibiotics as well [19]. A study by Karlowsky and colleagues [27] in 2003 examined this phenomenon. They found that 9.5% of *E coli* isolates resistant to TMP-SMX were also resistant to fluoroquinolones. They also found that 10.4% of ciprofloxacin-resistant isolates were resistant to nitrofurantoin.

As one can imagine, treatment failures not only increase the duration of the illness and increase patient suffering but increase the cost to the patient and health care system. There have been studies attempting to identify factors that are associated with an increased risk for having a uropathogen resistant to TMP-SMX. The following place the patient at increased risk for TMP-SMX treatment failure [6]:

- Diabetes
- Recent hospitalization
- Current use of any antibiotic
- Current or recent use of TMP-SMX (within the past 3 months)

Treatment

General considerations

Antibiotics are but one aspect of treating UTI. Supportive and symptomatic therapies are important as well. As discussed previously, patients presenting with UTI often experience nausea and vomiting in addition to suprapubic pain. Antiemetics may be indicated in addition to antibiotics, particularly if nausea results in the patient having difficulty in tolerating oral medications (see full discussion). Phenazopyridine, 200 mg, given three times a day can be given for dysuria, frequency, and urgency. A common side effect of this medication is discoloration of the urine or tears, and patients should be warned of this potential. Patients should be instructed to remove contact lenses while on this medication because it can lead to permanent discoloration. In patients who have pyelonephritis, nausea, vomiting, and flank and abdominal pain may be severe. If the patient is a candidate for outpatient treatment, oral analgesics and antiemetics should be prescribed if indicated.

Uncomplicated cystitis

Patients presenting to the emergency department with uncomplicated cystitis can be treated as outpatients with oral antibiotics. One of the first factors in choosing an antibiotic is institutional and geographic susceptibility. Most hospitals publish these data on a regular basis in the form of hospital antibiograms; however, clinicians must be cautious because of the selection bias in these susceptibility profiles. Having said that, because most patients who have uncomplicated cystitis do not have urine cultures performed and the choice of treatment is entirely empiric, the emergency physician should be cognizant of local trends in antibiotic resistance among the common uropathogens. If the local *E coli* resistance to TMP-SMX is less than 10% to 20%, a 3-day course of TMP-SMX (one double-strength tablet administered twice daily) would be a reliable empiric therapy [19].

If the resistance is greater than 20% and the patient is younger than 50 years of age, the clinician should consider a 7-day course of nitrofurantoin (100 mg twice a day) in the treatment of uncomplicated UTI. Resistance in *E coli* seems to remain low [27], and nitrofurantoin is active against *S saprophyticus*, most enterococcal isolates (including many VRE species), and group B streptococci. Nitrofurantoin allows the clinician to avoid fluoroquinolone use to treat a condition for which this antibiotic class is rarely necessary. Women older than 50 years of age have a higher incidence of *Proteus* and *Klebsiella*, which tend to be more resistant to nitrofurantoin [20]. In fact, many gram-negative pathogens are reliably resistant to nitrofurantoin, including *Pseudomonas, Enterobacter, Serratia, Morganella*, and *Acinetobacter* [28,29]. Therefore, this drug should never be used as empiric therapy in complicated cystitis, because these bacteria are seen more frequently. One drawback to the use of nitrofurantoin is possible lack of compliance to the 7 days necessary to treat the infection optimally. There is insufficient evidence at this time to support a 3-day course of this medication [19]. Another important consideration with nitrofurantoin use is its lack of efficacy in the upper urinary tract. Levels in the serum and most tissues are negligible [30,31] and are certainly lower than the minimum inhibitory concentration (MIC) of most organisms. The drug is concentrated in the urine [32], a fact that clinicians rely on in the treatment of cystitis. Because of these aspects of its distribution and excretion, however, nitrofurantoin should only be used in the treatment of cystitis and never in the treatment of pyelonephritis or in any patients who have renal failure (creatinine clearance <40).

In the patient in whom compliance is an issue or there is an allergy to TMP-SMX or nitrofurantoin, a 3-day course of ciprofloxacin (or an equivalent fluoroquinolone) can be prescribed. At the current time, the prevalence of resistance seems to remain significantly lower than that of TMP-SMX. Given the fact that the fluoroquinolones are used to treat a variety of serious and common conditions (eg, community-acquired pneumonia, intra-abdominal infections, pyelonephritis), however, it is wise to limit the inevitable increasing resistance by using these medications only when necessary [19]. If a patient presents with cystitis, the authors generally discourage the use of fluoroquinolones as first-line agents. This is not because of lack of efficacy but because of the potential to contribute further to resistance in the community (Table 1).

Acute uncomplicated pyelonephritis

Fluoroquinolones remain the initial choice of antibiotic class in patients who have pyelonephritis [18]. They are particularly favored for outpatient therapy, given their excellent oral bioavailability [33,34]. In fact, one of the first questions the emergency physician must consider is whether the patient is a candidate for outpatient therapy. Common indications for hospital admission are included in Box 1. Although not based on outcomes data, some consider the following to be relative indications for hospitalization: urinary tract abnormality or foreign body, significantly immunocompromised, age older than 60 years, and significant baseline debilitation.

If the patient can be treated as an outpatient, the antibiotic of choice is ciprofloxacin (500 mg twice daily for 7 days). Although levofloxacin is a viable alternative, it is important to remember that not all fluoroquinolones are equivalent in treating infections of the urinary tract. For example,

Table 1
Recommended antibiotics in acute uncomplicated cystitis

Drug	Dose
Nitrofurantoin[a]	100 mg twice a day for 7 days
TMP-SMX[b]	One DS tablet twice a day for 3 days
Ciprofloxacin	500 mg twice a day for 3 days

Abbreviation: DS, double-strength.

[a] Should not be used in patients who have suspected pyelonephritis, those older than 50 years of age, or those who have renal failure (creatinine clearance <40).

[b] Should only be used if local *E coli* resistance is less than 10% to 20%.

Box 1. Indications for hospitalization in patients who have acute pyelonephritis

- Inability to maintain oral hydration or take medications by mouth
- Uncertain diagnosis
- Suspected sepsis or other severe illness
- Urinary tract obstruction
- Progression of uncomplicated UTI
- Pregnancy
- Significant dehydration or acute renal insufficiency

---

moxifloxacin undergoes hepatic metabolism, and only approximately 20% of the drug is excreted unchanged into the urine [35]. Therefore, even if the isolate seems to be susceptible to fluoroquinolones, moxifloxacin would be a poor therapeutic choice. If the patient has an allergy to fluoroquinolones, a reasonable alternative would be oral amoxicillin or amoxicillin–clavulanic acid for 10 days if local susceptibility patterns indicate a low level of resistance in *E coli* in patients who have uncomplicated cystitis [2]. Another solution may be to admit the patient and treat with a third-generation cephalosporin. After antibiotic susceptibilities are reported, a definitive therapeutic decision can be made [18].

For patients requiring hospital admission for inpatient treatment, ciprofloxacin (400 mg administered intravenously every 12 hours), ceftriaxone (1 g administered intravenously every 24 hours), or ertapenem (1 g administered intravenously every 24 hours) is a reasonable empiric choice. An alternative would be gentamicin (5 mg/kg administered intravenously daily), although it is not optimal because of the potential for renal toxicity and ototoxicity. Changes to the antibiotic choice should, of course, be adjusted as cultures and sensitivities are reported (Table 2).

Acute complicated pyelonephritis

Patients who have complicated pyelonephritis should receive antimicrobial therapy directed toward the typical uropathogens but also toward *Pseudomonas*. Reasonable choices include cefepime, piperacillin-tazobactam, imipenem, meropenem, ampicillin plus tobramycin, or vancomycin plus tobramycin. These patients often require admission to the hospital for intravenous antibiotic therapy. Urine cultures should be obtained and therapy adjusted based on sensitivities (Table 3).

Recurrent urinary tract infections

Recurrent UTIs are commonly encountered in the emergency department setting. Reported recurrence rates vary depending on the population being

Table 2
Recommended empiric antibiotics in acute uncomplicated pyelonephritis

Oral	Dose
Oral	
Ciproflaxacin[a,b]	500 mg every 12 hours for 7 days
Amoxicillin	500 mg three times a day for 10 days
Amoxicillin–clavulanic acid	875 mg twice a day for 10 days
Cefpodoxime	200 mg every 12 hours for 14 days
Intravenous	
Ciprofloxacin[a,b]	400 mg every 12 hours for 7 days
Ceftriaxone	1 g every 24 hours for 14 days

Because of the increasing prevalence of resistance in *E coli*, TMP-SMX, ampicillin, and first-generation cephalosporins are generally not recommended for empiric therapy but may be an option when susceptibilities are known.

Doses provided are for patients who have normal renal function. Modified doses may be required in renal insufficiency.

Cephalosporins are ineffective for the treatment of *Enterococcus*.

[a] Some other fluoroquinolones may be suitable; however, moxifloxacin may not achieve adequate levels in the urine.

[b] Pregnancy category C.

studied but range from 27% to 40% [9]. In most situations, the uropathogen is different from the initial cause of infection. Risk factors for recurrent UTIs are vaginal intercourse, use of a diaphragm or spermicide, new sexual partner, maternal history of UTIs, and UTIs before the age of 15 years [9]. Patients who have a history of three or more symptomatic UTIs per year may benefit from prophylactic antibiotic therapy. In general, the patient's primary care physician can initiate this. The goal in the emergency department is to recognize the presence of recurrent UTI and provide the appropriate antimicrobial therapy. Agents commonly used include TMP-SMX, ciprofloxacin, and nitrofurantoin, with consideration given to previous cultures and susceptibilities. Another effective strategy is "self-start" therapy in which the patient is given a prescription for a short course (usually 3 days) of antibiotics. The patient begins therapy with the onset of symptoms. One study showed that using the self-start method, 86% of the cultures from the women initiating the antibiotics were positive. All were treated successfully with the antibiotic given [5].

Asymptomatic bacteriuria

Occasionally, urine cultures are collected in a patient who does not have symptoms of UTI. If a urine culture grows a significant quantity of a uropathogen in an asymptomatic person, this is referred to as asymptomatic bacteriuria. Based on previous studies, significant bacteriuria in the asymptomatic patient has been defined by the IDSA as 10^5 CFUs/mL or greater from a clean-catch specimen and 10^2 CFUs/mL or greater from a catheterized specimen [36]. The emergency physician should know

Table 3
Recommended empiric antibiotics in acute complicated pyelonephritis

Intravenous	Dose
Cefepime	1 g every 12 hours
Piperacilin/tazobactam[a,b]	4.5 g every 8 hours
Imipenem/cilastatin[c]	500 mg every 6 hours
Ertapenem[c]	1 g every 24 hours
Ampicillin (+ tobramycin)[b,d]	1–2 g every 6 hours (+5 mg/kg every 24 hours)
Vancomycin (+ tobramycin)[d,e]	15 mg/kg every 12 hours (+5 mg/kg every 24 hours)
Ciprofloxacin[f]	400 mg every 12 hours

Cephalosporins are ineffective for the treatment of *Enterococcus*.

Doses provided are for patients with normal renal function. Modified doses may be required in renal insufficiency.

[a] β-lactamase inhibitor (tazobactam) may provide broader coverage for some gram-negative enterics; however, if *Pseudomonas* is the known pathogen, high-dose piperacillin alone is preferred.

[b] Recommended if ampicillin-susceptible *Enterococcus* is suspected.

[c] Carbapenems are ideal empiric therapy if an extended-spectrum beta-lactamase–producer is suspected. Ertapenem does not cover *Pseudomonas* or reliably cover *Enterococcus*.

[d] Because of potential nephrotoxicity and ototoxicity, aminoglycosides should be avoided if possible. Check tobramycin level at 8 to 10 hours. If the level is less than 5 μg/mL, remain on once-daily dosing.

[e] Recommended if ampicillin-resistant *Enterococcus* is suspected.

[f] Because of high levels of resistance, ciprofloxacin is not the first choice for complicated pyelonephritis, which may commonly involve *Pseudomonas* or other resistant gram-negative antibiotics. Fluoroquinolones are pregnancy category C.

the indications regarding when to treat, and when not to treat, asymptomatic bacteriuria.

Prospective studies have shown that asymptomatic bacteriuria among young adult women is quite common, with an estimated prevalence of 3% to 8% [37,38]. Most healthy patients who have asymptomatic bacteriuria do not progress to UTI and derive no benefit from antibiotic treatment. Asymptomatic bacteriuria should, however, be treated in pregnant patients. Left untreated, it may lead to pyelonephritis, premature labor, pregnancy-induced hypertension, and low birth weight [39]. The antibiotic of choice is nitrofurantoin administered at a dosage of 100 mg twice a day for 3 days. An alternative would be cephalexin administered at a dosage of 250 to 500 mg four times a day for 3 days.

Pregnancy

The pregnant patient who has UTI can present the clinician with a particular challenge. This is attributable to the increased risk for complications in this population and to the fact that some of the most common antibiotics used for cystitis and pyelonephritis are contraindicated in the pregnant patient. In addition, some of the newer antibiotics do not have adequate data for safety in pregnancy to make a recommendation regarding their use. Nevertheless, there are some general evidence-based guidelines that should be followed.

As a class, β-lactam antibiotics are generally considered to be safe in pregnancy. This includes penicillins, cephalosporins, and carbapenems. Having said that, third-generation cephalosporins, such as ceftriaxone, may lead to kernicterus if given late in pregnancy because of the displacement of serum bilirubin and should be used with caution [40]. As for carbapenems, meropenem and ertapenem are considered to be pregnancy category B by the US Food and Drug Administration (FDA), and imipenem-cilastatin is FDA category C. Sulfonamides (eg, sulfisoxazole) are also considered safe; however, the authors recommend avoiding the use of trimethoprim in the first trimester because of its antimetabolic effects as a folic acid antagonist. Other options include nitrofurantoin [41] and fosfomycin [42]. The fluoroquinolones and tetracyclines are contraindicated in pregnancy because of their teratogenic potential.

The authors recommend treating cystitis in pregnancy with nitrofurantoin (100 mg twice daily or 50 mg four times daily) for 7 to 10 days because of the high prevalence of E coli resistance to amoxicillin in their community. If the prevalence of E coli resistance in your community is low, oral amoxicillin (500 mg twice daily) presents a potentially good empiric choice. An oral cephalosporin, such as cefpodoxime or cephalexin, for 3 to 7 days may be viable alternative [43].

For suspected pyelonephritis, one should never use nitrofurantoin because of negligible drug levels in serum and the renal parenchyma. Because of the increased risk for complications in pregnant women, the authors recommend hospitalization with initiation of intravenous therapy for patients who have pyelonephritis [44], although some studies have reported similar outcomes for selected women managed as outpatients with close follow-up [45,46]. An intravenously administered cephalosporin, such as ceftriaxone (1–2 g every 24 hours), is a reliable choice in most communities. If there is a high prevalence of cephalosporin resistance (greater than 10%–20%) in E coli in your community, however, the authors recommend including gentamicin (1–1.5 mg/kg administered intravenously every 8 hours) in the initial empiric regimen. The aminoglycoside should be discontinued because of the potential for toxicity if testing reveals susceptibility to a β-lactam. Patients usually improve within 24 to 48 hours and can be discharged home to complete a 10- to 14-day course or oral antibiotic therapy [44]. Clinical trials data are lacking with regard to the appropriate therapeutic choices and duration of therapy for pyelonephritis in pregnancy. These recommendations are based on clinical experience, extrapolation of data, and expert opinion.

Summary

Although the diagnosis and workup of UTIs have changed little over the years, the emergence of antibiotic resistance has forced us to reconsider our management strategies. It is clear that resistance to fluoroquinolones and TMP-SMX is increasing and is likely to continue to increase without intervention by clinicians. TMP-SMX still has a role in treatment of uncomplicated UTIs but only in situations in which local resistance is less than 10% to 20%. With uncomplicated UTIs in geographic areas in which resistance to TMP-SMX is greater than 10% to 20%, nitrofurantoin is recommended. It is important to remember that although useful in some situations, reliance on hospital antibiograms to treat uncomplicated UTIs is not recommended because of the selection bias toward complicated UTIs. The fluoroquinolones remain the treatment of choice for acute pyelonephritis, but there are other intravenous antibiotics available as well. The use of urine culture and sensitivities in this situation is helpful. Clinicians must recognize the situations that place the patient into the complicated UTI category and treat accordingly. An evidence-based approach to the diagnosis and management of UTIs as presented here should hopefully lead to fewer treatment failures and avoid overuse of important antibiotics with emerging resistance.

References

[1] Stamm WE, Hooton TM. Management of urinary tract infections in adults. N Engl J Med 1993;329(18):1328–34.
[2] Ramakrishnan K, Scheid DC. Diagnosis and management of acute pyelonephritis in adults. Am Fam Physician 2005;71(5):933–42.
[3] Marx J. Clinical practice of emergency medicine. In: Hockberger R, Walls R, editors. Rosen's emergency medicine: concepts and clinical practice. 6th edition. St. Louis (MO): Mosby, Inc; 2006. p. 428–34.
[4] Boie E, Goyal D, Sadosty A. Urinary tract infections. In: Wolfson A, editor. Clinical practice of emergency medicine. Philadelphia: Lippincott Williams & Wilkins; 2005.
[5] Krieger JN. Urinary tract infections: what's new? J Urol 2002;168(6):2351–8.
[6] Gupta K, Hooton TM, Stamm WE. Increasing antimicrobial resistance and the management of uncomplicated community-acquired urinary tract infections. Ann Intern Med 2001;135(1):41–50.
[7] Lipsky BA. Prostatitis and urinary tract infection in men: what's new; what's true? Am J Med 1999;106(3):327–34.
[8] Ronald A. The etiology of urinary tract infection: traditional and emerging pathogens. Am J Med 2002;113(Suppl 1A):14S–9S.
[9] Bass PF 3rd, Jarvis JA, Mitchell CK. Urinary tract infections. Prim Care 2003;30(1):41–61, v–vi.
[10] Bent S, et al. Does this woman have an acute uncomplicated urinary tract infection? JAMA 2002;287(20):2701–10.
[11] Rehmani R. Accuracy of urine dipstick to predict urinary tract infections in an emergency department. J Ayub Med Coll Abbottabad 2004;16(1):4–7.
[12] Lammers RL, et al. Comparison of test characteristics of urine dipstick and urinalysis at various test cutoff points. Ann Emerg Med 2001;38(5):505–12.
[13] Wiwanitkit V, Udomsantisuk N, Boonchalermvichian C. Diagnostic value and cost utility analysis for urine Gram stain and urine microscopic examination as screening tests for urinary tract infection. Urol Res 2005;33(3):220–2.

[14] Kass EH. Asymptomatic infections of the urinary tract. Trans Assoc Am Physicians 1956;69: 56–64.

[15] Gupta K, Scholes D, Stamm WE. Increasing prevalence of antimicrobial resistance among uropathogens causing acute uncomplicated cystitis in women. JAMA 1999;281(8):736–8.

[16] Stamm WE, et al. Diagnosis of coliform infection in acutely dysuric women. N Engl J Med 1982;307(8):463–8.

[17] McMurray BR, Wrenn KD, Wright SW. Usefulness of blood cultures in pyelonephritis. Am J Emerg Med 1997;15(2):137–40.

[18] Warren JW, et al. Guidelines for antimicrobial treatment of uncomplicated acute bacterial cystitis and acute pyelonephritis in women. Infectious Diseases Society of America (IDSA). Clin Infect Dis 1999;29(4):745–58.

[19] Hooton T, et al. Acute uncomplicated cystitis in an era of increasing antibiotic resistance: a proposed approach to empirical therapy. Clin Infect Dis 2004;39:75–80.

[20] Gupta K, et al. Antimicrobial resistance among uropathogens that cause community-acquired urinary tract infections in women: a nationwide analysis. Clin Infect Dis 2001; 33(1):89–94.

[21] Ansbach RK, Dybus K, Bergeson R. Uncomplicated E. coli urinary tract infection in college women: a follow-up study of E. coli sensitivities to commonly prescribed antibiotics. J Am Coll Health 2005;54(2):81–4 [discussion: 85–6].

[22] Livermore DM, et al. Trends in fluoroquinolone (ciprofloxacin) resistance in Enterobacteriaceae from bacteremias, England and Wales, 1990–1999. Emerg Infect Dis 2002;8(5): 473–8.

[23] Zhanel GG, et al. Antibiotic resistance in Escherichia coli outpatient urinary isolates: final results from the North American Urinary Tract Infection Collaborative Alliance (NAUTICA). Int J Antimicrob Agents 2006;27(6):468–75.

[24] Karlowsky JA, et al. Fluoroquinolone-resistant urinary isolates of Escherichia coli from outpatients are frequently multidrug resistant: results from the North American Urinary Tract Infection Collaborative Alliance-Quinolone Resistance study. Antimicrobial Agents Chemother 2006;50(6):2251–4.

[25] Killgore KM, March KL, Guglielmo BJ. Risk factors for community-acquired ciprofloxacin-resistant Escherichia coli urinary tract infection. Ann Pharmacother 2004;38(7–8): 1148–52.

[26] Gupta K, Hooton TM, Stamm WE. Isolation of fluoroquinolone-resistant rectal Escherichia coli after treatment of acute uncomplicated cystitis. J Antimicrob Chemother 2005;56(1): 243–6.

[27] Karlowsky JA, et al. Susceptibility of antimicrobial-resistant urinary Escherichia coli isolates to fluoroquinolones and nitrofurantoin. Clin Infect Dis 2003;36(2):183–7.

[28] Turck M, Ronald AR, Petersdorf RG. Susceptibility of Enterobacteriaceae to nitrofurantoin correlated with eradication of bacteriuria. Antimicrobial Agents Chemother (Bethesda) 1966;6:446–52.

[29] Barry AL. Nitrofurantoin susceptibility test criteria. J Antimicrob Chemother 1990;25(4): 711–3.

[30] Conklin JD. The pharmacokinetics of nitrofurantoin and its related bioavailability. Antibiot Chemother 1978;25:233–52.

[31] Schmidt FH. (On the decomposition of nitrofuran derivatives by mammalian tissue). Klin Wochenschr 1966;44(11):653–4 [in German].

[32] D'Arcy PF. Nitrofurantoin. Drug Intell Clin Pharm 1985;19(7–8):540–7.

[33] Dudley M. Pharmacokinetics of fluoroquinolones. In: Hooper DC, Rubinstein E, editors. Quinolone antimicrobial agents. 3rd edition. Washington (DC): ASM Press; 2003.

[34] Lode H, et al. Quinolone pharmacokinetics and metabolism. J Antimicrob Chemother 1990; 26(Suppl B):41–9.

[35] Stass H, Kubitza D. Pharmacokinetics and elimination of moxifloxacin after oral and intravenous administration in man. J Antimicrob Chemother 1999;43(Suppl B):83–90.

[36] Nicolle LE, et al. Infectious Diseases Society of America guidelines for the diagnosis and treatment of asymptomatic bacteriuria in adults. Clin Infect Dis 2005;40(5):643–54.
[37] Hooton TM, et al. A prospective study of asymptomatic bacteriuria in sexually active young women. N Engl J Med 2000;343(14):992–7.
[38] Bengtsson C, et al. Bacteriuria in a population sample of women: 24-year follow-up study. Results from the prospective population-based study of women in Gothenburg, Sweden. Scand J Urol Nephrol 1998;32(4):284–9.
[39] Engel JD, Schaeffer AJ. Evaluation of and antimicrobial therapy for recurrent urinary tract infections in women. Urol Clin North Am 1998;25(4):685–701, x.
[40] Wadsworth SJ, Suh B. In vitro displacement of bilirubin by antibiotics and 2-hydroxyben-zoylglycine in newborns. Antimicrobial Agents Chemother 1988;32(10):1571–5.
[41] Ben David S, et al. The safety of nitrofurantoin during the first trimester of pregnancy: meta-analysis. Fundam Clin Pharmacol 1995;9(5):503–7.
[42] Stein GE. Single-dose treatment of acute cystitis with fosfomycin tromethamine. Ann Phar-macother 1998;32(2):215–9.
[43] Vercaigne LM, Zhanel GG. Recommended treatment for urinary tract infection in preg-nancy. Ann Pharmacother 1994;28(2):248–51.
[44] ACOG educational bulletin. Antimicrobial therapy for obstetric patients. Number 245, March 1998 (replaces no. 117, June 1988). American College of Obstetricians and Gynecol-ogists. Int J Gynaecol Obstet 1998;61(3):299–308.
[45] Millar LK, et al. Outpatient treatment of pyelonephritis in pregnancy: a randomized con-trolled trial. Obstet Gynecol 1995;86(4 Pt 1):560–4.
[46] Wing DA, et al. Outpatient treatment of acute pyelonephritis in pregnancy after 24 weeks. Obstet Gynecol 1999;94(5 Pt 1):683–8.

ELSEVIER
SAUNDERS

Emerg Med Clin N Am
26 (2008) 431–455

EMERGENCY
MEDICINE
CLINICS OF
NORTH AMERICA

Community-Associated Methicillin-Resistant *Staphylococcus aureus*

Thomas R. Wallin, MD[a], H. Gene Hern, MD[b], Bradley W. Frazee, MD[b],*

[a]*Department of Emergency Medicine, Alameda County Medical Center-Highland Campus, 1411 East 31st Street, Oakland, CA 94602, USA*
[b]*Department of Emergency Medicine, Alameda County Medical Center-Highland Campus, University of California at San Francisco, 1411 East 31st Street, Oakland, CA 94602, USA*

Within a year of the introduction of semisynthetic antistaphylococcal penicillins in 1960, methicillin-resistant *Staphylococcus aureus* (MRSA) was discovered. Over the following three and a half decades, MRSA was a problem confined largely to hospitalized patients and to the occasional outpatient who had readily identified predisposing risk factors such as recent hospitalization, hemodialysis, or residence in a nursing home. In the late 1990s, the first United States reports appeared of so-called community-associated MRSA (CA-MRSA) infections, defined as MRSA infections occurring in patients who had no identifiable predisposing risk factors [1,2]. (The terms "community-acquired" and "community-onset" also are used.) These first cases occurred among children in the Midwest and included deaths from pneumonia. Subsequent studies have confirmed that CA-MRSA infections do occur commonly in otherwise healthy children and young adults. CA-MRSA pneumonia, however, has proven uncommon. It is now clear that CA-MRSA infections predominantly take the form of relatively minor skin and soft tissue infections [3,4]. Molecular genetic and microbiologic studies have revealed that CA-MRSA is associated with a novel genetic profile and phenotype that distinguish it from hospital-acquired MRSA (HA-MRSA). Unlike HA-MRSA of old, CA-MRSA is remarkably fit for spread within communities, is virulent, and is often susceptible to multiple narrow-spectrum antimicrobials. CA-MRSA has emerged very rapidly since it first appeared in the late 1990s, having been reported in virtually every geographic region, both urban and rural, in the United States [5–7].

---

* Corresponding author.
E-mail address: bradf_98@yahoo.com (B.W. Frazee).

0733-8627/08/$ - see front matter © 2008 Elsevier Inc. All rights reserved.
doi:10.1016/j.emc.2008.01.010
emed.theclinics.com

The emergence of CA-MRSA over the last decade is probably the most important development in infectious diseases to affect the routine practice of emergency medicine. Emergency departments (along with pediatric clinics) have been ground zero for the explosion of CA-MRSA skin and soft tissue infections (SSTIs). In studies conducted in 2004, CA-MRSA accounted for more than 75% of community-acquired S aureus isolates among children in Texas [8], and it was responsible for 59% of all SSTIs at a network of 11 emergency departments located across the United States [7]. Reports indicate that CA-MRSA also should be considered in cases of septic arthritis, osteomyelitis, pyomyositis, necrotizing fasciitis, and necrotizing pneumonia [9–12]. Thus, the emergence of CA-MRSA forces emergency physicians to reconsider what pathogen might be responsible for a range of infections, from the routine to the life-threatening. Recommended empiric treatment for these infections recently changed to account for CA-MRSA. This article reviews the important aspects of the microbiology and epidemiology of CA-MRSA, the types of clinical infections it causes, and the latest management strategies. It emphasizes the role of the emergency physician in proper evaluation and treatment. Controversies regarding antimicrobial treatment and the approach to infection control are covered.

Microbiology, pathophysiology and epidemiology

Microbiology and genetics

The genetic classification and molecular epidemiology of MRSA is complex, but some familiarity with the basics is essential. CA-MRSA is distinct from HA-MRSA, both genetically and phenotypically. Methicillin resistance, signifying resistance to all beta-lactam antibiotics, is mediated by the mecA gene, which codes for the penicillin-binding protein PBP2A. The mecA gene is located on a genetic island called the staphylococcal cassette chromosome mec (SCCmec), and differences in SCCmec are used to categorize MRSA. HA-MRSA strains carry SCCmec types I through III, whereas CA-MRSA strains carry SCCmec IV (and the more recently isolated SCCmec V). Hospital-associated SCCmec II and III are large genetic elements that also carry genes for resistance to non-beta-lactam antibiotics, whereas the small SCCmec IV carries only methicillin resistance. Thus, HA-MRSA tends to be multiresistant, whereas CA-MRSA tends to be susceptible to narrow-spectrum non-beta-lactams such as clindamycin, trimethoprim-sulfamethoxazole (TMP-SMX), and tetracyclines.

Another distinguishing genetic feature of CA-MRSA is that a high percentage of strains carry genes for Panton-Valentine leukocidin (PVL), an exotoxin that is lethal to leukocytes. Genes for PVL are largely absent from HA-MRSA strains. PVL, perhaps in combination with other exotoxins, appears to be responsible for the enhanced pathogenicity of CA-MRSA strains and instrumental in producing necrotic skin lesions and necrotizing pneumonia. Severe invasive disease, such as necrotizing pneumonia and necrotizing fasciitis, appears to be more common with CA-MRSA than methicillin-sensitive *S aureus* (MSSA) or HA-MRSA. Furthermore, unlike HA-MRSA, which is considered an opportunistic pathogen, CA-MRSA causes infection in healthy, predominantly young hosts who have no predisposing comorbidities [4].

Epidemiology

Perhaps the most remarkable feature of the CA-MRSA genotype is its evolutionary success, resulting in its rapid worldwide clonal emergence. The small SCCmec IV allele seems to carry little fitness cost, allowing CA-MRSA to thrive and spread readily outside the hospital environment, unlike HA-MRSA strains, which require the hospital milieu for sustained survival. Pulsed-field gel electrophoresis is used to classify CA-MRSA clones. Although there is worldwide variation, in the United States, most CA-MRSA isolates are from the USA 300 and USA 400 clonal families. The emergence of the USA 300 clone—first epidemic and now likely established as endemic—exemplifies the success of CA-MRSA. Not seen in California before 2000, by 2003, USA 300 had established itself as the major cause of SSTIs in Los Angeles and San Francisco prison inmates, and in emergency department patients in Oakland [13,14]. In a cross-sectional study of SSTIs conducted in August 2004 in 11 emergency departments across the United States, USA 300 was the cause of 59% of all infections and accounted for 97% of CA-MRSA isolates. Underscoring the apparent success of CA-MRSA in competing with other *S aureus* clones, SCCmec IV-containing MRSA strains have been identified increasingly in hospital-acquired infections [15,16]. Although some have theorized that the superadapted CA-MRSA phenotype is poised to replace MSSA in the community, there is evidence that CA-MRSA actually emerged alongside MSSA, without causing a reduction in MSSA colonization or infections [17,18].

Relatively little is known about CA-MRSA colonization patterns, how it is spread among individuals, or how these issues relate to infection. Based on the emerging evidence, it appears that here too CA-MRSA differs from MSSA and HA-MRSA. Colonization in the nares or elsewhere generally is considered a necessary precursor to infection with MSSA and HA-MRSA, but nasal colonization with CA-MRSA has been surprisingly low in recent community surveillance studies (where it was less than 1%) [19], and among patients who have active CA-MRSA infections (31% to 44%) [14,20]. There are numerous possible explanations for this finding and various theories about the alternative epidemiology of CA-MRSA. Other sites of colonization, such as the axilla, groin, or gastrointestinal (GI) tract, may be important. Fomites (such as wound dressings, towels, athletic equipment, and wooden sauna surfaces) might represent important reservoirs for spread between individuals, or CA-MRSA may employ a hit and run strategy, where direct contact with a draining skin lesion results in immediate infection without intervening colonization. In an illustrative case series involving the St. Louis Rams during the 2003 season, eight CA-MRSA infections (caused by a single clone) occurred in five St. Louis Rams linemen. A meticulous investigation revealed no nasal colonization among any players or trainers. It was theorized that CA-MRSA may have spread among lineman by direct contact between susceptible turf burns and draining infections, shared towels, or the unwashed hands of trainers [21].

Risk groups in which CA-MRSA outbreaks have occurred and demographic and clinical risk factors for CA-MRSA infection are listed in Box 1. It is apparent from this list that physical crowding and hygiene play significant roles in determining risk for CA-MRSA infection. Unfortunately, the utility of risk factors for identifying likely MRSA SSTIs appears limited in view of the very high overall MRSA prevalence in this infection type. On the other hand, for infections like community-acquired pneumonia (CAP), where CA-MRSA is an infrequent but possible pathogen, using risk factors to help identify patients who deserve empiric therapy for MRSA makes sense.

Antibiotic susceptibility

The usual antibiotic susceptibility pattern of CA-MRSA is summarized in Table 1. Treatment recommendations are covered in detail below under

---

Box 1. Risk factors associated with community-acquired methicillin-resistant *Staphylococcus aureus* infection and risk groups in which clusters of infection have been reported

Infection type being a furuncle
Household contacts of a confirmed case
Jail detainees
Military recruits
Children attending daycare centers
Participants in contact sports (eg, American football, fencing)
Urban dwellers of low socioeconomic status living in crowded
    conditions
Tattoo recipients
Homeless youth
Men who have sex with men
HIV-infected individuals
Pregnant and postpartum women
Healthy newborns
African Americans
Pacific Islanders
Native Americans

Table 1
Community-acquired methicillin-resistant *Staphylococcus aureus* antibiotic susceptibility
(12 communities; 1594 isolates; skin and soft tissue infections and invasive infections)

Antibiotic	Mean susceptibility rate (%)	Range (among communities; %)
Methicillin	0	0
Erythromycin	18	6–47
TMP-SMX	97	83–100
Tetracycline	88	89–91
Clindamycin	87	40–95
Rifampin	98	67–100
Vancomycin	100	99–100
Linezolid	96	92–100
Fluoroquinolones	65	40–95

Data from Fridkin SK, Hageman JC, Morrison M, et al. Methicillin-resistant *Staphylococcus aureus* disease in three communities. N Engl J Med 2005;352:1436; and Moran GJ, Krishnadasan A, Gorwitz RJ, et al. Methicillin-resistant *S aureus* infections among patients in the emergency department. N Engl J Med 2006;355:666.

infection type, but some general principles should be borne in mind. Methicillin resistance signifies resistance to all beta-lactam antibiotics. Because first-generation cephalosporins and antistaphylococcal penicillins long have been the first choice for SSTIs, it is not surprising that ineffective empiric antibiotic treatment of these infections has been documented in numerous recent studies. TMP-SMX and doxycycline are commonly recommended antibiotics for CA-MRSA SSTIs in adults; however, it should be recognized that outcome studies documenting their safety and efficacy remain lacking. TMP-SMX lacks activity against group A *Streptococcus* and therefore should be combined with a beta-lactam for initial treatment of SSTIs when the etiology is uncertain. Although clindamycin is a good choice for many types of CA-MRSA infections, the possibility of inducible clindamycin resistance must be recognized. Isolates initially reported susceptible to clindamycin (but resistant to erythromycin) may develop clindamycin resistance within days of beginning clindamycin treatment. Inducible resistance is a fairly uncommon problem, discovered in 2.4% to 10% of CA-MRSA isolates in United States studies [7,14,22]; however, resultant treatment failures have been reported [23]. Inducible clindamycin resistance is detected in the laboratory by the simple D-zone disk diffusion test, which now is performed routinely in most laboratories. Rifampin has good CA-MRSA activity and is used to promote decolonization, but it must be combined with another active antibiotic (usually TMP/SMX), because rifampin resistance develops rapidly when it is used alone. For infections requiring parenteral therapy, the role of vancomycin versus newer antibiotics such as linezolid and daptomycin is a source of controversy. For life-threatening infections, such as suspected MRSA pneumonia or necrotizing fasciitis, it is recommended that antibiotics such as clindamycin or linezolid, which might halt protein/toxin production, be included in the antibiotic regimen.

Skin and soft tissue infections

SSTIs are the predominant form of disease caused by CA-MRSA. In large studies involving adult and pediatric hospital isolates, SSTIs accounted for 77% to 96% of CA-MRSA infections [4,8]. The emergence of CA-MRSA in communities across the United States has taken the form of an epidemic of SSTIs. The bulk of these infections have presented to emergency departments and have been managed entirely in the outpatient setting. Recent data from emergency departments located across the United States indicate that CA-MRSA is by far the most common pathogen isolated from SSTIs [7,24]. Risk factors and risk groups for CA-MRSA infection have been identified (see Box 1). In view of the very high overall MRSA prevalence in SSTIs, however, the clinical utility of risk factors for identifying or excluding CA-MRSA seems limited.

CA-MRSA can cause a range of cutaneous manifestations, including virtually all of the infection types traditionally associated with *S aureus*. Although furuncles—superficial skin abscesses arising from infected hair follicles—are by far the most common infection type, CA-MRSA also causes folliculitis, impetigo, cellulitis, carbuncles, paronychia, deep subcutaneous abscesses, and necrotizing fasciitis [10,14,25,26]. Localized necrosis seems to be a very typical feature of CA-MRSA skin infections [25]. Although CA-MRSA cellulitis has been reported to complicate atopic dermatitis and other conditions that disrupt the skin barrier [26], it is more common for these infections to arise spontaneously on apparently unbroken skin. Spontaneous furuncles with a necrotic center often are mistaken by patients for spider bites (Fig. 1).

PVL production appears to be a key factor in the propensity of CA-MRSA to cause necrotic skin and soft tissue infections. Purified PVL injected into the skin of experimental animals causes tissue necrosis similar to that seen with infections from PVL-producing strains of *S aureus* [27]. Although representing less than 5% of all *S aureus* strains, PVL-producing strains caused 93% of furuncles in one study [28]. Compared with MSSA, CA-MRSA much more commonly carries genes for PVL production; 98% of CA-MRSA isolates from SSTIs were PVL-positive in a large emergency department surveillance study [7]. Thus, PVL production by CA-MRSA may in part explain the rising incidence of SSTIs that has been observed across the United States over the last decade [29].

The importance of CA-MRSA as a cause of cellulitis without purulence (typified by erysipelas) is unclear [30]. Studies of the etiology of pure cellulitis, which require punch biopsies, skin aspirates, or blood cultures, are difficult to perform. There have been no such studies published in the era of CA-MRSA. On the other hand, cellulitis surrounding an abscess or other focal, purulent lesion occurs frequently in CA-MRSA infections; all 116 cases of CA-MRSA cellulitis documented in one study were associated with a focal lesion such as an ulcer, abscess, or folliculitis [31]. What

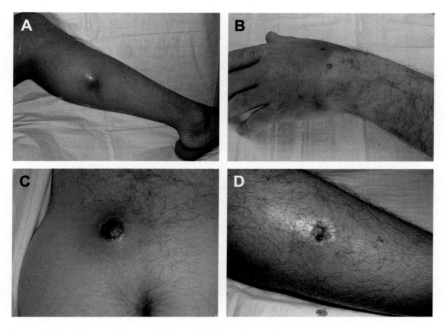

Fig. 1. Typical community-acquired methicillin-resistant *Staphylococcus aureus* skin and soft tissue infections. (*A*) Spontaneous furuncle on a shaved leg. (*B*) Folliculitis of the wrist. (*C, D*) Late stage furuncles demonstrating focal necrosis and surrounding hyperemia.

constitutes surrounding cellulitis (implying a need for antibiotics), as opposed to surrounding hyperemia (which should resolve with drainage of the abscess), has not been well delineated (see Fig. 1).

Diagnosis

The clinical evaluation of SSTIs varies according to severity, but it is often very straightforward. Furuncles usually present with fluctuance, spontaneous drainage, or focal skin necrosis, which points to the location for incision and drainage. Fluctuance may be subtle or absent when the abscess is deep or early in its course. Emergency department ultrasound has proved extremely useful in some cases: to identify small or deep fluid collections when skin signs are unrevealing, and to localize the fluid pocket before drainage [32].

Although culture of abscesses now is recommended widely [4,7,30,33], it is controversial whether cultures should be obtained routinely in the emergency department, particularly where the community prevalence of CA-MRSA is known. Abrahamian [34] argues that cultures should not be performed when the result is unlikely to change management, for example in uncomplicated abscesses clearly not requiring antibiotics or when antibiotics active against CA-MRSA will be given immediately. Abscess cultures are recommended to guide future antibiotic therapy in cases requiring admission, in immunocompromised patients, and in complicated abscesses. A complicated abscess generally is defined as one accompanied by fever, lymphangitis, or significant surrounding cellulitis. Nasal swab cultures to assess for CA-MRSA carriage rarely are indicated in the emergency department [30].

Treatment

Consensus documents covering treatment of CA-MRSA SSTIs have been published [30,33]; however recommendations remain vague, reflecting a lack of quality prospective data. A suggested approach to SSTI therapy in the setting of high community prevalence of CA-MRSA is summarized in Fig. 2. It must be emphasized that in most CA-MRSA SSTIs, the main therapeutic issue is aggressive surgical care, with the related issue of providing adequate anesthesia. For the typical uncomplicated CA-MRSA abscess, incision and drainage alone provide definitive therapy. Loculations should be broken up and necrotic tissue debrided, if necessary. Abscesses are packed, and a dressing is applied to prevent spread of infectious pus. For extremity infections, an elastic bandage is recommended to hold the gauze dressing in place. Patients generally are instructed to follow up in 24 to 48 hours for the first dressing change and to confirm that the infection is resolving. Thereafter, they should soak or wash the abscess cavity at least once a day and change and replace the packing loosely until cessation of drainage.

The need for antibiotic treatment following incision and drainage of uncomplicated abscesses has been the subject of four small prospective studies, all of which demonstrated no benefit with antibiotics [35–38]. In the most recent of these studies—the only one to involve CA-MRSA infections (88% of isolates)—cure rates were 84% in the cephalexin-treated group and

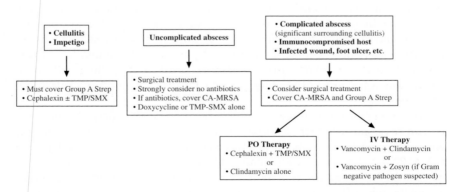

Fig. 2. Empiric treatment algorithm for skin and soft tissue infections.

90% in the placebo group [38]. Adjunctive antibiotics after incision and drainage are recommended in the following situations:

- Complicated abscesses (as defined previously)
- Rapidly progressive or severe local disease
- Abscess diameter greater than 5 cm
- Comorbid conditions or immune suppression
- Inability to completely drain an abscess cavity
- Extremes of age
- Failed prior incision and drainage

Among these indications for antibiotics, the issue of whether surrounding cellulitis is present is the most commonly encountered and the most problematic.

Interestingly, even for confirmed CA-MRSA SSTIs deemed to require antibiotics, the benefit of providing antibiotic therapy with activity against CA-MRSA remains unclear. Four retrospective studies of children and adults who had primarily uncomplicated SSTIs found no difference in outcomes between the majority who initially were prescribed a beta-lactam antibiotic and those who initially were prescribed an antibiotic with activity against CA-MRSA [4,39–41]. On the other hand, a recent retrospective cohort study of 531 cases of CA-MRSA SSTI (most of which underwent incision and drainage) found a significant difference in the rate of treatment failures—5% in those that received an antibiotic active against CA-MRSA versus 13% in those who received an ineffective antibiotic [31]. The authors examined the efficacy of a SSTI treatment algorithm (similar to Fig. 2) designed to promote appropriate use of antibiotics with activity against CA-MRSA [42]. In this small retrospective study conducted at the authors' institution, which has a very high prevalence of CA-MRSA, treatment failure occurred in only 3% of cases in which treatment conformed to the algorithm versus 62% of those in which treatment did not conform to the algorithm. The study design selected for complicated infections and patients with significant comorbidities, which might partially explain the apparent benefit of antibiotics with CA-MRSA activity [42]. Large prospective, randomized, controlled trials examining the efficacy of various antibiotics and surgical treatments in CA-MRSA SSTIs should be forthcoming.

Antibiotic choice and route of administration should be governed by severity of disease (see Fig. 2). For children under the age of eight, (in whom doxycycline is contraindicated) and adults who have complicated infections or significant comorbidities, oral clindamycin or the combination of TMP-SMX plus cephalexin (which covers group A *Streptococcus*) is recommended. For adult and adolescent outpatients following abscess incision and drainage, where the only issue is possible surrounding cellulitis, doxycycline is an excellent choice. Linezolid is another option for outpatient oral therapy, which the authors reserve for infections that have failed generic, narrow-spectrum antibiotics (Table 2). Seven days of therapy is usually

Table 2
Antibiotics used for treatment of community-acquired methicillin-resistant *Staphylococcus aureus* (CA-MRSA) infections

Antibiotic	Dosing	Comments
Trimethoprim sulfamethoxazole (TMP/SMX)	One double-strength tab twice daily	Does not cover group A *Streptococcus* Very little resistance among CA-MRSA to date
Clindamycin	150–450 mg po every 6 hours 600–900 mg iv every 8 h	Covers group A *Streptococcus* well Decreases toxin production Inducible resistance can occur
Doxycycline	100 mg p twice daily	Contraindicated in children less than 8 years old
Rifampin	300 mg po twice daily	Rapid resistance with monotherapy; combine with another antibiotic (TMP/SMX) Frequent drug–drug interactions
Linezolid	SSTI: 400 mg po or iv every12 h All other indications: 600 mg po or iv every 12 h	Generally reserved for treatment failure with narrow-spectrum antibiotics Preferred empiric therapy for possible CA-MRSA pneumonia Decreases toxin production
Vancomycin	15 mg/kg iv every 12 h	Traditional first-line intravenous therapy Combine with clindamycin for life-threatening infections
Daptomycin	4 mg/kg iv every 24 hours	Not recommended for empiric therapy
Dalbavancin	1 g iv on day 1, then 0.5 g iv on day 8	Approval pending Emergency department experience lacking
Mupirocin ointment	Apply to nares every 12 hours	Used for decolonization, efficacy unknown Resistance common in CA-MRSA

Abbreviations: po, by mouth; iv, intravenously.
Data from Gilbert DN, Moellering RC Jr, Elipoulos GM, et al. The Sanford guide to antimicrobial therapy. 36th edition. Sperryville (VA): Antimicrobial Therapy Incorporated; 2006.

adequate for abscesses that have been drained, although 10 to 14 days generally are recommended for true cellulitis.

Patients who have severe or complicated SSTIs requiring hospitalization should receive intravenous antibiotic therapy. Vancomycin remains first-line therapy for CA-MRSA. It often is combined with clindamycin, which is highly active against group A *Streptococcus*, covers anaerobes found in abscesses, and may halt exotoxin production. Clindamycin monotherapy, while commonly used in children, runs the risk of treatment failures because of inducible resistance. Linezolid is approved for severe SSTI in adults and has been used in children, but it is expensive and has significant potential adverse effects [30]. Linezolid may be a good first choice for empiric therapy in communities with a high rate of inducible clindamycin resistance among CA-MRSA. Daptomycin is a new parenteral antibiotic approved for severe MRSA SSTIs in adults. It is expensive, has a limited track record, and is not yet recommended for empiric therapy in the emergency department setting [33]. Dalbavancin, which has the unique property of once-weekly intravenous dosing [43], may be approved for use in MRSA SSTIs in the near future (see Table 2).

Community-acquired Staphylococcus aureus necrotizing fasciitis

Necrotizing fasciitis is an uncommon, rapidly progressive, life-threatening disease that requires prompt recognition and surgical debridement for cure. S aureus is a known pathogen in polymicrobial necrotizing fasciitis, and given the emergence of CA-MRSA as a cause of other SSTIs, it is not surprising that it has been reported to cause necrotizing fasciitis also. With only three reports in the literature so far [10,44,45], it remains unclear how important a manifestation of CA-MRSA this is. The first report to be published described 14 cases that occurred over 14 months in 2003 and 2004 at a single institution in California, where CA-MRSA made up 62% of all S aureus isolates. Twelve of 14 infections were monomicrobial for CA-MRSA. Risk factors and comorbidities included intravenous drug abuse in 43% of patients, prior MRSA infection in 21%, diabetes in 21%, and hepatitis C in 21%. The CA-MRSA necrotizing fasciitis described in this report seems to differ from typical necrotizing fasciitis in several ways. The disease was more indolent and mild than is typical, with an average of 6 days of symptoms before presentation and no deaths among the 14 cases. Furthermore, 8 of the 14 patients received an emergency department diagnosis of abscess, suggesting that there was a localized area of purulence or necrosis and that widespread induration and pain out of proportion to examination initially may have been absent. Additional reports of CA-MRSA necrotizing fasciitis include a report of seven adult cases at a single hospital in Taiwan from 2001 to 2005 and a case that occurred in an otherwise healthy 5-day-old neonate [44,45]. In the neonatal case, previously collected breast milk from the mother grew CA-MRSA identical to the child's surgical isolates.

In addition to immediate surgical debridement, treatment of necrotizing fasciitis requires broad-spectrum antibiotics, usually including clindamycin to reduce bacterial toxin production. Addition of vancomycin is recommended in cases occurring in intravenous drug users and in communities with a high prevalence of CA-MRSA (see Table 2) [10,46].

Deep infections

Musculoskeletal infections that are considered distinct from skin and soft tissue infections include septic arthritis, osteomyelitis and pyomyositis. These deeper musculoskeletal infections are far less common than SSTIs.

Their incidence, however, has been increasing over the last decade as the proportion of cases caused by CA-MRSA has risen.

Pyomyositis

Pyomyositis is an acute bacterial infection that causes the formation of intramuscular abscesses, most commonly in the large muscle groups of the thigh and pelvis. The proposed mechanism of infection is hematogenous seeding from transient bacteremia in the setting of underlying minor muscle damage caused by vigorous exercise, blunt trauma, or preceding viral infection [47]. Although there are several different causative bacteria, S aureus is the most common. At-risk populations include children and those who have immunosuppression because of HIV, diabetes, malignancy, or other factors. The onset is insidious, corresponding to the initial phase of myositis, with low-grade fever, local stiffness, and gradually increasing muscle pain that develops over the course of days. Development of pyomyositis, an actual muscle abscess, occurs after 1 to 3 weeks and is associated with high fevers and signs of localized infection. If untreated, pyomyositis can progress to sepsis and death [47–49].

Tropical pyomyositis, as the disease originally was known, accounts for 2% to 4% of surgical admissions in tropical areas, and S aureus is the causative organism in 75% to 95% of cases [47,50,51]. The first case of pyomyositis in the United States was reported in 1971 [52]. In a review of the 225 culture positive cases (not associated with HIV infection) reported in the United States from 1981 to 2002, 64% were caused by S aureus. In HIV-associated cases, S aureus is even more common [48]. The incidence of pyomyositis appears to have increased in recent years, linked to the emergence of CA-MRSA. For example, from 2000 to 2005 a single pediatric hospital identified 45 cases of bacterial myositis or pyomyositis among otherwise healthy children. CA-MRSA was the most common pathogen, isolated in 35% of cases [50]. Similarly, a cluster of CA-MRSA pyomyositis recently was reported in four adults over 6 months at a single facility. Three patients were under 50; one had diabetes; one had AIDS, and two of four had a recent history of skin furuncle. All four infections occurred in the thigh, with bacteremia in three [11].

Diagnosis and treatment

Early clinical diagnosis of pyomyositis is difficult, because nonspecific symptoms may suggest other more common entities such as muscle strain or osteomyelitis. Unlike viral or necrotizing myositis, creatine kinase levels are most often normal or only slightly elevated [48,50]. MRI with gadolinium is the most sensitive imaging modality for diagnosis. CT and ultrasound are less sensitive than MRI for detection of muscle inflammation but can be useful for identifying and localizing an abscess in the later stages of disease [48,50]. Early infection may be treated successfully with intravenous antibiotics alone, but once an intramuscular abscess forms, definitive treatment consists of percutaneous or open drainage plus intravenous antibiotics [48,53]. Given the high proportion of cases caused by CA-MRSA, initial empiric antibiotics should include vancomycin, clindamycin, or linezolid [50]. Coverage of gram-negative organisms is recommended in patients who are immunosuppressed (see Table 2) [48].

Septic arthritis and osteomyelitis

Septic arthritis usually is caused by transient bacteremia and seeding of an already abnormal joint. Risk factors include joint prosthesis, prior joint damage or osteoarthritis, rheumatologic joint disease, and immunosuppression [54]. Loss of skin barrier integrity, as in psoriasis or eczema, is also a purported risk factor; however, an identifiable source of infection is evident in less than 50% of cases [55]. S aureus is the most common pathogen, accounting for 44% of cases in one series [56]. S aureus septic arthritis carries a mortality of 7% to18% and results in osteomyelitis or loss of joint function in 27% to 46% of cases [57,58]. Osteomyelitis can be grouped into three subtypes by etiology: direct inoculation of an open fracture, spread of infection from a contiguous soft tissue source (typically a foot ulcer), and hematogenous seeding. Localized spread is more common in adults who have diabetes or peripheral vascular disease, while hematogenous seeding is more common in the elderly and children [59,60]. S aureus is the dominant pathogen in all three infection types and across all age groups, which may be related to its expression of various receptors for bone proteins and its ability to survive after phagocytosis by osteoblasts [59]. Osteomyelitis is difficult to treat once established. Inflammation of surrounding bone cuts off the vascular supply, leading to areas of bone necrosis and poor antibiotic delivery [61].

Although published data are still limited, it appears that CA-MRSA has become a common cause of both septic arthritis and osteomyelitis in the United States. One population study (including adults) from 2001 to 2002 found that among 1647 total CA-MRSA infections, there were 15 cases of septic arthritis (0.9%) and 24 cases of osteomyelitis (1.5%) [4]. Of 193 invasive pediatric S aureus infections in a recent study, 82 were cases of osteomyelitis, of which 54 (61%) were caused by CA-MRSA [60]. In another study of 158 cases of osteomyelitis and septic arthritis at a single pediatric referral center from 2000 to 2004, 52% of culture positive cases were caused by CA-MRSA. Over the 4-year study period, the proportion of osteoarticular infections from MRSA climbed from 4% to 40%, while the proportion caused by MSSA remained stable, at just over 10% [12]. Given the rising prevalence of CA-MRSA in osteoarticular infections, the authors recommend that CA-MRSA coverage routinely be included in empiric antibiotic therapy for these infections.

Osteoarticular infections caused by CA-MRSA appear to be somewhat more severe than infections caused by MSSA and other pathogens, as measured by an increased number of febrile days [62] and a greater likelihood of subperiosteal abscess [12]. Osteomyelitis cases in which there was bacteremia with PVL-positive CA-MRSA had increased levels of inflammatory markers, required longer ICU care, and had an increased rate of concomitant myositis or pyomyositis [63]. Children who had PVL-positive musculoskeletal infections were also more likely to develop complications such as deep venous thrombosis or chronic osteomyelitis [62].

CA-MRSA septic arthritis involving newly placed prosthetic joints also appears to be an emerging problem. A recent study at one institution found that five of nine prosthetic joint infections over 13 months were caused by CA-MRSA [64]. The authors have seen a similar rise in orthopedic postoperative infections caused by CA-MRSA at their institution (Larry Lambert, MPH, unpublished data, 2007). As a result, the authors now recommend vancomycin in place of cefazolin for all orthopedic surgery involving hardware, including joint replacement, in which preoperative prophylaxis is needed.

Diagnosis

The emergency department diagnosis of suspected septic arthritis begins with arthrocentesis and joint fluid analysis. Synovial aspirate can be inoculated directly into blood culture bottles for a higher yield [54]. Blood cultures, which are positive in up to one-third of cases [54], should be obtained before administration of antibiotics. The traditional threshold for the diagnosis and empiric treatment of septic arthritis—50,000 white blood cells (WBC)/mm in joint fluid—may be too stringent. Greater than one-third of patients who had culture-proven septic arthritis in a recent study fell below this threshold [65], and immunosuppressed patients may mount little or no leukocytosis in response to joint infection.

In established osteomyelitis, erythrocyte sedimentation rate and C-reactive protein levels almost always are elevated, but their utility for initial diagnosis is limited by poor specificity [61]. Blood cultures are a very important step in the initial evaluation, because they may identify an etiologic organism in 20% to 30% of cases. Additionally, if the patient is clinically stable, it may be appropriate to delay antibiotic treatment until bone cultures are obtained by needle aspiration or debridement. Plain radiographs are a reasonable first diagnostic step, but are unlikely to show bony changes until 10 to 14 days after the onset of infection [60]. MRI has supplanted nuclear bone scan in most centers as the best imaging modality for detecting osteomyelitis. MRI has high sensitivity for early inflammatory changes of bone and soft tissue.

Treatment

Optimal treatment of septic arthritis involves both intravenous antibiotics and repeated joint drainage and irrigation. Osteomyelitis can be treated with intravenous antibiotics alone, although surgical debridement of diseased bone and drainage of subperiosteal abscesses may be required. Vancomycin or clindamycin are recommended for empiric intravenous therapy of septic arthritis and osteomyelitis, to cover *S aureus* including CA-MRSA. Both agents also provide coverage of *Streptococcus pyogenes* and *Streptococcus pneumoniae*, which occasionally cause both osteomyelitis and septic arthritis. Clindamycin should be used with caution in communities with high rates of inducible clindamycin resistance in local CA-MRSA strains. Immunocompromised patients, those who have sickle cell disease, and injection drug users, also should receive appropriate gram-negative coverage. Although possibly effective in CA-MRSA bone and joint infections, linezolid and daptomycin have been studied very little in this setting and are not approved as empiric therapy (see Table 2) [12,46,54,60,62].

Community-acquired pneumonia

MRSA is a major cause of hospital-acquired and ventilator-acquired pneumonia; however, most of these nosocomial pneumonias are caused by multidrug resistant MRSA strains that are distinct from CA-MRSA. MSSA, on the other hand, is a well-recognized, although uncommon, cause of CAP, representing between 1% and 5% of cases [66]. Cases of lethal CAP in children, caused by CA-MRSA, were among the first CA-MRSA infections to be reported in the United States [2]. Although CA-MRSA CAP has proven to be quite rare, representing at most 2% of CA-MRSA infections [4], increasing reports of severe CA-MRSA pneumonia in young, healthy adults and children [9,67–72] have paralleled the increasing incidence of CA-MRSA SSTIs.

In communities where CA-MRSA has become endemic, it seems that a cycle exists involving CA-MRSA colonization (nasal and elsewhere), purulent skin infections, and spread between close contacts. This cycle occasionally gives rise to serious invasive infections such as pneumonia when host conditions are conducive. In support of this concept is the association, seen in multiple case reports, between CA-MRSA pneumonia and a prior history of CA-MRSA SSTI or close contact with an infected or colonized person [2,9,70,71]. A similar association between *S aureus* pneumonia and recent SSTI or nasal colonization was seen during the 1958 influenza epidemic [73].

Another major risk factor, and possibly a prerequisite, for CA-MRSA pneumonia is recent or concomitant influenza-like illness. *S aureus* pneumonia historically has been associated closely with viral respiratory infections, especially influenza A [73–75]. CA-MRSA pneumonia clusters have been related temporally to influenza A outbreaks [70,71], and in most cases reported thus far, CA-MRSA pneumonias have had a preceding influenza-like illness or proven influenza A infection [9,69,70]. It is believed that viral respiratory infections result in denuded respiratory epithelium to which PVL-positive *S aureus*, which demonstrates adherence to bronchial epithelial basement membrane, can attach [76,77]. Whether CA-MRSA pneumonia occurs at all in the absence of viral infection, for example in the summer, is not known.

CA-MRSA CAP frequently presents with hemoptysis and chest radiograph evidence of necrosis and carries a very high mortality rate. Panton-Valentine leukocidin appears to be central to the increased virulence and mortality seen in CA-MRSA CAP. Historically, less than 5% of *S aureus* strains have been PVL-positive [28,76], but even before the emergence of CA-MRSA, it was noted that 85% of *S aureus* isolates from necrotizing pneumonia were PVL-positive [28,70]. Autopsy in PVL-positive cases reveals *S aureus* adherent to bronchial epithelium, with underlying ulceration and tissue necrosis. Interstitial and alveolar hemorrhage is present, and cavities may erode into larger vessels, resulting in massive pulmonary hemorrhage [28,76]. In addition to causing lung necrosis and hemoptysis, when compared with PVL-negative *S aureus*, PVL-positive strains (MSSA and MRSA) tend to affect younger, healthier patients who have a history of preceding influenza-like illness [28,76].

The addition of the gene for PVL to PVL-negative *S aureus* renders it capable of causing a pneumonia-like illness in mice that resembles the necrotizing pneumonia seen in people [78]. Other pathogenic proteins, which appear to play a role in mortality in mouse models of *S aureus* pneumonia, also are up-regulated by PVL-producing strains [78]. The effects of PVL on neutrophils are postulated to underlie the characteristic necrosis, hemoptysis, and leukopenia seen in CA-MRSA pneumonia. Release of PVL causes neutrophil chemotaxis, activation, and release of cytotoxic elements, resulting in local tissue damage and neutrophil lysis [72,76,79].

Diagnosis

The clinical features of CA-MRSA pneumonia can include:

- Prodrome of influenza-like illness (or confirmed influenza A), onset in winter months
- Prior CA-MRSA SSTI, or contact with case
- Hemoptysis
- Hypotension
- Leukopenia
- Chest radiograph infiltrates with cavitation or ARDS-like pattern

The typical presentation of CA-MRSA pneumonia includes a prodrome of an influenza-like illness, and concomitant influenza A infection often can be confirmed. CA-MRSA pneumonia thus far has been reported only in the fall and winter months. The pneumonia is rapidly progressive, presenting with high fever, tachypnea, tachycardia, hypotension, and hemoptysis. Leukopenia is common [76]. Initial chest radiographic findings include uni- or multilobar infiltrates and an acute respiratory distress syndrome

(ARDS)-like pattern caused by alveolar hemorrhage [67,69]. Later in the course of disease, effusions and characteristic coalescing cavitary lesions may appear on chest radiograph because of necrosis of lung tissue. In most reported cases, septic shock develops. Mortality among case reports to date stands at 42% [2,9,68–71]. Clinicians should consider CA-MRSA in any case of severe pneumonia, pneumonia accompanied by hemoptysis or leukopenia, or pneumonia that occurs during influenza season.

Treatment

In addition to standard measures recommended in CAP guidelines for patients requiring hospitalization, such as blood cultures and rapid antibiotic administration, emergency department evaluation of suspected CA-MRSA CAP should include sputum Gram's stain and culture and rapid influenza A testing. Presence of gram-positive cocci in clusters in sputum can lead to early diagnosis and promote appropriate antibiotic choice [80]. The importance of sputum culture is underscored by one recent series in which CA-MRSA was recovered only from sputum samples in 30% of CA-MRSA pneumonia cases [71].

If CA-MRSA is considered a significant possibility, and the pneumonia is severe enough to require ICU level care, empiric therapy against MRSA should be administered immediately. The 2007 IDSA/ATS guidelines recommend adding either vancomycin or linezolid to standard ICU therapy for suspected CA-MRSA pneumonia, noting there are insufficient data to recommend one drug over the other [80]. In fact, there is significant controversy about whether vancomycin provides effective therapy for invasive CA-MRSA infections, particularly pneumonia [81]. Case reports have documented instances of vancomycin treatment failure in CA-MRSA CAP, followed by improvement after switching to linezolid [69]. Unlike linezolid, vancomycin is not concentrated in alveolar fluid and may not remain above minimum inhibitory concentration (MIC) in lung tissue long enough to be effective [82]. Linezolid and clindamycin significantly reduce PVL production, whereas vancomycin has no effect on protein synthesis [83,84]. On the other hand, linezolid is far more expensive than vancomycin and has been associated with serious adverse effects, such as myelosuppression and serotonin syndrome. One author has recommended the combination of clindamycin plus linezolid as preferred therapy for PVL-positive *S aureus* pneumonia based on the ability of each of these agents to reduce exotoxin production [72]. TMP-SMX is another available parenteral treatment option in patients unable to tolerate vancomycin or linezolid, although there is little experience with its use in this setting (see Table 2) [80].

To date, there are no pediatric pneumonia treatment guidelines addressing CA-MRSA CAP. Given the limited clinical experience with linezolid in children, however, vancomycin plus clindamycin probably remains the preferred treatment at this time for pediatric CA-MRSA CAP.

Because most patients who have CA-MRSA CAP are young and otherwise healthy, upon initial pneumonia severity assessment, they may meet criteria for a lower level of care or even outpatient therapy. However, ICU-level care should be considered strongly in any case of suspected CA-MRSA CAP that is treated with anti-MRSA therapy.

Infection control in the community and the emergency department

How to prevent recurrent CA-MRSA infections and how to control their spread in the community, hospital, and emergency department environments are critical questions. As noted previously in the section on epidemiology, there are only limited data so far addressing these questions. It is unclear to what extent lessons learned about decolonization and infection control in HA-MRSA can be applied to CA-MRSA. The epidemiology of CA-MRSA may more closely resemble that of MSSA than HA-MRSA, with crowding, repeated physical contact, inadequate hygiene, and skin trauma being the main conditions leading to colonization and infection. These conditions are found on sports teams, in correctional facilities, and among military recruits in basic training, where outbreaks have occurred [85–87]. Transmission of CA-MRSA may occur readily by means of fomites, such as the surface of wood saunas or shared towels [6,21], which has important implications for community and hospital infection control. The relationship between nasal colonization with CA-MRSA and infection is uncertain. There is some longitudinal evidence that, like MSSA, CA-MRSA colonization comes and goes over time among individuals, unrelated to antibiotic exposure or decolonization therapy [87]. Although CA-MRSA nasal colonization appears to substantially increase the risk of a CA-MRSA SSTI, nasal colonization is also frequently absent from patients who have CA-MRSA infections [14,87]. The likelihood that CA-MRSA colonizes other areas of the body such as the axilla and groin should be considered when prescribing decolonization measures and argues against relying on a positive nares culture as a criterion for decolonization.

Decolonization

Despite uncertainty about CA-MRSA epidemiology and infection control strategies, there are situations where emergency physicians may wish to attempt to decolonize a patient or eradicate CA-MRSA from all members of a household. Although there are limited published recommendations on this topic [30], it seems reasonable to attempt decolonization in the following settings:

- Patients who have experienced multiple CA-MRSA SSTIs over a 1-year period
- Households in which multiple members have been infected
- Households with very young, very old, or immunosuppressed members

Outbreaks in larger cohorts, such as schools or sports teams, should be managed by local health departments. In prescribing a decolonization strategy, first and foremost, patients should be educated about nonpharmacologic measures to eradicate CA-MRSA and prevent its spread. Measures to remove and prevent the spread of CA-MRSA in the community setting include:

- Keep draining wounds covered with a clean bandage.
- Wash hands frequently with soap and water or alcohol-based hand gel and always wash after touching infected wounds or soiled bandages.
- Maintain good general hygiene with regular bathing.
- Launder clothing that is contaminated by wound drainage.
- Do not share contaminated items like towels, bedding, clothing, and razors.
- While there is wound drainage, do not participate in activities involving skin-to-skin contact or in contact sports.
- Clean contaminated environmental surfaces and equipment with a detergent or disinfectant that specifies *S aureus* on the label.

Secondly, it is important to recognize that studies of various pharmacologic decolonization strategies for MRSA have demonstrated only limited efficacy, with most placebo-controlled trials showing no significant long-term benefit in the active treatment arm [88]. There are no published trials of CA-MRSA decolonization. Successful sustained decolonization of an individual or a cohort probably requires a multifaceted approach aimed at intranasal and extranasal sites [89] and environmental cleaning. It is unclear whether systemic antibiotics are necessary once active infections are treated. Finally, short treatment courses (3 to 7 days), which can be repeated if necessary at monthly intervals, are recommended to prevent development of resistance.

At the authors' institution, in the rare case when decolonization seems warranted and compliance likely, the authors have prescribed a combination of intranasal mupirocin ointment, chlorhexidine body washes, and oral rifampin plus TMP-SMX, all twice daily for 5 days. Intranasal mupirocin ointment is recommended by most sources [30,33]. It also can be applied under fingernails. Unfortunately, widespread use of mupirocin has led to the emergence of mupirocin-resistant CA-MRSA in Australia and Canada [90,91]. Chlorhexidine soap is expensive; bathing with dilute bleach is an inexpensive but unproven alternative. Tea tree oil-containing soaps and ointments have been advocated as an alternative to mupirocin and chlorhexidine. Tea tree oil has in vitro MRSA activity but has undergone only limited clinical testing [92]. Rifampin is used for systemic decolonization therapy, because it penetrates the nasal mucosa well. Rifampin monotherapy, however, results in rapid development of resistance, so it should be combined with another inexpensive, narrow-spectrum twice-a-day antibiotic like TMP-SMX or doxycycline (see Table 2).

Hospital infection control

Developing rational strategies to prevent the spread of CA-MRSA in the emergency department and hospital environment is a considerable challenge. At public hospitals where CA-MRSA is prevalent, such efforts easily could overwhelm scarce resources. The traditional hospital infection control paradigm of nasal swab screening for MRSA, isolation of colonized patients, and decolonization therapy is not suited well to the control of CA-MRSA. It may make more sense to screen emergency department and hospitalized patients for active SSTIs, and to isolate these patients, even without nasal swab or wound culture data. On the other hand, traditional measures used to limit hospital spread of MRSA by means of contaminated hands and fomites may apply well to CA-MRSA. Hand hygiene means using gloves, changing them between patients, and washing hands between patients even when gloves are used. Good hand hygiene is considered the most important barrier to nosocomial MRSA transmission [93]. Hospital fomites such as gurney surfaces, computer terminals, and mops can be colonized with MRSA, and these are believed to be another important vehicle for MRSA spread within the hospital [93]. Transmission by means of fomites has been implicated in community outbreaks of CA-MRSA [6], and CA-MRSA has been found on emergency department curtains, charts, and door keypads [94,95].

The emergency department environment presents a unique set of infection control challenges. Patients presenting with CA-MRSA SSTIs frequently have lesions that are draining and uncovered. While waiting to be seen, these patients share chairs, bathrooms, and vending machines with uninfected patients. In a high-volume emergency department, there may be inadequate resources to decontaminate blood pressure cuffs and stethoscopes between patients in triage, let alone to frequently decontaminate surfaces in a public waiting area. Moreover, patients who have typical CA-MRSA SSTIs may return to the emergency department multiple times for postsurgical care. Processes should be developed to rapidly identify and effectively isolate these cases. In the emergency department, isolation might mean simply ensuring maximal distance between patient gurneys and strict adherence to universal precautions, or it might involve cohorting of SSTI cases.

Finally, there is the issue of whether emergency staff are at increased risk of acquiring CA-MRSA (as identified genetically or by antibiotic susceptibility pattern). Health care worker colonization with MRSA is well-documented, and this phenomenon has been implicated in the spread of HA-MRSA within ICUs [93]. CA-MRSA infections have occurred occasionally in emergency department personnel [96], and it has been assumed the infections were acquired at work. Preliminary studies examining CA-MRSA colonization in emergency department personnel, however, have found rates of only 0% to 5% [97–99], similar to rates from community surveillance. These data suggest that routine universal precautions protect health care workers from acquiring

CA-MRSA in the workplace, and that patient-to-patient spread by means of colonized emergency department personnel is unlikely to occur.

Summary

The emergence of CA-MRSA has had—and will continue to have—a major impact on the practice of emergency medicine. The deluge of CA-MRSA SSTIs presenting to emergency departments requires that efficient, evidence-based management strategies be adopted. Because CA-MRSA is now a possible cause of necrotizing fasciitis, musculoskeletal infections, and severe pneumonia, recommended empiric treatment of all of these infections has changed. Research is underway to investigate optimal treatment and infection control strategies and to develop new antibiotics and a vaccine. Clinicians will have to stay abreast of the literature and modify practice as new evidence comes on line.

References

[1] Herold BC, Immergluck LC, Maranan MC, et al. Community-acquired methicillin-resistant Staphylococcus aureus in children with no identified predisposing risk. JAMA 1998;279:593–8.
[2] From the Centers for Disease Control and Prevention. Four pediatric deaths from community-acquired methicillin-resistant Staphylococcus aureus–Minnesota and North Dakota, 1997–1999. JAMA 1999;282:1123–5.
[3] Naimi TS, LeDell KH, Como-Sabetti K, et al. Comparison of community- and health care-associated methicillin-resistant Staphylococcus aureus infection. JAMA 2003;290:2976–84.
[4] Fridkin SK, Hageman JC, Morrison M, et al. Methicillin-Resistant Staphylococcus aureus Disease in Three Communities. N Engl J Med 2005;352:1436–44.
[5] Community-associated methicillin-resistant Staphylococcus aureus infections in Pacific Islanders–Hawaii, 2001–2003. MMWR Morb Mortal Wkly Rep 2004;53:767–70.
[6] Baggett HC, Hennessy TW, Rudolph K, et al. Community-Onset Methicillin-Resistant Staphylococcus aureus Associated with Antibiotic Use and the Cytotoxin Panton-Valentine Leukocidin during a Furunculosis Outbreak in Rural Alaska. J Infect Dis 2004;189:1565–73.
[7] Moran GJ, Krishnadasan A, Gorwitz RJ, et al. Methicillin-resistant S. aureus infections among patients in the emergency department. N Engl J Med 2006;355:666–74.
[8] Kaplan SL, Hulten KG, Gonzalez BE, et al. Three-year surveillance of community-acquired Staphylococcus aureus infections in children. Clin Infect Dis 2005;40:1785–91.
[9] Francis JS, Doherty MC, Lopatin U, et al. Severe community-onset pneumonia in healthy adults caused by methicillin-resistant Staphylococcus aureus carrying the Panton-Valentine leukocidin genes. Clin Infect Dis 2005;40:100–7.
[10] Miller LG, Perdreau-Remington F, Rieg G, et al. Necrotizing Fasciitis Caused by Community-Associated Methicillin-Resistant Staphylococcus aureus in Los Angeles. N Engl J Med 2005;352:1445–53.
[11] Ruiz ME, Yohannes S, Wladyka CG. Pyomyositis Caused by Methicillin-Resistant Staphylococcus aureus. N Engl J Med 2005;352:1488–9.
[12] Arnold SR, Elias D, Buckingham SC, et al. Changing patterns of acute hematogenous osteomyelitis and septic arthritis: emergence of community-associated methicillin-resistant Staphylococcus aureus. J Pediatr Orthop 2006;26:703–8.
[13] Pan ES, Diep BA, Carleton HA, et al. Increasing prevalence of methicillin-resistant Staphylococcus aureus infection in California jails. Clin Infect Dis 2003;37:1384–8.

[14] Frazee BW, Lynn J, Charlebois ED, et al. High prevalence of methicillin-resistant Staphylococcus aureus in emergency department skin and soft tissue infections. Ann Emerg Med 2005;45:311–20.

[15] Donnio PY, Preney L, Gautier-Lerestif AL, et al. Changes in staphylococcal cassette chromosome type and antibiotic resistance profile in methicillin-resistant Staphylococcus aureus isolates from a French hospital over an 11 year period. J Antimicrob Chemother 2004;53: 808–13.

[16] Seybold U, Kourbatova EV, Johnson JG, et al. Emergence of community-associated methicillin-resistant Staphylococcus aureus USA300 genotype as a major cause of health care-associated blood stream infections. Clin Infect Dis 2006;42:647–56.

[17] Ala'Aldeen D. A non-multiresistant community MRSA exposes its genome. Lancet 2002; 359:1791–2.

[18] Hota B, Ellenbogen C, Hayden MK, et al. Community-associated methicillin-resistant Staphylococcus aureus skin and soft tissue infections at a public hospital: do public housing and incarceration amplify transmission? Arch Intern Med 2007;167:1026–33.

[19] Graham PL 3rd, Lin SX, Larson EL. A U.S. population-based survey of Staphylococcus aureus colonization. Ann Intern Med 2006;144:318–25.

[20] Zafar U, Johnson LB, Hanna M, et al. Prevalence of nasal colonization among patients with community-associated methicillin-resistant Staphylococcus aureus infection and their household contacts. Infect Control Hosp Epidemiol 2007;28:966–9.

[21] Kazakova SV, Hageman JC, Matava M, et al. A clone of methicillin-resistant Staphylococcus aureus among professional football players. N Engl J Med 2005;352:468–75.

[22] Sattler CA, Mason EO Jr, Kaplan SL. Prospective comparison of risk factors and demographic and clinical characteristics of community-acquired, methicillin-resistant versus methicillin-susceptible Staphylococcus aureus infection in children. Pediatr Infect Dis J 2002;21:910–7.

[23] Frank AL, Marcinak JF, Mangat PD, et al. Clindamycin treatment of methicillin-resistant Staphylococcus aureus infections in children. Pediatr Infect Dis J 2002;21:530–4.

[24] Hasty MB, Klasner A, Kness S, et al. Cutaneous community-associated methicillin-resistant staphylococcus aureus among all skin and soft-tissue infections in two geographically distant pediatric emergency departments. Acad Emerg Med 2007;14:35–40.

[25] Daum RS. Skin and Soft-Tissue Infections Caused by Methicillin-Resistant Staphylococcus aureus. N Engl J Med 2007;357:380–90.

[26] Cohen PR. Community-acquired methicillin-resistant Staphylococcus aureus skin infections : implications for patients and practitioners. Am J Clin Dermatol 2007;8:259–70.

[27] Ward PD, Turner WH. Identification of staphylococcal Panton-Valentine leukocidin as a potent dermonecrotic toxin. Infect Immun 1980;28:393–7.

[28] Lina G, Piemont Y, Godail-Gamot F, et al. Involvement of Panton-Valentine leukocidin-producing Staphylococcus aureus in primary skin infections and pneumonia. Clin Infect Dis 1999;29:1128–32.

[29] Egan DJ, Pelletier AJ, Hooper DC, et al. 183: Trends in U.S. Emergency Department Visits for Skin and Soft Tissue Infections in the Age of Methicillin-Resistant Staphylococcus aureus, 1993–2004. Annals of Emergency Medicine 2007;50:S58.

[30] Gorwitz RJ, Jernigan DB, Powers JH, et al. Strategies for clinical management of MRSA in the community: Summary of an experts' meeting convened by the Centers for Disease Control and Prevention. 2006.

[31] Ruhe JJ, Smith N, Bradsher RW, et al. Community-Onset Methicillin-Resistant Staphylococcus aureus Skin and Soft-Tissue Infections: Impact of Antimicrobial Therapy on Outcome. Clin Infect Dis 2007;44:777–84.

[32] Squire BT, Fox JC, Anderson C. ABSCESS: applied bedside sonography for convenient evaluation of superficial soft tissue infections. Acad Emerg Med 2005;12:601–6.

[33] Stevens DL, Bisno AL, Chambers HF, et al. Practice guidelines for the diagnosis and management of skin and soft-tissue infections. Clin Infect Dis 2005;41:1373–406.

[34] Abrahamian FM, Shroff SD. Use of routine wound cultures to evaluate cutaneous abscesses for community-associated methicillin-resistant Staphylococcus aureus. Ann Emerg Med 2007;50:66–7.

[35] Rutherford WH, Hart D, Calderwood JW, et al. Antibiotics in surgical treatment of septic lesions. Lancet 1970;1:1077–80.

[36] Llera JL, Levy RC. Treatment of cutaneous abscess: a double-blind clinical study. Ann Emerg Med 1985;14:15–9.

[37] Hankin A, Everett WW. Are antibiotics necessary after incision and drainage of a cutaneous abscess? Ann Emerg Med 2007;50:49–51.

[38] Rajendran PM, Young D, Maurer T, et al. Randomized, Double-Blind, Placebo-Controlled Trial of Cephalexin for Treatment of Uncomplicated Skin Abscesses in a Population at Risk for Community-Acquired Methicillin-Resistant Staphylococcus aureus Infection. Antimicrob Agents Chemother 2007;51:4044–8.

[39] Lee MC, Rios AM, Aten MF, et al. Management and outcome of children with skin and soft tissue abscesses caused by community-acquired methicillin-resistant Staphylococcus aureus. Pediatr Infect Dis J 2004;23:123–7.

[40] Fergie JE, Purcell K. Community-acquired methicillin-resistant Staphylococcus aureus infections in south Texas children. Pediatr Infect Dis J 2001;20:860–3.

[41] Young DM, Harris HW, Charlebois ED, et al. An epidemic of methicillin-resistant Staphylococcus aureus soft tissue infections among medically underserved patients. Arch Surg 2004;139:947–51, discussion 51–3.

[42] Chuck EA, Frazee BW, Lambert L, et al. Benefit of Algorithmic Empiric Treatment of Community-Acquired Methicillin-resistant Staphylococcus aureus Skin and Soft Tissue Infections. J Emerg Med 2008 (in press).

[43] Micek ST. Alternatives to vancomycin for the treatment of methicillin-resistant Staphylococcus aureus infections. Clin Infect Dis 2007;45(Suppl 3):S184–90.

[44] Dehority W, Wang E, Vernon PS, et al. Community-associated methicillin-resistant Staphylococcus aureus necrotizing fasciitis in a neonate. Pediatr Infect Dis J 2006;25:1080–1.

[45] Lee YT, Lin JC, Wang NC, et al. Necrotizing fasciitis in a medical center in northern Taiwan: emergence of methicillin-resistant Staphylococcus aureus in the community. J Microbiol Immunol Infect 2007;40:335–41.

[46] Gilbert DN, Moellering RC Jr, Eliopoulos GM, et al. The Sanford Guide to Antimicrobial Therapy, 2006. 36th edition. Sperryville, VA: Antimicrobial Therapy, Inc.; 2006.

[47] Nizet V. Myositis and Pyomyositis. In: Long SS, Pickering LK, Prober CG, editors. Principles and Practice of Pediatric Infectious Diseases. 2nd edition. Philadelphia: Churchill Livingstone; 2003.

[48] Crum NF. Bacterial pyomyositis in the United States. Am J Med 2004;117:420–8.

[49] Pasternack MS, Swartz MN. Myositis. In: Mandell GM, Bennett JE, Dolin R, editors. Mandell, Douglas, and Bennett's: Principles and Practice of Infectious Diseases. 6th edition. Philadelphia: Churchill Livingstone; 2005.

[50] Pannaraj PS, Hulten KG, Gonzalez BE, et al. Infective pyomyositis and myositis in children in the era of community-acquired, methicillin-resistant Staphylococcus aureus infection. Clin Infect Dis 2006;43:953–60.

[51] Chiedozi LC. Pyomyositis. Review of 205 cases in 112 patients. Am J Surg 1979;137:255–9.

[52] Levin MJ, Gardner P. "Tropical" pyomyositis: an unusual infection due to Staphylococcus aureus. N Engl J Med 1971;284:196–8.

[53] Spiegel DA, Meyer JS, Dormans JP, et al. Pyomyositis in children and adolescents: report of 12 cases and review of the literature. J Pediatr Orthop 1999;19:143–50.

[54] Ross JJ. Septic arthritis. Infect Dis Clin North Am 2005;19:799–817.

[55] Sharp JT, Lidsky MD, Duffy J, et al. Infectious arthritis. Arch Intern Med 1979;139:1125–30.

[56] Ross JJ, Saltzman CL, Carling P, et al. Pneumococcal septic arthritis: review of 190 cases. Clin Infect Dis 2003;36:319–27.

[57] Weston VC, Jones AC, Bradbury N, et al. Clinical features and outcome of septic arthritis in a single UK Health District 1982–1991. Ann Rheum Dis 1999;58:214–9.

[58] Goldenberg DL, Cohen AS. Acute infectious arthritis. A review of patients with nongonococcal joint infections (with emphasis on therapy and prognosis). Am J Med 1976;60:369–77.

[59] Berbari EF, Steckelberg JM, Osmon DR. Osteomyelitis. In: Mandell GM, Bennett JE, Dolin R, editors. Mandell, Douglas, and Bennett's: Principles and Practice of Infectious Diseases. 6th edition. Philadelphia: Churchill Livingstone; 2005.

[60] Kaplan SL. Osteomyelitis in children. Infect Dis Clin North Am 2005;19:787–97, vii.

[61] Lew DP, Waldvogel FA. Osteomyelitis. Lancet 2004;364:369–79.

[62] Martinez-Aguilar G, Avalos-Mishaan A, Hulten K, et al. Community-acquired, methicillin-resistant and methicillin-susceptible Staphylococcus aureus musculoskeletal infections in children. Pediatr Infect Dis J 2004;23:701–6.

[63] Bocchini CE, Hulten KG, Mason EO Jr, et al. Panton-Valentine leukocidin genes are associated with enhanced inflammatory response and local disease in acute hematogenous Staphylococcus aureus osteomyelitis in children. Pediatrics 2006;117:433–40.

[64] Kourbatova EV, Halvosa JS, King MD, et al. Emergence of community-associated methicillin-resistant Staphylococcus aureus USA 300 clone as a cause of health care-associated infections among patients with prosthetic joint infections. Am J Infect Control 2005;33:385–91.

[65] Li SF, Henderson J, Dickman E, et al. Laboratory tests in adults with monoarticular arthritis: can they rule out a septic joint? Acad Emerg Med 2004;11:276–80.

[66] Bartlett JG, Mundy LM. Community-acquired pneumonia. N Engl J Med 1995;333: 1618–24.

[67] Boussaud V, Parrot A, Mayaud C, et al. Life-threatening hemoptysis in adults with community-acquired pneumonia due to Panton-Valentine leukocidin-secreting Staphylococcus aureus. Intensive Care Med 2003;29:1840–3.

[68] Frazee BW, Salz TO, Lambert L, et al. Fatal community-associated methicillin-resistant Staphylococcus aureus pneumonia in an immunocompetent young adult. Ann Emerg Med 2005;46:401–4.

[69] Micek ST, Dunne M, Kollef MH. Pleuropulmonary complications of Panton-Valentine leukocidin-positive community-acquired methicillin-resistant Staphylococcus aureus: importance of treatment with antimicrobials inhibiting exotoxin production. Chest 2005;128:2732–8.

[70] Hageman JC, Uyeki TM, Francis JS, et al. Severe community-acquired pneumonia due to Staphylococcus aureus, 2003–04 influenza season. Emerg Infect Dis 2006;12:894–9.

[71] Severe methicillin-resistant Staphylococcus aureus community-acquired pneumonia associated with influenza–Louisiana and Georgia, December 2006-January 2007. MMWR Morb Mortal Wkly Rep 2007;56:325–9.

[72] Morgan MS. Diagnosis and treatment of Panton-Valentine leukocidin (PVL)-associated staphylococcal pneumonia. Int J Antimicrob Agents 2007;30:289–96.

[73] Goslings WR, Mulder J, Djajadiningrat J, et al. Staphylococcal pneumonia in influenza in relation to antecedent staphylococcal skin infection. Lancet 1959;2:428–30.

[74] Chickering HT, Park JH. Staphylococcus aureus pneumonia. JAMA 1919;72:617–26.

[75] Schwarzmann SW, Adler JL, Sullivan RJ Jr, et al. Bacterial pneumonia during the Hong Kong influenza epidemic of 1968–1969. Arch Intern Med 1971;127:1037–41.

[76] Gillet Y, Issartel B, Vanhems P, et al. Association between Staphylococcus aureus strains carrying gene for Panton-Valentine leukocidin and highly lethal necrotising pneumonia in young immunocompetent patients. Lancet 2002;359:753–9.

[77] de Bentzmann S, Tristan A, Etienne J, et al. Staphylococcus aureus isolates associated with necrotizing pneumonia bind to basement membrane type I and IV collagens and laminin. J Infect Dis 2004;190:1506–15.

[78] Labandeira-Rey M, Couzon F, Boisset S, et al. Staphylococcus aureus Panton-Valentine leukocidin causes necrotizing pneumonia. Science 2007;315:1130–3.

[79] Deresinski S. Methicillin-resistant Staphylococcus aureus: an evolutionary, epidemiologic, and therapeutic odyssey. Clin Infect Dis 2005;40:562–73.

[80] Mandell LA, Wunderink RG, Anzueto A, et al. Infectious Diseases Society of America/ American Thoracic Society consensus guidelines on the management of community-acquired pneumonia in adults. Clin Infect Dis 2007;44(Suppl 2):S27–72.

[81] Deresinski S. Counterpoint: Vancomycin and Staphylococcus aureus–an antibiotic enters obsolescence. Clin Infect Dis 2007;44:1543–8.

[82] Scheetz MH, Wunderink RG, Postelnick MJ, et al. Potential impact of vancomycin pulmonary distribution on treatment outcomes in patients with methicillin-resistant Staphylococcus aureus pneumonia. Pharmacotherapy 2006;26:539–50.

[83] Dumitrescu O, Boisset S, Badiou C, et al. Effect of antibiotics on Staphylococcus aureus producing Panton-Valentine leukocidin. Antimicrob Agents Chemother 2007;51:1515–9.

[84] Stevens DL, Ma Y, Salmi DB, et al. Impact of antibiotics on expression of virulence-associated exotoxin genes in methicillin-sensitive and methicillin-resistant Staphylococcus aureus. J Infect Dis 2007;195:202–11.

[85] Methicillin-resistant Staphylococcus aureus infections in correctional facilities—Georgia, California, and Texas, 2001–2003. MMWR Morb Mortal Wkly Rep 2003;52:992–6.

[86] Methicillin-resistant staphylococcus aureus infections among competitive sports participants–Colorado, Indiana, Pennsylvania, and Los Angeles County, 2000–2003. MMWR Morb Mortal Wkly Rep 2003;52:793–5.

[87] Ellis MW, Hospenthal DR, Dooley DP, et al. Natural history of community-acquired methicillin-resistant Staphylococcus aureus colonization and infection in soldiers. Clin Infect Dis 2004;39:971–9.

[88] Loeb M, Main C, Walker-Dilks C, et al. Antimicrobial drugs for treating methicillin-resistant Staphylococcus aureus colonization. Cochrane Database Syst Rev 2003;CD003340.

[89] Simor AE, Phillips E, McGeer A, et al. Randomized controlled trial of chlorhexidine gluconate for washing, intranasal mupirocin, and rifampin and doxycycline versus no treatment for the eradication of methicillin-resistant Staphylococcus aureus colonization. Clin Infect Dis 2007;44:178–85.

[90] Torvaldsen S, Roberts C, Riley TV. The continuing evolution of methicillin-resistant Staphylococcus aureus in Western Australia. Infect Control Hosp Epidemiol 1999;20:133–5.

[91] Simor AE, Stuart TL, Louie L, et al. Mupirocin-resistant, methicillin-resistant Staphylococcus aureus strains in Canadian hospitals. Antimicrob Agents Chemother 2007;51: 3880–6.

[92] Flaxman D, Griffiths P. Is tea tree oil effective at eradicating MRSA colonization? A review. Br J Community Nurs 2005;10:123–6.

[93] Henderson DK. Managing methicillin-resistant staphylococci: a paradigm for preventing nosocomial transmission of resistant organisms. Am J Med 2006;119:S45–52, discussion S62–70.

[94] Huang R, Mehta S, Weed D, et al. Methicillin-resistant Staphylococcus aureus survival on hospital fomites. Infect Control Hosp Epidemiol 2006;27:1267–9.

[95] Kei J, Richards JR. 188: The Prevalence of Methicillin-Resistant Staphylococcus aureus on Frequently Touched Objects in an Urban Emergency Department. Annals of Emergency Medicine 2007;50:S59–60.

[96] Storch J, Jacoby JL, Heller M. Community-Associated Methicillin Resistant Staphylococcus Aureus in an Emergency Medicine Resident: Lessons Learned. Annals of Emergency Medicine 2005;46:384–5.

[97] Hern G Jr, Singh A, Frazee B. 102: Low Rate of MRSA Colonization Among Residents. Acad Emerg Med 2007;14:S46.

[98] Nardi A, Hansen KN, Witting M, et al. 189: Low Levels of MRSA Nasal Carriage in Emergency Physicians and their Household Contacts. Annals of Emergency Medicine 2007; 50:S60.

[99] Suffoletto B, Cannon E, Ilkhanipour K, et al. 100: The Local Prevalence of Nasal Colonization of Methicillin-Resistant Staphylococcus Aureus in Emergency Department Personnel. Acad Emerg Med 2007;14:S45-a-.

ELSEVIER
SAUNDERS

Emerg Med Clin N Am
26 (2008) 457–473

EMERGENCY
MEDICINE
CLINICS OF
NORTH AMERICA

Management of Oral and Genital Herpes in the Emergency Department

Howard K. Mell, MD, MPH[a,b,*]

[a]Department of Emergency Medicine, College of Medicine,
The Ohio State University, Columbus, OH, USA
[b]The Ohio State University Medical Centers, Center for Emergency Medical Services,
141 Means Hall, 1654 Upham Drive, Columbus, OH 43210–1228, USA

The herpes family of viruses (or Herpesviridae) comprises double-stranded DNA viruses whose capsids display icosahedral symmetry (similar to a soccer ball) and are wrapped in a bilipid layered envelope [1]. These viruses are responsible for several medically important infections. Members of this family include: herpes simplex virus 1 (HSV-1), herpes simplex virus 2 (HSV-2), varicella-zoster virus (VZV), cytomegalovirus (CMV), Epstein-Barr virus (EBV), human herpesvirus 6 (HHV-6), human herpesvirus 7 (HHV-7), and human herpesvirus 8 (HHV-8) [2]. Although there are more than 80 identified herpesviruses, only 8 are thought to infect humans commonly [2], and a ninth (herpesvirus simiae) has caused fatal or severely debilitating encephalomyelitis after zoonotic infection in untreated individuals [3]. A list of the common illnesses caused by human herpesvirus infections is included in Table 1.

The epidemiology of oral and genital herpes has changed dramatically over the past several years [7–12]. This is especially important to the practice of emergency medicine, because between 5% and 10% of patients seeking care for a sexually transmitted disease (STD) do so in an emergency department [13]. In 2006, the Centers for Disease Control and Prevention (CDC) released new guidelines regarding the treatment of STDs [12]. The CDC makes specific recommendations concerning the screening, confirmatory testing, treatment, and counseling of patients who have oral or genital herpes infections [12]. Other literature suggests changes to common practices regarding herpes, given its changing epidemiology.

---

* Department of Emergency Medicine, Center for Emergency Medical Services, 141 Means Hall, 1654 Upham Drive, Columbus, OH 43210–1228.

E-mail address: howard.mell@osumc.edu

0733-8627/08/$ - see front matter © 2008 Elsevier Inc. All rights reserved.
doi:10.1016/j.emc.2008.02.001

458   MELL

Table 1
Common illnesses caused by human herpesviruses by type

Common name	Abbreviation	Human herpesvirus	Common illness
Herpes simplex virus-1	HSV-1	HHV-1	Mucosal lesions (oral and genital)
Herpes simplex virus-2	HSV-2	HHV-2	Mucosal lesions (oral and genital)
Varicella zoster virus	VZV	HHV-3	Chickenpox and shingles
Epstein-Barr virus	EBV	HHV-4	Infectious mononucleosis, lymphoproliferative disorders [4]
Cytomegalovirus	CMV	HHV-5	Febrile hepatitis [5]
Roseolovirus		HHV-6 (subtypes a and b)	Roseola, undifferentiated febrile illness
		HHV-7	Roseola, undifferentiated febrile illness (higher incidence of febrile seizure [6])
Kaposi's sarcoma–associated herpesvirus	KSHV	HHV-8	Lymphoproliferative disorders [4]

Pathophysiology of herpes

Infection with a Herpesviridae virus is a multistep process. Specific glycoproteins on the viral envelope interact with specific cell membrane receptors [14–18]. Differences in these cell membrane receptors may play a significant role in the expression of the disease [14,17,18]. Once bound to the host cell, the viral DNA and capsid are internalized and the viral DNA migrates to the cell nucleus. Once inside the nucleus, viral DNA is replicated and viral genes are transcribed. One viral gene encodes for latency-associated transcripts (LATs) [16]. Once replicated, these LATs can accumulate in a host cell and persist in the host in a latent state [19]. Reactivation of LATs results in several organic diseases. Although primary infection can be accompanied by a period of clinical illness, long-term latency is symptom-free. If reactivated, transcription of specific signaling genes contained in the LATs occurs and virus production restarts [20]. Often, reactivation leads to host cell death and clinical symptoms (ie, lymphadenopathy, fever, headache, malaise, rash). Reactivation can result from local trauma (ie, surgery, dental procedures, burns [21], fever [2], or sunlight [21]).

This latency and reactivation are unique characteristics of the Herpesviridae viruses [2]. Viral invasion of epithelial cells and intracellular viral replication at the site of primary exposure frequently occur after exposure to a herpesvirus [2]. After the primary infection, which may be devoid of clinical symptoms, herpesviruses ascend in a retrograde manner along sensory nerve sheaths to the trigeminal, cervical, lumbosacral, or autonomic ganglia [2]. There, the virus replicates—undetected by the host's immune surveillance—and persists in a dormant state, often for the life of the host [2].

The Herpesviridae viruses are differentiated into subgroups based on their expression of specific genes [1,2]. These α, β, and γ genes, respectively, control translation of the viral genome, transcription of the proteins essential for viral DNA synthesis, and the collection and exit of viral particles from the infected cell [2]. Expression of these genes defines each herpesvirus as a member of the α, β, or γ subgroup.

Human herpesviruses in the α subfamily (HSV-1, HSV-2, and VZV) exert a cytopathic effect on infected host cells [2]. This cell destruction leads to the characteristic vesicular lesions of infection with α subgroup Herpesviridae viruses through the separation of the epithelium and blister formation [2,22]. The infected cells become multinucleated giant cells and demonstrate ballooning degeneration [22], which may be seen on a Tzanck smear taken from a lesion. A Tzanck smear may also reveal intranuclear inclusion bodies in infected cells [23]. Viruses of other Herpesviridae subgroups (eg, CMV [β subgroup], EBV [γ subgroup]) are also cytopathic but markedly less so. The α-subfamily viruses are transmitted by a variety of mechanisms, including sexual, close contact, and airborne (by means of respiratory secretions) [24]. Herpes α-subfamily viruses often produce infections that reactivate after a period of latency [25–27]. These reactivations may be accompanied by symptoms or may be clinically silent [25–27].

The incubation period for a primary infection with an α subfamily herpesviridae ranges between 2 and 12 days [28]. Vesicles generally erupt 6 to 48 hours after the onset of a prodrome [2,28,29] regardless of whether they result from primary infection or reactivation. Lesions associated with primary infections generally take longer to form and persist for a greater length of time [2,28,29] but rarely persist for longer than 2 weeks. Viral shedding can continue for days to weeks after clinical resolution [28,30].

Epidemiology

HSV-1 is an α-subfamily herpesvirus that has traditionally been associated with orofacial herpes or "cold sores." HSV-1 is most often transmitted during childhood in a nonsexual manner, and the overall seropositive rate in the United States population is 65.3% (95% confidence interval [CI]: 62.6–68.0) by the fourth decade of life [7].

HSV-1 infections are generally asymptomatic, and the primary infection may go unnoticed. When they do become clinically relevant, infections usually manifest as orolabial or facial vesicular lesions [7]. These lesions are vesicular and painful, described as burning and intensely itching. Recurrent lesions are generally preceded by 6 hours of local burning or numbness and lymphadenopathy [2]. In primary infections, the prodrome is often more severe, including fever, malaise, myalgias, loss of appetite, and headache, and can last from 24 to 48 hours [2,30].

Primary and recurrent HSV-1 infections can involve the facial, nasal, ocular, or genital mucosa or digits [31]. An infected individual may "autoinoculate" or self-infect by spreading the virus from one infected anatomic area to another when the virus is being shed [32]. (In one study, 67% of patients presenting with herpes simplex labialis [HSL] were found to have to have HSV-1 on their hands [33]). Autoinoculation is more likely to occur with primary (as opposed to recurrent) infections and is more likely in HSV-1 as opposed to HSV-2 infections [31,32]. Patients seen in the emergency department with suspected or confirmed HSV-1 primary infections should be warned of this possibility and instructed regarding fastidious personal hygiene. Sharing of kitchen utensils, kissing, and other oral contacts, including oral-genital sexual activity, should be avoided [25]. Patients should be encouraged to wash their hands frequently [25]. Viral shedding (therefore contagion) begins with the prodrome and can continue for as long as several weeks after a primary infection or for as short as 3 to 5 days after a recurrence [28,30]. There is some concern that an infected health care worker could be a source of nosocomial herpes infection [34]. Literature suggests that HSV-1 and HSV-2 can persist on inanimate surfaces for between 4.5 hours and 8 weeks [34]. Therefore, without proper hand washing, nosocomial transmission is theoretically possible.

HSV-2 is an α-subfamily herpesvirus that has traditionally been associated with genital herpes. HSV-2 is almost always transmitted by means of sexual contact [12], and the overall seropositive rate in the US population is 26.4% (95% CI: 24.3–28.7) by the fourth decade of life, with women far more likely than men to be infected (33.9% versus 18.6%; $P = .001$) [7]. In an analysis of the US National Health and Nutrition Examination Surveys (NHANES) database from 1999 through 2004, HSV-2 was found to be associated with "persons who were divorced, separated, or widowed; those living below the poverty level; who had ever used cocaine; and who had sex for the first time at the age of 17 years or younger" [7].

HSV-2 infection is difficult to differentiate from HSV-1 infection based on clinical presentation alone [12]. It is important to differentiate the two to educate patients properly regarding the likely source of their disease, however, and to make decisions regarding the need for suppression therapy. Because nearly all HSV-2 infections are sexually transmitted, the presence of type-specific HSV-2 antibody implies anogenital infection [12]. The CDC recommends that all patients who test positive for type-specific HSV-2 antibodies be provided with counseling as though they have genital herpes, even in the absence of clinical symptoms [12].

Recently, HSV-1 has played a larger role in genital herpes infections in developing countries [8–11], especially in young adults [35]. It has been suggested that HSV-1 may now be more prevalent than HSV-2 in first episodes of genital herpes [36,37]. The presumed mechanism for these infections is oral-genital contact [38]. This has a significant impact on the effort extended toward herpes prevention. The public perception of genital herpes is that it is solely an STD arising from sexual intercourse with an infected partner. In fact, autoinoculation is a possible etiology [2], as is oral-genital inoculation [38] by a partner who may be unaware of his or her own HSV-1 infection. The public needs to be educated on the contagious nature of HSV-1, efficacy of barrier techniques (ie, condoms, dental dams) in preventing disease transmission, possibility of asymptomatic viral shedding, and utility of prophylactic antiviral therapy [2].

Despite the prevalence of HSV-1 within the population, recurrent orofacial herpes is relatively infrequent. Only 15% to 40% of seropositive persons have a recrudescence of orofacial herpes after their primary infection [2] (recurrent orofacial herpes rarely results from HSV-2 infection [39]). Many factors, including genetic susceptibility, immune status, age, anatomic site of infection, and initial dose of inoculum, have been suggested to influence the occurrence and frequency of recrudescence [2]. Recurrent orofacial herpes symptoms are generally milder and of shorter duration than those of primary infections [39,40] and rarely lead to systemic symptoms [40]. Recurrences can be characterized by a range of symptoms from mild discomfort to lesions on the lips, cheeks, nose, or nasal septum, or they may be clinically silent [29]. Many patients outgrow these outbreaks by the age of 35 years [2]. Most patients who have recurrent attacks have less than two per year, but as many as 10% have six or more recrudescences annually [41].

Recurrence of genital herpes is more common in those persons infected with HSV-2 than in those infected with HSV-1 [28]. Persons infected with HSV-2 are five times more likely than those infected with HSV-1 to have a recurrence (with or without symptoms) [42,43]. Regardless of viral typology, these recurrences are generally less severe than primary infections and heal in 5 to 10 days without antiviral therapy [44]. Although HSV-1 and HSV-2 recurrences tend to diminish in frequency over time, HSV-1 recurrences diminish more rapidly [42]. HSV-2 infection frequently leads to intermittent asymptomatic viral shedding, even in persons with long-standing disease. It is believed this asymptomatic shedding may be responsible for transmission originating from those with known disease who were asymptomatic at the time of transmission [43].

Serologic testing and screening

There are several methods to test for HSV infection. Viral cultures can be used, but their sensitivity is relatively low, given the intermittent nature of viral shedding [12]. Polymerase chain reaction (PCR) testing of fluid or scrapings from lesions for HSV DNA is more sensitive than viral culture [45], but it is not approved by the US Food and Drug Administration (FDA) for genital swabs and may not be widely available [12]. A Tzanck smear can be performed on fluid from a fresh lesion or ulcer, but this is also not effectively sensitive (because it only demonstrates characteristic cytopathic changes to host cells) and cannot provide viral typing [12]. Serologic tests assessing for the presence of immunoglobulin specific to HSV glycoproteins are available and are fairly sensitive and quite specific [12,45].

Viral cultures have been the main method of confirming HSV infection over the past several decades [45]. At best (collection from vesicular or pustular lesions), herpes isolation rates on culture (therefore sensitivity) approach 90% [45]. As the lesions mature to ulcers and then crusted sores, the culture isolation rates drop to 70% and 27%, respectively [45]. Cultures cannot be accurately performed on clinically asymptomatic patients. Additionally, viral culture as a means of emergency department testing is hindered by the need to keep the culture material on ice (4°C is preferred) and the processing time (some changes may be recognizable after 24 hours but can take as long as 5 days to develop) [45]. Once the virus is isolated, it can be typed (HSV-1 or HSV-2) [45].

Assessing for the presence of HSV DNA in samples taken from lesions using PCR testing is another means to confirm herpes infection [12,45]. The available literature places the sensitivity of PCR testing for HSV at between 59% and 89% [45]. This seemingly low sensitivity likely results from the intermittent nature of viral shedding. Additionally, it should be noted that according to the CDC, "PCR tests are not FDA-cleared for testing of genital specimens" [12]. Although the CDC recommendations do note that clinical laboratories that have independently developed their own HSV PCR tests and performed a Clinical Laboratory Improvement Amendment (CLIA) verification study may use PCR testing for genital samples [12], it is unlikely that these exist in large enough numbers to be of general use to emergency physicians at large. PCR testing, although more sensitive than viral culture, is similarly limited to use when active viral shedding is known to be occurring.

The most accurate tests are ELISAs for the presence of immunoglobulin G (IgG) to the HSV-specific glycoprotein G2 (HSV-2) and glycoprotein G1 (HSV-1) [12] in samples of the patient's serum. The ELISAs for IgG to glycoprotein G2 (HSV-2) vary in sensitivity from 80% to 98% (by brand) and have a specificity of 96% or greater [12]. The 2006 CDC guidelines also suggest that older and less accurate tests remain on the market, however. The CDC recommends that ELISA testing be performed in the following settings [12]:

1. Recurrent genital symptoms or atypical symptoms with negative HSV cultures
2. A clinical diagnosis of genital herpes without laboratory confirmation
3. A partner with genital herpes

Thus, any patient presenting to the emergency department in whom there is a strong clinical suspicion for genital herpes should have an ELISA test. A patient whose clinical picture is consistent with a primary genital herpes infection should have an ELISA test performed to ascertain if the patient is infected with HSV-1 or HSV-2 [12]. If HSV-2 infection is confirmed, suppression therapy should be initiated [12] (see recommendations). If HSV-1 is the causative agent, the primary infection (or current recrudescence) can be treated but suppression therapy is not indicated [12]. In the patient with recurrent symptoms or atypical symptoms, an ELISA test provides confirmation of herpes infection and appropriate therapy can be started [12]. In the patient exposed to a sexual partner with genital herpes, ELISA testing provides confirmation of a potentially asymptomatic yet contagious infection [12]. The CDC guidelines are clear on the need for the clinical diagnosis of genital herpes to be confirmed by laboratory testing [12]. Given the low sensitivity of PCR and viral cultures, the emergency physician should seriously consider use of ELISA tests as the primary means of confirming genital herpes infections. Table 2 summarizes the limitations and uses of the available tests.

One systematic review suggests that HSV serologic testing should be included in a comprehensive evaluation for STDs in HIV-infected patients and "patients at risk for sexually transmitted disease/HIV" [46]. That review additionally found "that universal screening would not be useful to pregnant women and should generally not be offered" [46]. Opponents to universal screening of pregnant women argue that the risk for transmission is low, the prophylactic therapies have not been proved to be of benefit, and the costs of treating all seropositive women (estimated to be one in four) would be enormous [47]. Additionally, those testing positive would bear that stigmata for the rest of their lives [47]. Experts have suggested that offering voluntary screening to all persons as part of routine preventative care might be of benefit in preventing transmission and is of little psychosocial risk [48,49].

In addition to following the CDC guidelines, emergency physicians should consider adding type-specific HSV serology screening when assessing for STDs (even in patients without current clinical signs or symptoms of herpes infection), especially in the setting of known HIV infection [46]. Data and expert consensus do not support the routine testing of pregnant women.

Clinical presentation

Genital herpes is classically described as painful vesicles on the labia minora, introitus, and urethra meatus in women and on the shaft and glans of the penis in men that rupture to form irregular crusted ulcerations [2]. In primary infections, these lesions heal over 2 to 6 weeks [50] (recurrent infections may resolve more rapidly). Primary infections may be preceded by a 24- to 48-hour prodrome of localized pain, tingling, or a burning sensation [50]. Additionally, a headache, fever, malaise, or inguinal lymphadenopathy may be noted [51]. The vesicles erupt within approximately 6 days of sexual contact with an infected partner [50]. The vesicles may also be present on the perineum, thighs, and buttocks of either gender [51], but women may be

Table 2
Overview of available herpes simplex virus tests

Test	Optimal time of use	Sensitivity	Advantages	Limitations
Viral culture	Vesicular lesions present	27%–90%	Most recognized course of testing (best known to clinicians)	Frequent false-negative results [45] Long processing time Samples must be kept cold (4°C) [45] Cannot be used if lesions not present [12]
PCR	Any lesions present	59%–89%	More accurate than viral culture [45] and does not require phlebotomy	Frequent false-negative results [45] Not approved by FDA for genital swabs [12] Cannot be used if lesions not present [12]
ELISA	May be used at any time (rare false-negative results are most likely early in infection)	80%–98%	Type specific False-negative results are extremely rare (NPV ∼99%–100%) [45] Can be used even if lesions not present	Older less sensitive assays still on the market [12] Requires phlebotomy

Abbreviation: NPV, negative predictive value.

predisposed to more severe clinical manifestations because of the involvement of a larger body surface area by means of the facilitation of viral spread over moist female genitalia [50]. Women are also more prone to complications, such as aseptic meningitis (which occurs in 10% of men and 30% of women during primary HSV infection [52]). Women are four times more likely to be infected from a male sexual partner (as opposed to men from a female sexual partner) [53]. This may be the result of an anatomic predisposition to HSV infection in women [54]. Regardless of gender, an asymptomatic patient may shed virus and be a source of infection [2,12,30]. In fact, the CDC suggests that "the majority of genital herpes infections are transmitted by persons unaware that they have the infection or who are asymptomatic when transmission occurs" [12].

Unfortunately, the diagnosis of genital herpes by clinical presentation alone is insensitive and nonspecific [12]. The classically described lesions may not be present in all patients [12,55]. It can be difficult to differentiate genital ulcers arising from other etiologies (eg, syphilis, chancroid) from those of herpes [55]. Although one study suggested that swallow depth, tenderness, and presence of multiple lesions could exclude syphilis and chancroid with 94% specificity, the constellation remained only 35% sensitive to the diagnosis of HSV infection [55]. The potential for internal (therefore difficult to visualize) lesions may further complicate the diagnosis in some women. Although, clinically, there is no difference between the appearance of HSV-1 and HSV-2 genital herpes [56], there is evidence that recurrent episodes and subclinical viral shedding are far more common in HSV-2 infections [42,57]. Specific viral etiology (HSV-1 versus HSV-2) has importance in prognosis and patient counseling [12] and in the decision to initiate suppressive therapy [12]. Thus, the CDC recommends that "the clinical diagnosis of genital herpes should be confirmed by laboratory testing. Both virologic and type-specific serologic tests for HSV should be available in clinical settings that provide care for patients with STDs or those at risk for STDs" [12].

When assessing oral herpes, intraoral lesions are suggestive of a primary lesion [28]. Primary herpetic gingivostomatitis (PHGS) is a common clinically apparent form of primary oral herpes infection, occurring in 12% of infections [58]. PHGS usually occurs in children and is most often (~90% of cases) associated with the HSV-1 virus [58]. Patients present with a 24- to 48-hour prodrome of fever, anorexia, irritability, malaise, and headache [50]. In adolescents, the prodrome is described as "mononucleosis-like," characterized by pharyngitis, fever, malaise, and lymphadenopathy [29]. The syndrome advances to small round vesicles on the involved buccal mucosa, tongue, posterior pharynx, and any gingival or palatal mucosae, which quickly erupt, creating shallow irregular ulcerations covered by a yellowish membrane. At this stage, submandibular lymphadenitis, halitosis, and painful swallowing and refusal to drink are often present [58]. These lesions generally resolve in 5 to 7 days, but more severe cases may

The CDC recommends that patients who have recurrent genital herpes be treated with daily suppressive therapy to reduce the chance of disease transmission and to provide symptom relief [12]. The recommended regimes are acyclovir, 400 mg, given orally twice a day; famciclovir, 250 mg, given orally twice a day; valacyclovir, 500 mg, given orally once a day; or valacyclovir, 1 g, given orally once a day. The higher valacyclovir dose is recommended for those having more than 10 recrudescences per year.

Other investigators have suggested that a "prescription in the pocket" approach may also be effective. In this approach, the patient is provided with a prescription for antiviral medication to be taken at the first symptom of a prodrome [62,63]. These approaches have shown promise in suppressing and shortening recrudescences (acyclovir and famciclovir by 2 days each, although valacyclovir failed to shorten the course [64]) but have not yet been demonstrated to prevent the asymptomatic shedding of virus. If an emergency physician uses this approach with patients experiencing recurrent genital herpes, counseling regarding the likelihood of spreading the disease by means of sexual contact should be provided. Suppressive, as opposed to episodic, therapy should be used if the patient remains sexually active with a noninfected partner or outside of a monogamous relationship to prevent transmission during periods of asymptomatic shedding.

There are several treatment considerations for the emergency physician when dealing with PHGS. Antiviral therapy is suggested to alleviate symptoms more rapidly (Table 4). In children, acyclovir, 15 mg/kg, given orally five times daily is recommended for 5 to 7 days [65]. Ideally, treatment should be started within the first 3 days of disease onset. A mixture of Maalox and diphenhydramine "swish and swallow" or viscous lidocaine applied topically with a swab may help to alleviate the pain of these lesions [66]. Valacyclovir, 1 g, given orally twice daily or famciclovir, 500 mg, given orally twice daily for 5 to 7 days is recommended for adults presenting with acute herpetic gingivostomatitis [67]. Valacyclovir and famciclovir are not approved by the FDA for pediatric use, but there may be some utility in their use in adolescent patients [68]. Acyclovir remains the mainstay of pediatric therapy.

Dehydration secondary to reduced oral intake is a frequent problem in young children presenting with PHGS [69]. This should be treated as with any other pediatric dehydration (20 mL/kg intravenous fluid bolus). If, after the administration of local analgesia (eg, Maalox and diphenhydramine or

Table 4
Treatment of primary herpetic gingivostomatitis

Population	Drug	Dose	Frequency	Duration
Pediatric	Acyclovir	15 mg/kg	Five times a day	5–7 days
Adult	Valacyclovir	1 g	BID	5–7 days
	Famciclovir	500 mg	BID	5–7 days

Abbreviation: BID, two times daily.

viscous lidocaine), the patient is still unable to tolerate oral fluid intake, admission should be considered [58,69].

To be effective, treatment of a recrudescence of oral herpes must begin as soon as possible [25,56]. Ideally, therapy begins during the prodrome [56]. Oral and topical therapies have been shown to shorten the course of symptoms by 1 day [56]. Various topical solutions, such as docosanol 10% cream, penciclovir 1% cream, and idoxuridine 15% solution, [25] may be used to ameliorate symptoms (these should be continued for the duration of symptoms). Oral valacyclovir, 500 mg, taken twice daily for 1 week may also be helpful if initiated early in the symptom course [25,56]. A single-day course of valacyclovir, 2 g, taken twice daily may also be effective [70]. Suppression therapy (with the same agents as used in recurrent genital infections) can be used in cases of extremely frequent outbreaks [2,12].

The immunocompromised patient

Herpes infections in the immunocompromised patient are generally slow to respond to antiviral therapies [56]. The lesions are usually more extensive and are often extremely painful [12]. In the setting of a low CD4 count, their ulcers may be extensive, deeply ulcerated, and necrotic, persisting longer than the usual HSV course [59]. There is a synergy between HIV-1 and HSV-2 infection that is becoming well described in the literature [59] and seems to lead to increased viral shedding in patients who have HIV disease [12,59]. The immunocompromised patient is more likely to have systemic complications of the infection [12,56]. The virus may spread to multiple visceral organs [56]. This can lead to a variety of symptoms. HSV hepatitis can lead to leukopenia, thrombocytopenia, and disseminated intravascular coagulopathy (DIC) [71]. Esophagitis, colitis, pneumonia, and encephalitis can also occur [71]. Interestingly, visceral involvement is usually diagnosed postmortem [71]. Unfortunately, systemic herpes in the immunocompromised patient is usually fatal, despite antiviral therapy [71]. If extensive cutaneous disease is present, or if there are concerns of systemic involvement, the patient should be admitted for antiviral therapy. The emergency physician should also recognize that lesions in the immunocompromised patient can be exquisitely painful [55], and admission for intravenous analgesia may be required.

The CDC recommends that acyclovir, 400 to 800 mg, given orally two to three times a day; famciclovir, 500 mg, given orally twice a day; or valacyclovir, 500 mg, given orally twice a day be used for daily suppression therapy in HIV-positive patients who are seropositive for HSV-2 infection [12]. If episodic therapy is used, the CDC recommends acyclovir, 400 mg, given orally three times a day for 5 to 10 days; famciclovir, 500 mg, given orally twice a day for 5 to 10 days; or valacyclovir, 1 g, given orally twice a day for 5 to 10 days [12]. In the event of severe systemic disease, acyclovir, 5 to 10 mg/kg, given intravenously every 8 hours is recommended [12]. If the clinical course seems to be resistant to antiviral therapy, foscarnet, 40 mg/kg, given intravenously every 8 hours should be initiated and antiviral susceptibilities obtained to guide therapy [12,72].

Summary

The epidemiology of oral and genital herpes has dramatically changed over the past decade. New guidelines from the CDC and recent scientific literature suggest that emergency physicians should be adapting their practices to respond to these changes. As more patients use the emergency department as a means of primary care, emergency physicians should be familiar with the medications used to treat and suppress these chronic infections.

References

[1] Cardone G, Winkler DC, Trus BL, et al. Visualization of the herpes simplex virus portal in situ by cryo-electron tomography. Virology 2007;361(2):426–34.

[2] Fatahzadeh M, Schwartz RA. Human herpes simplex virus infections: epidemiology, pathogenesis, symptomatology, diagnosis, and management. J Am Acad Dermatol 2007;57(5): 737–63.

[3] CDC. Guidelines for prevention of Herpesvirus simiae (B virus) infection in monkey handlers. MMWR Morb Mortal Wkly Rep 1987;36:680–2, 687–9.

[4] Seliem RM, Griffith RC, Harris NL, et al. HHV-8+, EBV+ multicentric plasmablastic microlymphoma in an HIV+ man: the spectrum of HHV-8+ lymphoproliferative disorders expands. Am J Surg Pathol 2007;31(9):1439–45.

[5] Just-Nübling G, Korn S, Ludwig B, et al. Primary cytomegalovirus infection in an outpatient setting—laboratory markers and clinical aspects. Infection 2003;31(5):318–23.

[6] Jackson MA, Sommerauer JF. Human herpesviruses 6 and 7. Pediatr Infect Dis J 2002;21(6): 565–6.

[7] Xu F, Sternberg MR, Kottiri BJ, et al. Trends in herpes simplex virus type 1 and type 2 seroprevalence in the United States. JAMA 2006;296(8):964–73.

[8] Lowhagen GB, Tunback P, Andersson K, et al. First episodes of genital herpes in a Swedish STD population: a study of epidemiology and transmission by the use of herpes simplex virus (HSV) typing and specific serology. Sex Transm Infect 2000;76:179–82.

[9] Nilsen A, Myremel H. Changing trends in genital herpes simplex virus infection in Bergen, Norway. Acta Obstet Gynecol Scand 2000;79:693–6.

[10] Tran T, Druce JD, Catton MC, et al. Changing epidemiology of genital herpes simplex virus infection in Melbourne, Australia, between 1980 and 2003. Sex Transm Infect 2004;80: 277–9.

[11] Scoular A, Norrie J, Gillespie G, et al. Longitudinal study of genital infection by herpes simplex virus type 1 in Western Scotland over 15 years. BMJ 2002;324:1366–7.

[12] CDC. Sexually transmitted diseases treatment guidelines, 2006. MMWR 2002; 55(No. RR-11).

[13] Brackbill RM, Sternberg MR, Fishbein M. Where do people go for treatment of sexually transmitted diseases? Fam Plann Perspect 1999;31(1):10–5.

[14] Taylor JM, Lin E, Susmarski N, et al. Alternative entry receptors for herpes simplex virus and their roles in disease. Cell Host Microbe 2007;2(1):19–28.

[15] Krummenacher C, Baribaud F, Ponce de Leon M, et al. Comparative usage of herpesvirus entry mediator A and nectin-1 by laboratory strains and clinical isolates of herpes simplex virus. Virology 2004;322(2):286–99.

[16] Margolis TP, Imai Y, Yang L, et al. Herpes simplex virus type 2 (HSV-2) establishes latent infection in a different population of ganglionic neurons than HSV-1: role of latency-associated transcripts. J Virol 2007;81(4):1872–8.

[17] Spear PG, Manoj S, Yoon M, et al. Different receptors binding to distinct interfaces on herpes simplex virus gD can trigger events leading to cell fusion and viral entry. Virology 2006; 344(1):17–24.

[18] Reske A, Pollara G, Krummenacher C, et al. Understanding HSV-1 entry glycoproteins. Rev Med Virol 2007;17(3):205–15.

[19] Barton ES, White DW, Cathelyn JS, et al. Herpesvirus latency confers symbiotic protection from bacterial infection. Nature 2007;447(7142):326–9.

[20] Sinclair J, Sissons P. Latency and reactivation of human cytomegalovirus. J Gen Virol 2006; 87(Pt 7):1763–79.

[21] Nikkels AF, Pièrard GE. Treatment of mucocutaneous presentations of herpes simplex virus infections. Am J Clin Dermatol 2002;3(7):475–87.

[22] Syrjänen S, Mikola H, Nykänen M, et al. In vitro establishment of lytic and nonproductive infection by herpes simplex virus type 1 in three-dimensional keratinocyte culture. J Virol 1996;70(9):6524–8.

[23] Polis MA, Haile-Mariam T. Viruses. In: Marx, editor. Rosen's emergency medicine: concepts and clinical practice. 6th edition. St. Louis (MO): Mosby; 2006.

[24] Abendroth A, Arvin A. Varicella-zoster virus immune evasion. Immunol Rev 1999;168: 143–56.

[25] Fatahzadeh M, Schwartz RA. Human herpes simplex labialis. Clin Exp Dermatol 2007; 32(6):625–30.

[26] Knaup B, Schünemann S, Wolff MH. Subclinical reactivation of herpes simplex virus type 1 in the oral cavity. Oral Microbiol Immunol 2000;15(5):281–3.

[27] Wolff MH, Schmitt J, Rahaus M, et al. Clinical and subclinical reactivation of genital herpes virus. Intervirology 2002;45(1):20–3.

[28] Whitley RJ, Roizman B. Herpes simplex virus infections. Lancet 2001;357(9267):1513–8.

[29] Whitley RJ, Gnann JW. The epidemiology and clinical manifestations of herpes simplex virus infections. In: Roizman B, Whitley RJ, Lopez C, editors. The human herpesviruses. New York: Raven Press; 1993. p. 69–105.

[30] Nadelman CM, Newcomer VD. Herpes simplex virus infections. Postgrad Med 2000;107: 189–200.

[31] Esmann J. The many challenges of facial herpes simplex virus infection. J Antimicrob Chemother 2001;47:17–27.

[32] Marcus B, Lipozencic J, Mafz H, et al. Herpes simplex: autoinoculation versus dissemination. Acta Dermatovenerol Croat 2005;13:237–41.

[33] Turner R, Shehab Z, Osborne K, et al. Shedding and survival of herpes simplex virus from "fever blisters." Pediatrics 1982;70:547–9.

[34] Kramer A, Schwebke I, Kampf G. How long do nosocomial pathogens persist on inanimate surfaces? A systematic review. BMC Infect Dis 2006;6:130.

[35] Roberts CM, Pfister JR, Spear SJ. Increasing proportion of herpes simplex virus type 1 as a cause of genital herpes infection in college students. Sex Transm Dis 2003;30(10): 797–800.

[36] Mertz GJ, Rosenthal SL, Stanberry LR. Is herpes simplex virus type 1 (HSV-1) now more common than HSV-2 in first episodes of genital herpes? Sex Transm Dis 2003;30(10): 801–2 [comment on: Sex Transm Dis. 2003 Oct;30(10):797–800].

[37] Samra Z, Scherf E, Dan M. Herpes simplex virus type 1 is the prevailing cause of genital herpes in the Tel Aviv area, Israel. Sex Transm Dis 2003;30:794–6.

[38] Nieuwenhuis RF, van Doornum GJ, Mulder PG, et al. Importance of herpes simplex virus type-1 (HSV-1) in primary genital herpes. Acta Derm Venereol 2006;86(2):129–34.

[39] Bader C, Crumpacker CS, Schnipper LE, et al. The natural history of recurrent facial oral infection with herpes simplex virus. J Infect Dis 1978;138:897–905.

[40] Glick M. Clinical aspects of recurrent oral herpes simplex virus infection. Compend Contin Educ Dent 2002;23(Suppl 2):4–8.

[41] Rooney JF, Straus SE, Mannix ML, et al. Oral acyclovir to suppress frequently recurrent herpes labialis. Ann Intern Med 1993;118:268–72.

[42] Engelberg R, Carrell D, Krantz E, et al. Natural history of genital herpes simplex virus type 1 infection. Sex Transm Dis 2003;30(2):174–7.

[43] Sen P, Barton SE. Genital herpes and its management. BMJ 2007;334(7602):1048–52.

[44] Gupta R, Warren T, Wald A. Genital herpes. Lancet 2007;370(9605):2127–37.

[45] Scoular A. Using the evidence base on genital herpes: optimising the use of diagnostic tests and information provision. Sex Transm Infect 2002;78(3):160–5.

[46] Guerry SL, Bauer HM, Klausner JD, et al. Recommendations for the selective use of herpes simplex virus type 2 serological tests. Clin Infect Dis 2005;40(1):38–45.

[47] Urato AC, Caughey AB. Universal prenatal herpes screening is a bad idea in pregnancy. Lancet 2006;368(9539):898–9.

[48] Richards J, Scholes D, Caka S, et al. HSV-2 serologic testing in an HMO population: uptake and psychosocial sequelae. Sex Transm Dis 2007;34(9):718–25.

[49] Miyai T, Turner KR, Kent CK, et al. The psychosocial impact of testing individuals with no history of genital herpes for herpes simplex virus type 2. Sex Transm Dis 2004;31(9):517–21.

[50] Beauman JG. Genital herpes: a review. Am Fam Physician 2005;72:1527–34.

[51] Lautenschlager S, Echmann A. The heterogenous clinical spectrum of genital herpes. Dermatology 2001;202:211–9.

[52] Corey L, Adams H, Brown Z, et al. Genital herpes simplex virus infections: clinical manifestations, course and complications. Ann Intern Med 1983;98:958–72.

[53] Brown TJ, McCrary M, Tyring SK. Antiviral agents: nonantiviral drugs. J Am Acad Dermatol 2002;47:581–99.

[54] Frenkel L, Garratty E, Shen J, et al. Clinical reactivation of herpes simplex virus type 2 infection in seropositive pregnant women with no history of genital herpes. Ann Intern Med 1993;118:414–8.

[55] Lingappa JR, Celum C. Clinical and therapeutic issues for herpes simplex virus-2 and HIV co-infection. Drugs 2007;67(2):155–74.

[56] Brady RC, Bernstein DI. Treatment of herpes simplex virus infections. Antiviral Res 2004; 61(2):73–81.

[57] Benedetti JK, Corey L, Ashley R. Recurrence rates in genital herpes after symptomatic first-episode infection. Ann Intern Med 1994;121:847–54.

[58] Kolokotronis A, Doumas S. Herpes simplex virus infection, with particular reference to the progression and complications of primary herpetic gingivostomatitis. Clin Microbiol Infect 2006;12(3):202–11.

[59] DiCarlo RP, Martin DH. The clinical diagnosis of genital ulcer disease in men. Clin Infect Dis 1997;25(2):292–8.

[60] Sciubba JJ. Herpes simplex and aphthous ulcerations: presentation, diagnosis and management—an update. Gen Dent 2003;51:510–6.

[61] McMillan JA, Weiner LB, Higgins AM, et al. Pharyngitis associated with herpes simplex virus in college students. Pediatr Infect Dis J 1993;12(4):280–4.

[62] Fife KH, Almekinder J, Ofner S. A comparison of one year of episodic or suppressive treatment of recurrent genital herpes with valacyclovir. Sex Transm Dis 2007;34(5):297–301.

[63] Aoki FY, Tyring S, Diaz-Mitoma F, et al. Single-day patient initiated famciclovir therapy for recurrent genital herpes: a randomized, double-blind, placebo-controlled trial. Clin Infect Dis 2006;42:8–13.

[64] Spruance S, Aoki FY, Tyring S, et al. Short-course therapy for recurrent genital herpes and herpes labialis. J Fam Pract 2007;56(1):30–6.
[65] Amir J. Clinical aspects and antiviral therapy in primary herpetic gingivostomatitis. Paediatr Drugs 2001;3(8):593–7.
[66] Faden H. Management of primary herpetic gingivostomatitis in young children. Pediatr Emerg Care 2006;22(4):268–9.
[67] Chauvin PJ, Ajar AH. Acute herpetic gingivostomatitis in adults: a review of 13 cases, including diagnosis and management. J Can Dent Assoc 2002;68(4):247–51.
[68] Dekker CL, Prober CG. Pediatric uses of valacyclovir, penciclovir and famciclovir. Pediatr Infect Dis J 2001;20(11):1079–81.
[69] Amir J, Harel L, Smetana Z, et al. The natural history of primary herpes simplex type 1 gingivostomatitis in children. Pediatr Dermatol 1999;16:259–63.
[70] Spruance SL, Jones TM, Blatter MM, et al, the Valacyclovir Cold Sore Study Group. High-dose, short-duration, early valacyclovir therapy for episodic treatment of cold sores: results of two randomized, placebo-controlled, multicenter studies. Antimicrob Agents Chemother 2003;47:1072–80.
[71] Herget GW, Riede UN, Schmitt-Gräff A, et al. Generalized herpes simplex virus infection in an immunocompromised patient—report of a case and review of the literature. Pathol Res Pract 2005;201(2):123–9.
[72] Chilukuri S, Rosen T. Management of acyclovir-resistant herpes simplex virus. Dermatol Clin 2003;21:311–20.

ELSEVIER
SAUNDERS

Emerg Med Clin N Am
26 (2008) 475–497

EMERGENCY
MEDICINE
CLINICS OF
NORTH AMERICA

Foodborne Illness

David C. Pigott, MD

*Department of Emergency Medicine, The University of Alabama at Birmingham,
619 South 19th Street, JTN 266, Birmingham, AL 35249-7013, USA*

As the blaring newspaper headlines and 24-hour news cycle continue to emphasize, foodborne illness has rarely achieved such a prominent role in our national consciousness. Every day, it seems that another processed or prepackaged food has sent dozens of unwitting consumers to the hospital with gastrointestinal complaints or worse. A recent *New York Times* article pointed out that 16 recalls for *Escherichia coli* beef contamination have occurred in 2007 alone [1]. For emergency physicians or other health care providers encountering these patients, differentiating those who may be managed with simple hydration and reassurance from those who require a more in-depth approach, including antibiotics, hospitalization, or other interventions, has never been more important. Through a discussion of the most common causes of foodborne illness, as well as a few of the more dangerous but rare organisms, this article aims to provide a rational approach to the evaluation and management of patients presenting with foodborne illness.

According to the Centers for Disease Control and Prevention (CDC), an estimated 76 million cases of foodborne illness are reported in the United States each year, leading to approximately 5,000 deaths [2]. In the developing world, the deaths of an estimated 2 million young children are attributable to diarrheal illness caused by contaminated food and water every year. In the United States, just as in underdeveloped countries, the most common cause of foodborne illness is viral or bacterial contamination. While the cleanliness of public water supplies in industrialized countries tends to prevent most foodborne illness, inadvertent contamination of food products during the harvesting, processing, or packaging stages can lead to widespread outbreaks of foodborne illness. This is particularly true for products that may be shipped nationwide, leading to multistate outbreaks of similar illness, such as the recent outbreak of *E. coli* O157:H7, attributed to the

---

E-mail address: dpigott@uabmc.edu

consumption of fresh spinach [3]. These outbreaks of foodborne illness are the subject of ongoing epidemiologic studies by the CDC and other state and local agencies, through collaborative efforts such as FoodNet.

FoodNet, the Foodborne Disease Active Surveillance Network, is an ongoing multidisciplinary project that tracks outbreaks of foodborne illness and coordinates epidemiologic studies. As the primary foodborne illness component of the CDC's Emerging Infections Program (EIP), FoodNet collects data from ten EIP sites nationwide, as well as from the United States Department of Agriculture and the Food and Drug Administration (FDA) [4]. FoodNet investigators have recently studied the overall burden of acute diarrheal illness in the United States, estimating that 5% of the population may be affected at any given time, 20% of whom seek medical attention, and 7% of whom receive antibiotics [5]. The most recent FoodNet data from 2006 reveal that while foodborne infections from a number of common pathogens continue to decline, including *Campylobacter*, *Listeria*, *Shigella*, and *Yersinia*, infections caused by Shiga toxin-producing *E. coli* O157:H7 (STEC) and *Vibrio* infections have remained constant or increased [6]. In addition to FoodNet, there are several other specialty-specific networks that track outbreaks of foodborne illness both nationally and worldwide.

Coordinated by the CDC and the National Center for Infectious Diseases, these organizations serve as provider-based, emerging infections sentinel networks that are designed to detect and study conditions and patterns of illness that may otherwise go unnoticed by existing health department surveillance systems. EMERGEncy ID NET is one such organization, a multicenter emergency department-based network for research on emerging infectious diseases, including foodborne illness [7]. Similarly dedicated to the detection of emerging infections, the Global Emerging Infections Sentinel Network, or GeoSentinel, is charged with tracking outbreaks of infectious disease on a worldwide basis, primarily through tropical and travel medicine clinics [8]. Sponsored by the International Society of Travel Medicine (ISTM) and the CDC, the GeoSentinel network records data from over 1,500 ISTM sites worldwide.

An initial approach to foodborne illness

Foodborne illness is typically caused by micro-organisms or their toxins and most often manifests itself through gastrointestinal illness, which can vary markedly in severity and duration. In addition to microscopic foodborne pathogens, such as bacteria, viruses, fungi, and parasites, foodborne illness may also be caused by toxic contaminants, such as heavy metals, chemicals, and pesticides. Toxic substances present in food naturally may also play a role, as in the case of toxic mushrooms, plants, fish, or shellfish. Given the multitude of potential causes for a given patient's symptoms of undifferentiated gastroenteritis, it may seem a hopeless task to determine the specific pathogen responsible, particularly in an Emergency Department

(ED)-based or primary care setting where definitive diagnostic testing is likely to be unavailable. Even given these limitations, however, a reasoned approach to the patient with suspected foodborne illness can provide clues to the most likely cause for the patient's illness and the most appropriate treatment strategy.

As always, the dictum that "If you don't consider the diagnosis, you'll never find it" applies to the detection of foodborne illness in the ED setting. Having a high initial level of suspicion for the presence of foodborne illness is essential in the evaluation and management of these patients. Even the so-called "24-hour flu" is likely to represent a brief episode of foodborne illness, such as that caused by *Clostridium perfringens* [9]. Although most patients present with relatively mild to moderate symptoms of diarrheal illness, the clinician must be prepared to encounter patients with more acute presentations caused by severe volume depletion, including impending shock, metabolic acidosis, and circulatory collapse. Particularly for those health care providers working in the developing world or who may encounter ill travelers from nonindustrialized settings, the degree of dehydration in patients suffering from foodborne gastrointestinal illness must not be underestimated. A study of pediatric diarrheal deaths in India found that those patients with moderate to severe dehydration or suffering from *Shigella* infection were significantly more likely to have a fatal outcome [10].

During the initial assessment of patients with suspected foodborne illness, a proper history is invaluable in determining the most likely etiology for the patient's symptoms. Important questions to consider include time of onset and duration of symptoms, history of recent travel or antibiotic use, as well as the presence of blood or mucus in the stool. While relevant information about recent meals, including types of food, cooking and refrigeration methods, and a history of others affected with similar symptoms can be helpful, in the majority of outbreaks of foodborne illness, no specific offending food item can be identified [11].

After historical information regarding the patient's symptoms has been obtained, a careful physical examination should be performed, with special attention paid to the patient's vital signs, degree of dehydration, and abdominal examination. A digital rectal examination for the presence of gross or occult blood, mucus, or pus should also be completed. A recent study attempted to evaluate whether the digital rectal examination is necessary for the detection of fecal occult blood or if guaiac examination of spontaneously passed stool is sufficient. The researchers found no difference in the method of stool collection, with both groups demonstrating a colonic source of occult bleeding in approximately 21% to 22% of subjects [12]. While the presence of fever, systemic symptoms, bloody diarrhea, or rectal bleeding should clearly suggest invasive diarrheal illness, in patients with nonbloody diarrhea, a negative test for fecal occult blood has been shown to have a negative predictive value for invasive illness greater than 90% [13]. The presence of diarrhea, however, should not be interpreted as pathognomonic for the diagnosis of gastroenteritis or nonsurgical gastrointestinal illness. A recent review of 200 pediatric and adult patients with confirmed appendicitis revealed that over 20% also had diarrhea as part of their presentation [14].

Therapy

Initial therapy for patients with foodborne illness should focus on reversal of dehydration, either through oral rehydration therapy (ORT), especially in the pediatric population, or through intravenous infusion of isotonic crystalloids. In children, the use of ORT in patients with mild-to-moderate dehydration because of gastroenteritis has been shown to be as effective as intravenous rehydration [15]. In developing countries, the World Health Organization (WHO) Oral Rehydration Solution (ORS), a glucose-based oral solution designed to treat or prevent diarrhea in both adults and children, has provided an inexpensive and effective therapy for populations where diarrheal foodborne disease is endemic and health care resources are scarce [16]. In 2002, a low-osmolar version of the WHO ORS replaced the original formulation, after pediatric data suggested a reduction in stool output and vomiting, as well as decreased need for supplemental intravenous therapy [17,18].

Although WHO ORS has primarily been used in developing countries, a United States study comparing the use of WHO ORS to a commercially-prepared ORS solution showed that caregivers were more satisfied with the WHO ORS than the commercial product and more likely to use it in the future [19]. Similar efforts have demonstrated the effectiveness of various oral rehydration solutions for adults in the United States. One study comparing well known adult and child commercial rehydration products and a new oral rehydration solution for the treatment of United States adults with viral gastroenteritis found similar effectiveness in each group, although the adult commercial rehydration product group had higher rates of hypokalemia [20]. There is currently no compelling evidence for withholding breastfeeding or formula for more than 4 hours for infants with diarrhea, as only 5% to 10% of infants have lactose intolerance [21].

The role for antibiotic therapy in patients with foodborne illness is controversial, although most sources favor the use of antibiotics in patients with invasive diarrheal illness, such as *Shigella*, or in patients with severe disease. It should be noted that in mild-to-moderate cases of nontyphoidal *Salmonella* infection, antibiotic use may not be helpful and may actually lead to a prolonged carrier state [22]. This asymptomatic carrier state can last for weeks, exposing others to the infection as well [23]. A single dose of a fluoroquinolone (eg, ciprofloxacin, 500 mg) has been shown to be effective in the treatment of traveler's diarrhea [24]. The use of empiric antibiotics in patients with suspected STEC infection should be discouraged because of the increased risk for development of the hemolytic-uremic syndrome

(HUS) in STEC patients who receive antibiotics, a process thought to be secondary to antimicrobial induction of Shiga-toxin production [25,26].

Although the use of further diagnostic testing, such as stool evaluation for fecal leukocytes, stool culture, and ova and parasite assays are typically beyond the reach of most ED evaluations, for selected patients with persistent symptoms (ie, those with symptoms lasting longer than 3 weeks), these tests may be indicated. In the setting of a suspected or confirmed multiple patient outbreak of foodborne illness, stool cultures for *Shigella*, *Campylobacter*, and *Salmonella* should be sent and empiric therapy initiated. It also should be noted that in many hospitals, stool analysis for the presence of Shiga-toxin for patients with suspected *E. coli* O157:H7 infection must be ordered separately from routine stool cultures. Research into rapid-detection methods for enteric pathogens is ongoing, with some polymerase chain reaction assays showing promising results in the detection of *Campylobacter*, *Salmonella* and *E. coli* O157:H7 (Table 1) [27].

Staphylococcus aureus

One of the most common causes of foodborne illness, *Staphylococcus aureus* is a gram-positive coccoid bacterium that produces a heat-stable enterotoxin during the growth of *S. aureus* in food [28]. These enterotoxins, of which there are seven known subtypes, are responsible for the clinical picture typically seen in patients with foodborne illness caused by *S. aureus*. Additional enterotoxins generated by *S. aureus* are responsible for the various other manifestations of staphylococcal disease, including toxic shock syndrome and staphylococcal scalded skin syndrome. Patients with *S. aureus*-related gastrointestinal symptoms most often present with nausea, crampy abdominal pain, and vomiting, usually within 1 to 6 hours of ingestion of contaminated foods [29]. Diarrhea is often present but tends to be less characteristic of patients with *S. aureus* food poisoning. The duration of symptoms is generally less than 2 days. The ingestion of a preformed toxin leads to the rapid onset of symptoms without a prolonged incubation period, as is typically seen in patients with Salmonellosis. While *S. aureus* must multiply in contaminated food to form enough toxin to cause illness (greater than 10^6 colony-forming units per gram), its incubation period is relatively short, from 30 minutes to 8 hours, with an average of 1 to 6 hours.

The most common cause of *S. aureus* food contamination is through direct contact with food workers carrying the bacterium or through contaminated dairy products. It is estimated that the prevalence of nasal colonization with *S. aureus* in the general population is up to 25% [30]. Food products that have been typically responsible for *S. aureus*-related foodborne illness include meat and meat products; poultry and egg products; salads such as egg, tuna, potato, and macaroni; foods that are handled directly; cream-filled pastries; and casseroles. A 1997 outbreak of staphylococcal food poisoning was associated with precooked ham served at

Table 1
Causes of food-borne illness

Etiology	Incubation period	Signs and symptoms	Duration	Associated foods	Laboratory testing	Treatment
Staph aureus	1–6 hours	Severe nausea and vomiting	24–48 hours	Unrefrigerated meats, potato or egg salad, cream-filled pastries	Normally a clinical diagnosis	Supportive care
Salmonella	1–3 days	Diarrhea, fever, abdominal cramps, vomiting	4–7 days	Contaminated eggs, poultry, unpasteurized milk or juice	Routine stool cultures	Supportive care. Antibiotics generally not indicated unless there is extraintestinal spread, or the risk of extraintestinal spread. Consider ampicillin, gentamicin, trimethoprim-sulfamethoxazole (TMP-SMX), or quinolones.
Clostridium perfringens	8–16 hours	Watery diarrhea, nausea, abdominal cramps	24–48 hours	Meats, poultry, gravy, time- or temperature-abused food	Stool for enterotoxin and quantitative culture	Supportive care
Campylobacter jejuni	2–5 days	Diarrhea (may be bloody), cramps, fever, and vomiting	2–10 days	Raw and undercooked poultry, unpasteurized milk, contaminated water	Routine stool cultures	Supportive care. For severe cases, erythromycin or quinolones may be indicated early in the diarrheal disease

Organism	Onset Time	Symptoms	Duration	Source	Diagnosis	Treatment
Shigella	24–48 hours	Abdominal cramps, fever and diarrhea. Diarrhea may contain blood or mucus	4–7 days	Food or water contaminated with human fecal material. Ready-to-eat foods touched by infected food workers.	Routine stool cultures	Supportive care. TMP-SMX indicated in the United States if organism is susceptible. Quinolones may be indicated for resistant organisms.
E. coli O157:H7	1–8 days	Severe diarrhea, often bloody, abdominal pain and vomiting. Little or no fever.	5–10 days	Undercooked beef, especially hamburger, unpasteurized milk and juice, raw fruits and vegetables	Stool culture. If *E. coli* O157:H7 is suspected, specific testing must be requested	Supportive care, monitor renal function, hemoglobin and platelets closely. Associated with HUS, which can cause lifelong complications. Antibiotics may promote the development of HUS.
Enterotoxigenic *E. coli*	1–3 days	Watery diarrhea, abdominal cramps, some vomiting.	3 to > 7 days	Water or food contaminated with human feces.	Stool culture. Specific testing must be requested.	Supportive care. Antibiotics rarely needed except in severe cases. TMP-SMX or quinolones.
Vibrio parahaemolyticus	2–48 hours	Watery diarrhea, abdominal cramps, nausea and vomiting	2–5 days	Undercooked or raw seafood, such as fish, shellfish	Stool cultures	Supportive care. Antibiotics are recommended in severe cases: tetracycline, doxycycline, gentamicin and cefotaxime

(continued on next page)

Table 1 (*continued*)

Etiology	Incubation period	Signs and symptoms	Duration	Associated foods	Laboratory testing	Treatment
Vibrio vulnificus	1–7 days	Vomiting, diarrhea, abdominal pain, bacteremia and wound infections. Can be fatal in patients with liver disease and who are immuno-compromised	2–8 days	Undercooked or raw shellfish, especially oysters, other contaminated seafood, wounds exposed to sea water	Stool, wound or blood cultures	Supportive care and antibiotics; tetracycline, doxycycline and ceftazidime are recommended.
Scombroid (histamine)	1 min to 3 hours	Flushing, rash, burning sensation of skin, mouth and throat, dizziness, urticaria, paresthesias	3–6 hours	Fish: bluefin, tuna, mackerel, marlin, mahi mahi	Demonstration of histamine in food or clinical diagnosis	Supportive care, antihistamines.
Ciguatera fish poisoning (ciguatera toxin)	2–6 hours	Gastrointestinal: abdominal pain, nausea, vomiting, diarrhea	Days to weeks to months	A variety of large reef fish. Grouper, red snapper, amberjack, and barracuda (most common).	Radioassay for toxin in fish or a consistent history	Supportive care, intravenous mannitol.
	3 hours	Neurologic: parethesias, reversal of hot and cold, pain, weakness				
	2–5 days	Cardiovascular: bradycardia, hypotension				

	Onset	Signs and symptoms	Duration	Associated foods	Laboratory testing	Treatment
Paralytic shellfish poisoning	30 minutes to 3 hours	Diarrhea, nausea, vomiting, leading to paresthesias of mouth, lips, weakness, respiratory paralysis	Days	Scallops, mussels, clams	Detection of toxin in food or water where fish are located; high-pressure liquid chromatography	Life-threatening, may need respiratory support.
Clostridium botulinum (preformed toxin)	12–72 hours	Vomiting, diarrhea, blurred vision, diplopia, dysphagia, and descending muscle weakness.	Variable (from days to months). Can be complicated by respiratory failure and death.	Home-canned foods with low acid content, improperly canned commercial foods.	Stool, serum and food can be tested for toxin. Stool and food can also be culture for the organism.	Supportive care. Botulinum antitoxin helpful if given early in the course of the illness. Contact the state health department.

Data from the American Medical Association; American Nurses Association-American Nurses Foundation; Centers for Disease Control and Prevention; Center for Food Safety and Applied Nutrition, Food and Drug Administration; Food Safety and Inspection Service, US Department of Agriculture. Diagnosis and management of foodborne illnesses: a primer for physicians and other health care professionals. MMWR Recomm Rep 2004;53(RR-4): 1–33; with permission.

a retirement party. Of 18 people who fell ill after the party, 17 (94%) had eaten the ham [28]. Unsanitary preparation techniques as well as improper storage temperatures were implicated in this outbreak.

Treatment for patients with *S. aureus* food poisoning is generally supportive, with antiemetics and intravenous fluids if indicated. Admission is rarely needed in these patients. While the diagnosis of staphylococcal food poisoning is generally clinical, in the setting of larger outbreaks, epidemiologic investigations may be undertaken by public health officials, including questionnaires to document food histories, symptoms and illness, as well as collection of leftover food for laboratory analysis.

Salmonella

Salmonella infection, caused by a gram-negative rod-shaped bacterium, is characterized by fever, abdominal pain, and diarrhea that occur between 12 and 72 hours after ingestion of contaminated foods [31]. It can also be transmitted through contact with infected animals. *Salmonella enterica* bacteria occur in more than 2,500 pathogenic serotypes and cause an estimated 1.2 million infections yearly in the United States [32]. The most common serotypes in the United States are *Salmonella* serotype Typhimurium and serotype Enteritidis. *Salmonella Typhi*, the etiologic agent for typhoid fever, while common in the developing world, is rare in the United States, with an estimated 400 cases per year, 75% of which occur in international travelers [33].

Recently, an overall increase in foodborne *Salmonella* infections has been seen, including multistate outbreaks caused by contaminated pot pies, peanut butter, raw tomatoes, and fruit salad [34–37]. Salmonella bacteria normally inhabit the intestinal tracts of human beings and animals, including birds, and human infection is usually caused by contact with animal feces or with infected animals, such as reptiles. Although any food can be contaminated with *Salmonella*, complete cooking kills the bacterium. Consumption of raw animal products that may harbor *Salmonella*, such as raw eggs, undercooked chicken, and beef, should be avoided. A 2007 outbreak of *Salmonella Typhimurium* infection was attributed to the consumption of raw (ie, unpasteurized) milk from a Pennsylvania dairy [38]. Before the advent of widespread pasteurization of dairy products in the early twentieth century, infections from raw milk or cheese accounted for up to 25% of the foodborne infections in the United States [39]. Despite the clear health risks, some consumers continue to consume raw milk and raw milk products, either for taste or for perceived health benefits.

Characterized by fever, abdominal cramps, and diarrhea, which may be bloody, *Salmonella* infection tends to be self-limited and most individuals infected with *Salmonella* recover within 5 to 7 days with supportive care. The need for hospital admission is uncommon in these patients. Rarely, individuals with *Salmonella* infection may develop localized infection, such as septic arthritis or sepsis. Treatment for patients with more severe infections, including the elderly or immunocompromised, should include antibiotics such as trimethoprim-sulfamethoxazole (TMP/SMX) or ciprofloxacin, although some fluoroquinolone-resistant *Salmonella* strains have been reported [40].

Clostridium perfringens

Like other Clostridia species, *Clostridium perfringens* is an anaerobic, gram-positive, spore-forming bacterium. These heat-activated spores grow in food, particularly meat and poultry, subsequently producing an enterotoxin in the small intestine when ingested [41]. Symptoms include profuse watery diarrhea, accompanied by severe abdominal cramping and gas. The time of onset is usually delayed approximately 8 to 16 hours after ingestion of contaminated foods.

Most outbreaks of *C. perfringens* are related to poor temperature control of cooked or reheated foods, especially meats, meat products, and gravy. *C. perfringens* spores can resist high temperatures, then germinate during cooling, leading to live vegetative forms of the organism that can be ingested if foods are not properly reheated before serving. Two large outbreaks of *C. perfringens* food poisoning that occurred on St. Patrick's Day, 1993 in Ohio and Virginia, related to improperly reheated corned beef, affecting over 100 patients [42].

The disease course for *C. perfringens* foodborne illness tends to be self-limited, requiring only supportive care, and resolving within 12 to 24 hours. As previously noted, there is some thought that the common "24-hour flu" may actually be caused by *C. perfringens* gastroenteritis [9]. The diagnosis is clinical, except in the case of multiple patient outbreaks where stool cultures or analysis of leftover foods may be obtained.

Other causes of invasive gastroenteritis

Campylobacter jejuni

Among industrialized nations, *Campylobacter jejuni* is the most common cause of bacterial gastroenteritis, affecting an estimated 2.4 million people yearly in the United States [43]. A gram-negative curved, rod-shaped enteric bacterium, *Campylobacter* is typically acquired through contact with contaminated food, particularly poultry, but can also be transmitted through contact with infected animals. *Campylobacter* infection causes a gastroenteritis characterized by fever, abdominal cramps, and diarrhea, which may be bloody. Symptoms usually last 1 week and resolve without specific therapy, although it may cause life-threatening sepsis in immunocompromised patients. Despite an increased incidence of macrolide- and fluoroquinolone-resistant *Campylobacter*, current recommendations for antibiotic therapy include a 5 to 7 day course of erythromycin, azithromycin, or ciprofloxacin for severe or persistent cases, which may shorten the duration of illness [44].

Shigella sonnei

Like *Salmonella* and *Campylobacter*, *Shigella* infection may cause an invasive gastroenteritis associated with fever, crampy abdominal pain, and diarrhea, which may be bloody and contain mucus. Seizures may occur in children with *Shigella* infection, although the exact mechanism is unclear. Because only a small inoculum of the gram-negative, rod-shaped bacteria (10–200 organisms) is sufficient to cause infection, Shigellosis is easily transmissible through fecal-oral contamination [45]. Following a 24- to 48-hour incubation period, the duration of illness is generally 4 to 7 days. In the United States, *Shigella sonnei* is the predominant species, while in developing countries, *S. flexneri* is more common. In the developing world, extensive outbreaks of Shigellosis are not uncommon because of poor hygiene practices and the highly infectious nature of *Shigella* [46].

Treatment of *Shigella* infection is usually with antibiotics, including TMP/SMX, ciprofloxacin, or ampicillin. The course of treatment is generally 5 to 7 days and can shorten the duration of symptoms. Recently, however, several outbreaks of multidrug-resistant *Shigella* infection in United States day care centers have been reported. Transmission in these cases was thought to be secondary to inadequate handwashing and hygiene practices [47]. Although sequelae of *Shigella* infection are rare, development of Reiter's syndrome has been reported after *Shigella* infection. Research into live-attenuated *Shigella* vaccines is ongoing, although no vaccine is currently available [48].

E. coli *O157:H7*

Largely because of several recent multistate outbreaks, *E. coli* O157:H7 has achieved a certain notoriety as a highly pathogenic foodborne illness. Outbreaks involving fresh spinach, fast food restaurants, and ground beef patties have caused dozens of consumers to fall ill and several deaths, primarily because of the subsequent development of HUS [3,49,50]. *E. coli* O157:H7, a Shiga-toxin producing strain of *E. coli* (STEC), is a gram-negative rod-shaped enteric bacterium that typically causes a gastroenteritis-type picture characterized by bloody diarrhea, abdominal cramps, and little if any fever. An infectious colitis can also result from STEC infection, characterized on computed tomographic imaging by abnormal colonic wall thickening and pericolonic stranding (Fig. 1) [51]. STEC infection is most often transmitted by fecal-oral contamination, as is the case with other enteric pathogens such as *Salmonella*, *Campyliobacter*, or *Shigella* [45].

One of the largest and best-studied recent outbreaks of *E. coli* O157:H7 involved a 2006 outbreak attributed to prepackaged, fresh spinach. Based

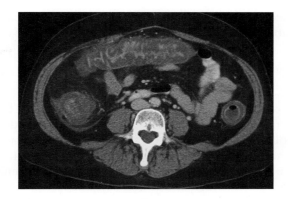

Fig. 1. Abdominal and pelvic CT scan of patient with colitis secondary to Shiga-toxin-producing *E. coli*. Note the presence of abnormal colonic wall thickening and pericolonic stranding. (*Courtesy of* David C. Pigott, MD, Birmingham, AL.)

on reporting to the CDC, 183 patients from 26 states were infected with the outbreak strain of *E. coli* O157:H7, with 29 patients (16%) developing HUS, and one death reported [3]. Subsequent epidemiologic investigations by the CDC and FDA narrowed the source of contaminated spinach to three California counties and led to a temporary FDA consumer advisory to avoid fresh bagged spinach.

As previously noted, the development of the hemolytic-uremic syndrome has been closely associated with *E. coli* O157:H7 infection. HUS, a syndrome characterized by microangiopathic hemolytic anemia, acute renal failure, and thrombocytopenia, is classically seen in patients with preceding STEC infection [52]. The pathophysiologic mechanism by which HUS develops in these patients is thought to be caused by action of Shiga toxin on the renal endothelium, leading to the development of an ongoing inflammatory reaction, acute renal failure, and disseminated intravascular coagulation. HUS is more common in the pediatric and elderly population. Recently, it has been shown that the administration of antibiotics to patients with STEC infection is highly associated with the subsequent development of HUS. A study evaluating the link between STEC and HUS by Wong and colleagues [26], found a markedly elevated relative risk (17.3, 95% confidence intervals 2.2 to 137) for the development of HUS in those patients with STEC infection who received antibiotics.

Therapy for patients with STEC infection should emphasize supportive care and close monitoring for signs of HUS, including renal function, hemoglobin, and platelet levels [53]. Most people recover from STEC without specific treatment within 5 to 10 days. Despite major public health efforts focused on the prevention of *E. coli* O157:H7 infection, multiple outbreaks have continued to occur. Precautions, such as completely cooking ground beef and hamburger, avoiding unpasteurized milk, juice, or cider, and washing all vegetables before consumption can further reduce the risk of STEC infection.

Enterotoxigenic E. coli (Traveler's diarrhea)

Far more common than STEC is enterotoxigenic *E. coli* (ETEC) infection, the cause of traveler's diarrhea. This non-Shiga-toxin-producing form of *E. coli* is ubiquitous in developing countries and also has been the cause of several outbreaks of foodborne illness in the United States [54,55]. Like other forms of *E. coli*, ETEC is transmitted via fecal-oral contamination of food and water. In nonindustrialized settings where contamination of water resources by sewage effluent may occur, ETEC tends to be endemic. Although most patients with ETEC infection have watery diarrhea, usually without fever, bloody diarrhea may occur. Symptoms are generally self-limited, lasting from 3 days to 1 week or more, following an incubation period of 1 to 3 days.

While treatment is generally supportive, TMP/SMX or fluoroquinolones may be used in more severe cases. The duration of therapy, whether a single dose or a 3- to 5-day course, does not appear to impact the duration of symptoms; all regimens appear to reduce the duration of illness by an average of 1 to 3 days [56]. Interestingly, several placebo-controlled studies have demonstrated that the prophylactic use of bismuth preparations by international travelers can reduce the incidence of traveler's diarrhea by up to 60% [57,58]. This modality is likely underused by travelers at risk for this disease. While antibiotic prophylaxis is also effective in preventing traveler's diarrhea, routine antibiotic use is not recommended for international travelers because of the potential for the selection of resistant organisms [59]. In patients with traveler's diarrhea who do receive antibiotics, there are several options as noted above. In addition to TMP/SMX or fluoroquinolones, some newer agents and strategies for the treatment of traveler's diarrhea have proven effective.

Rifaximin, a nonabsorbed, rifamycin-based antibiotic, was approved by the FDA in 2004 for the treatment of diarrhea caused by *E. coli*. A recent randomized trial has shown that a regimen of rifaximin combined with loperamide was more effective against traveler's diarrhea than treatment with either agent alone [60]. The use of probiotics, living bacterial cultures that inhibit bacterial colonization, is another emerging modality for the prevention and treatment of traveler's diarrhea. In a group of international travelers at risk for traveler's diarrhea, the use of the probiotic *Lactobacillus GG* reduced the expected incidence of the illness by 47% [61]. A recent meta-analysis of probiotic use for the prevention of acute diarrhea demonstrated efficacy in the prevention of antibiotic-associated diarrhea but a lack of data on the use of probiotics for patients with nonantibiotic-associated diarrhea [62].

Vibrio *species*

Vibrio is a genus of gram-negative curved rod-shaped bacteria that includes several species that are highly pathogenic to humans. *Vibrio cholerae*, the causative agent of cholera, is likely the most well known; however, *Vibrio vulnificus* and *V. parahaemolyticus* also cause serious outbreaks of foodborne disease. As live marine animals such as crabs or shellfish may carry *Vibrio*, the consumption of raw or undercooked shellfish is the most commonly reported cause of *Vibrio* infection. Following Hurricane Katrina in August 2005, 18 cases of wound-associated *Vibrio* infection were reported in Gulf Coast states, as well as several cases of nonwound-associated *Vibrio* infection [63].

Vibrio vulnificus may cause either wound-associated infection or foodborne illness. Symptoms of foodborne *V. vulnificus* infection include gastroenteritis symptoms in healthy individuals, as well as a potentially lethal sepsis syndrome in immunocompromised patients, especially those with chronic liver disease. The typical clinical course of patient with *V. vulnificus* infection is 2 to 8 days in duration, following an incubation period of 1 to 7 days. A 12-year review of *V. vulnificus* infection in Florida associated with eating raw oysters reported 125 patients, 44 of whom (35%) died. Two-thirds of those who died had pre-existing liver disease [64]. Multiple outbreaks of *V. vulnificus* and *V. parahaemolyticus* infection have been attributed to the consumption of raw oysters, particularly during warmer months [65]. Therapy for *V. vulnificus* should include inpatient admission and rapid administration of antibiotics because of the potential for overwhelming sepsis. Current antibiotic recommendations for the treatment of *V. vulnificus* include a 7- to 14-day course of doxycycline in conjunction with a third-generation cephalosporin, such as ceftazidime, although monotherapy with a fluoroquinolone has also been shown to be effective [66,67]. With proper antibiotic therapy, recovery is usually complete.

Fish and shellfish poisoning

The consumption of certain types of fish and shellfish can present significant risk for foodborne illness, including scombroid poisoning, ciguatera poisoning, as well as various types of shellfish poisoning. In many of these cases, heat-stable toxins are generated that may still be present despite adequate cooking. Alternatively, natural toxins that may be inherent in certain marine animals, such as tetrodotoxin in puffer fish, have the potential to cause serious or even lethal illness upon consumption.

Scombroid fish poisoning

Scombroid fish poisoning occurs after the consumption of fish containing high levels of histamine or other vasoactive amines. These biogenic amines are heat-stable and are not eliminated by cooking. Typically, improperly stored or refrigerated dark-meat fish such as tuna, mackerel, or mahimahi are responsible for outbreaks of scombroid poisoning. Histidine on the surface of improperly stored fish can produce histamine and histamine-like substances through the action of histamine decarboxylase. The clinical picture seen with scombroid poisoning consists of facial flushing, rash, itching, abdominal pain, and diarrhea, associated with a peppery or metallic taste in the mouth. Scombroid fish poisoning is typically a clinical diagnosis. Treatment is generally supportive and symptoms tend to resolve spontaneously, although antihistamines may also be effective. More severe cases may present with facial or tongue swelling, blurry vision and respiratory distress. A recent case involving an elderly female was associated with near fatal cardiovascular collapse that resolved after treatment with crystalloids and antihistamines [68].

In 2006, two outbreaks of scombroid fish poisoning that occurred in Texas and Florida were associated with eating tuna steaks. An FDA investigation revealed that imported tuna shipments from Indonesia and Vietnam were responsible, but no clearly identifiable breach in temperature control was found [69]. Although scombroid poisoning is generally quite rare in the United States, preventive measures, such as proper refrigeration are important to maintain. Given that most fish consumed in the United States is imported, maintenance of proper refrigeration at less than or equal to 40°F (less than or equal to 4.4°C) is essential to prevent scombroid poisoning [69]. In the event that scombroid poisoning is suspected or confirmed, the responsible restaurant, if known, as well as local and state public health officials, should be notified, as outbreaks involving multiple patients are typical in scombroid poisoning, often caused by contaminated fish served in restaurants or at public gatherings.

Ciguatera fish poisoning

Ciguatera fish poisoning is caused by the ingestion of certain fish that contain high concentrations of a toxin produced by a one-celled organism, the dinoflagellate *Gambierdiscus toxicus*. This toxin, known as ciguatoxin, is heat-stable, odorless and tasteless. Larger predatory reef fish such as barracuda, grouper, snapper and shark are most often implicated in outbreaks of ciguatera poisoning. Symptoms associated with ciguatera toxicity include gastrointestinal and neurologic manifestations. Nausea, vomiting, abdominal pain, and diarrhea often occur within the first few hours after ingestion, later followed by neurologic symptoms, including severe weakness, paresthesias, pain, pruritus, tooth pain, or feelings that teeth are loose. A sensation of hot-cold temperature sensation reversal is characteristic of ciguatera poisoning but is not always present [70]. Cardiovascular symptoms, such as hypotension, bradycardia, or dysrhythmia may occur, usually 1 to 3 days following ingestion.

Diagnosis is based on the clinical picture of ciguatoxic symptoms following fish ingestion. Therapy is generally supportive, as most patients recover spontaneously within a few weeks, although patients with ciguatera toxicity may have persistent neurologic symptoms lasting for weeks or months. Some investigators have recommended the use of mannitol for the neurologic manifestations of ciguatera poisoning, although the only randomized trial comparing its use to placebo failed to show any effect [71].

Paralytic shellfish poisoning

Systemic toxicity caused by the ingestion of toxic shellfish is rare but may have serious consequences. Paralytic shellfish poisoning (PSP), diarrheic, neurotoxic, and amnesic shellfish poisoning have all been reported, all of which are caused by toxic microscopic marine organisms that become concentrated in certain shellfish. Paralytic shellfish poisoning is caused by saxitoxin ingestion, usually through the consumption of contaminated bivalve shellfish, such as clams, oysters, and mussels. Saxitoxins are produced by various marine dinoflagellates, particularly *Alexandrium tamarense*. Often PSP is associated with large "algal blooms," surface aggregations of reddish-brown microscopic phytoplankton which may occur in such large numbers as to cause the ocean surface to appear red or brown in color, hence the term "red tide." These large algal blooms may be toxic to multiple forms of sea life including marine mammals, such as whales [72].

Clinical manifestations of PSP include numbness and tingling of the face and neck, headache, nausea, and muscle weakness, which can lead to respiratory failure. The mechanism of action is thought to be related to rapid sodium channel blockade. Symptoms typically occur within minutes of ingestion of contaminated shellfish. A recent cluster of cases involving a family in Maine was traced to the ingestion of contaminated mussels that had been harvested off the Maine coast. Shortly after ingestion, family members developed symptoms of PSP, ultimately resulting in hospitalization for four family members, including two family members in critical condition. Samples of mussels taken from the home were highly contaminated with saxitoxins [73].

Treatment of PSP is primarily supportive, including close observation for signs of respiratory failure requiring mechanical ventilation. Patients may also present in a deeply comatose state. A patient who presented ambulatory to an Alaska hospital with PSP rapidly became unresponsive soon after arrival, leading clinicians to briefly entertain a diagnosis of brain death before the clinical picture of PSP caused by the ingestion of contaminated mussels was ultimately discovered [74]. Epidemiologic investigations using quantitative enzyme-linked immunoassays for saxitoxin may provide useful information for tracking PSP outbreaks and developing anti-saxitoxin therapies [75].

Botulism

Botulism is a potentially life-threatening paralytic illness caused by a neurotoxin produced by the bacterium *Clostridium botulinum*. The etiologic agent, *Clostridium botulinum*, is a spore-forming bacterium found in soil as well as contaminated food, growing particularly well in low oxygen conditions. The neurotoxin produced by *C. botulinum*, is considered the most lethal toxin known to mankind and has been categorized as a Category A agent by the CDC, as one of the most potentially dangerous bioterrorism agents [76–78]. Foodborne botulism is caused by the consumption of food containing the botulism toxin, often from home-canned foods. Symptoms of botulism include a prodrome characterized by abdominal cramps, nausea, vomiting, and possibly diarrhea. Following an incubation period of 12 to 72 hours, patients may go on to develop progressive neurologic symptoms, including diplopia, blurred vision, ptosis, and difficulty swallowing, followed by muscle weakness and eventually respiratory failure secondary to paralysis of the muscles of respiration. Botulinum toxin exerts its effects through the blockage of acetylcholine release from motor neurons because of the rapid and irreversible binding of botulinum toxin to receptors on the motor nerve terminals. It is the irreversible nature of this effect on neurons that causes the long-lasting clinical effects of botulism seen in patients with foodborne botulism. Respiratory failure in these patients may be weeks or months in duration, because of the need for the development of new motor axons to innervate paralyzed muscle fibers [76].

Although rare, outbreaks of foodborne botulism can have devastating public health consequences. A recent outbreak of foodborne botulism was traced to a commercially canned chili sauce. In July 2007, four cases of suspected foodborne botulism were traced to the consumption of canned hot dog chili sauce, all of whom developed cranial nerve palsies and a symmetric descending paralysis, requiring mechanical ventilation [79]. Investigations by the CDC and state departments of health identified botulinum toxin type A in leftover samples of the chili mixture. Ultimately, the FDA and the chili sauce manufacturer issued a nationwide recall of more than 90 canned products. This episode was reportedly the first episode of foodborne botulism associated with a commercial canning facility in over 30 years.

As noted above, initial therapy for patients with botulism is primarily supportive, with mechanical ventilation being the mainstay of treatment. Definitive treatment with botulinum antitoxin, however, should not be delayed. This antitoxin is a horse-derived product containing antibodies to botulism toxins type A, B, and E. This antitoxin binds any free botulinum toxin, preventing it from exerting its paralytic effect on motor nerve terminals. It should be noted however, that the antitoxin has no effect once the toxin has bound to these motor neurons, as this binding is irreversible. In addition to botulinum antitoxins, research efforts are ongoing into a recombinant botulism vaccine as well as immunotherapies targeting specific domains of the botulinum toxin protein [80,81].

Summary

Given the widespread consumption of prepackaged and processed foods, as well as importation of foods from nonindustrialized nations where quality controls and hygienic practices may be substandard, outbreaks of foodborne illness are likely to continue to occur in the United States with some regularity. Clinicians should be familiar with the various syndromes associated with foodborne illness occurring from contaminated food and water, and be particularly vigilant with regard to those foodborne illnesses with the potential for causing severe illness and death, particularly in susceptible populations.

References

[1] Drew C, Martin A. "Many red flags preceded a recall". New York Times October 23, 2007. Available at: http://www.nytimes.com. Accessed December 3, 2007.
[2] Centers for Disease Control and Prevention. Preliminary FoodNet data on the incidence of infection with pathogens transmitted commonly through food—selected sites, United States, 2003. MMWR Morb Mortal Wkly Rep 2004;53(16):338–43.
[3] Centers for Disease Control and Prevention. Ongoing multistate outbreak of Escherichia coli serotype O157:H7 infections associated with consumption of fresh spinach—United States, September 2006. MMWR Morb Mortal Wkly Rep 2006;55(38):1045–6.
[4] Jones TF, Scallan E, Angulo FJ. FoodNet: overview of a decade of achievement. Foodborne Pathog Dis 2007;4(1):60–6.
[5] Jones TF, McMillian MB, Scallan E, et al. A population-based estimate of the substantial burden of diarrhoeal disease in the United States; FoodNet, 1996–2003. Epidemiol Infect 2007;135(2):293–301.
[6] Centers for Disease Control and Prevention (CDC). Preliminary FoodNet data on the incidence of infection with pathogens transmitted commonly through food—10 states, 2006. MMWR Morb Mortal Wkly Rep 2007;56(14):336–9.
[7] Talan DA, Moran GJ, Mower WR, et al. EMERGEncy ID NET: an emergency department-based emerging infections sentinel network. The EMERGEncy ID NET Study Group. Ann Emerg Med 1998;32(6):703–11.
[8] Freedman DO, Kozarsky PE, Weld LH, et al. GeoSentinel: the global emerging infections sentinel network of the International Society of Travel Medicine. J Travel Med 1999;6(2): 94–8.
[9] Thielman NM, Guerrant RL. Clinical practice. Acute infectious diarrhea. N Engl J Med 2004;350(1):38–47.
[10] Uysal G, Sökmen A, Vidinlisan S. Clinical risk factors for fatal diarrhea in hospitalized children. Indian J Pediatr 2000;67(5):329–33.
[11] Jones TF, Imhoff B, Samuel M, et al, Emerging Infections Program FoodNet Working Group. Limitations to successful investigation and reporting of foodborne outbreaks: an analysis of foodborne disease outbreaks in FoodNet catchment areas, 1998–1999. Clin Infect Dis 2004;38(Suppl 3):S297–302.
[12] Bini EJ, Rajapaksa RC, Weinshel EH. The findings and impact of nonrehydrated guaiac examination of the rectum (FINGER) study: a comparison of 2 methods of screening for

colorectal cancer in asymptomatic average-risk patients. Arch Intern Med 1999;159(17): 2022–6.

[13] Bardhan PK, Beltinger J, Beltinger RW, et al. Screening of patients with acute infectious diarrhoea: evaluation of clinical features, faecal microscopy, and faecal occult blood testing. Scand J Gastroenterol 2000;35(1):54–60.

[14] Guss DA, Richards C. Comparison of men and women presenting to an ED with acute appendicitis. Am J Emerg Med 2000;18(4):372–5.

[15] Spandorfer PR, Alessandrini EA, Joffe MD, et al. Oral versus intravenous rehydration of moderately dehydrated children: a randomized, controlled trial. Pediatrics 2005;115(2): 295–301.

[16] Avery ME, Snyder JD. Oral therapy for acute diarrhea. The underused simple solution. N Engl J Med 1990;323(13):891–4.

[17] Santosham M, Fayad I, Abu Zikri M, et al. A double-blind clinical trial comparing World Health Organization oral rehydration solution with a reduced osmolarity solution containing equal amounts of sodium and glucose. J Pediatr 1996;128(1):45–51.

[18] World Health Organization. Reduced Osmolarity Oral Rehydration Salts (ORS) Formulation. New York: UNICEF House; July 18, 2001, 2001. WHO/FCH/CAH/01.22.

[19] Ladinsky M, Duggan A, Santosham M, et al. The World Health Organization oral rehydration solution in US pediatric practice: a randomized trial to evaluate parent satisfaction. Arch Pediatr Adolesc Med 2000;154(7):700–5.

[20] Rao SS, Summers RW, Rao GR, et al. Oral rehydration for viral gastroenteritis in adults: a randomized, controlled trial of 3 solutions. JPEN J Parenter Enteral Nutr 2006;30(5):433–9.

[21] Turck D. Prevention and treatment of acute diarrhea in infants. Arch Pediatr 2007;14(11): 1375–8.

[22] Sirinavin S, Garner P. Antibiotics for treating Salmonella gut infections. Cochrane Database Syst Rev 2000;(2):CD001167.

[23] Sirinavin S, Pokawattana L, Bangtrakulnondh A. Duration of nontyphoidal Salmonella carriage in asymptomatic adults. Clin Infect Dis 2004;38(11):1644–5.

[24] De Bruyn G, Hahn S, Borwick A. Antibiotic treatment for travellers' diarrhoea. Cochrane Database Syst Rev 2000;(3):CD002242.

[25] Zhang X, McDaniel AD, Wolf LE, et al. Quinolone antibiotics induce Shiga toxin-encoding bacteriophages, toxin production, and death in mice. J Infect Dis 2000;181:664–70.

[26] Wong CS, Jelacic S, Habeeb RL, et al. The risk of the hemolytic-uremic syndrome after antibiotic treatment of Escherichia coli O157:H7 infections. N Engl J Med 2000;342(26): 1930–6.

[27] Abubakar I, Irvine L, Aldus CF, et al. A systematic review of the clinical, public health and cost-effectiveness of rapid diagnostic tests for the detection and identification of bacterial intestinal pathogens in faeces and food. Health Technol Assess 2007;11(36):23–58.

[28] Centers for Disease Control and Prevention. Outbreak of staphylococcal food poisoning associated with precooked ham—Florida, 1997. MMWR Morb Mortal Wkly Rep 1997; 46(50):1189–91.

[29] Murray RJ. Recognition and management of Staphylococcus aureus toxin-mediated disease. Intern Med J 2005;35(Suppl 2):S106–19.

[30] Rim JY, Bacon AE 3rd. Prevalence of community-acquired methicillin-resistant Staphylococcus aureus colonization in a random sample of healthy individuals. Infect Control Hosp Epidemiol 2007;28(9):1044–6.

[31] Brenner FW, Villar RG, Angulo FJ, et al. Salmonella nomenclature. J Clin Microbiol 2000; 38(7):2465–7.

[32] Voetsch AC, Van Gilder TJ, Angulo FJ, et al, Emerging Infections Program FoodNet Working Group. FoodNet estimate of the burden of illness caused by nontyphoidal Salmonella infections in the United States. Clin Infect Dis 2004;38(Suppl 3):S127–34.

[33] Ryan CA, Hargrett-Bean NT, Blake PA. Salmonella typhi infections in the United States, 1975–1984: increasing role of foreign travel. Rev Infect Dis 1989;11(1):1–8.

[34] United States Department of Agriculture, Food Safety and Inspection Service. Missouri firm recalls frozen pot pie products for possible Salmonella contamination. Recall Release Oct 11, 2007. Available at: http://www.fsis.usda.gov/news/Recall_044_2007_Release/index.asp. Accessed December 4, 2007.

[35] Centers for Disease Control and Prevention. Multistate outbreak of Salmonella serotype Tennessee infections associated with peanut butter—United States, 2006–2007. MMWR Morb Mortal Wkly Rep 2007;56(21):521–4.

[36] Centers for Disease Control and Prevention. Multistate outbreaks of Salmonella infections associated with raw tomatoes eaten in restaurants—United States, 2005–2006. MMWR Morb Mortal Wkly Rep 2007;56(35):909–11.

[37] Centers for Disease Control and Prevention. Salmonella Oranienburg infections associated with fruit salad served in health-care facilities—northeastern United States and Canada, 2006. MMWR Morb Mortal Wkly Rep 2007;56(39):1025–8.

[38] Centers for Disease Control and Prevention. Salmonella typhimurium infection associated with raw milk and cheese consumption—Pennsylvania, 2007. MMWR Morb Mortal Wkly Rep 2007;56(44):1161–4.

[39] Center for Food Safety and Applied Nutrition. Grade "A" pasteurized milk ordinance: 2001 revision. US Department of Health and Human Services, Food and Drug Administration, Center for Food Safety and Applied Nutrition; 2002.

[40] Giraud E, Baucheron S, Cloeckaert A. Resistance to fluoroquinolones in Salmonella: emerging mechanisms and resistance prevention strategies. Microbes Infect 2006;8(7): 1937–44.

[41] Shandera WX, Tacket CO, Blake PA. Food poisoning due to Clostridium perfringens in the United States. J Infect Dis 1983;147:167–70.

[42] Centers for Disease Control and Prevention. Clostridium perfringens gastroenteritis associated with corned beef served at St. Patrick's Day meals—Ohio and Virginia, 1993. MMWR Morb Mortal Wkly Rep 1994;43(8):137, 143–4.

[43] Nachamkin I, Blaser MJ, editors. Campylobacter. 2nd edition. Washington: ASM Press; 2000.

[44] Engberg J, Aarestrup FM, Taylor DE, et al. Quinolone and macrolide resistance in Campylobacter jejuni and C. coli: resistance mechanisms and trends in human isolates. Emerg Infect Dis 2001;7(1):24–34.

[45] Musher DM, Musher BL. Contagious acute gastrointestinal infections. N Engl J Med 2004; 351(23):2417–27.

[46] Greig JD, Todd EC, Bartleson CA, et al. Outbreaks where food workers have been implicated in the spread of foodborne disease. Part 1. Description of the problem, methods, and agents involved. J Food Prot 2007;70(7):1752–61.

[47] Centers for Disease Control and Prevention. Outbreaks of multidrug-resistant Shigella sonnei gastroenteritis associated with day care centers—Kansas, Kentucky, and Missouri, 2005. MMWR Morb Mortal Wkly Rep 2006;55(39):1068–71.

[48] Venkatesan MM, Ranallo RT. Live-attenuated Shigella vaccines. Expert Rev Vaccines 2006; 5(5):669–86.

[49] United States Food and Drug Administration. FDA investigating E. coli O157 infections associated with Taco Bell restaurants in Northeast. FDA Statement. December 6, 2006. Available at: http://www.fda.gov/bbs/topics/NEWS/2006/NEW01517.html. Accessed December 4, 2007.

[50] United States Department of Agriculture, Food Safety and Inspection Service. New Jersey Firm Recalls Ground Beef Products For Possible E. coli O157:H7 Contamination. Recall Release September 25, 2007. Available at: http://www.fsis.usda.gov/News_&;_Events/ Recall_040_2007_release/index.asp. Accessed December 4, 2007.

[51] Miller FH, Ma JJ, Scholz FJ. Imaging features of enterohemorrhagic Escherichia coli colitis. AJR Am J Roentgenol 2001;177(3):619–23.

[52] Siegler RL. The hemolytic uremic syndrome. Pediatr Clin North Am 1995;42(6):1505–29.

[53] Tarr PI, Gordon CA, Chandler WL. Shiga-toxin-producing *Escherichia coli* and haemolytic uraemic syndrome. Lancet 2005;365(9464):1073–86.

[54] Dalton CB, Mintz ED, Wells JG, et al. Outbreaks of enterotoxigenic *Escherichia coli* infection in American adults: a clinical and epidemiologic profile. Epidemiol Infect 1999;123(1): 9–16.

[55] Devasia RA, Jones TF, Ward J, et al. Endemically acquired foodborne outbreak of enterotoxin-producing *Escherichia coli* serotype O169:H41. Am J Med 2006;119(2):168.e7–e10.

[56] DuPont HL. Travelers' diarrhea: antimicrobial therapy and chemoprevention. Nat Clin Pract Gastroenterol Hepatol 2005;2(4):191–8.

[57] Steffen R, DuPont HL, Heusser R, et al. Prevention of traveler's diarrhea by the tablet form of bismuth subsalicylate. Antimicrob Agents Chemother 1986;29(4):625–7.

[58] DuPont HL, Ericsson CD, Johnson PC, et al. Prevention of travelers' diarrhea by the tablet formulation of bismuth subsalicylate. JAMA 1987;257(10):1347–50.

[59] Tellier R, Keystone JS. Prevention of traveler's diarrhea. Infect Dis Clin North Am 1992; 6(2):333–54.

[60] Dupont HL, Jiang ZD, Belkind-Gerson J, et al. Treatment of travelers' diarrhea: randomized trial comparing rifaximin, rifaximin plus loperamide, and loperamide alone. Clin Gastroenterol Hepatol 2007;5(4):451–6.

[61] Hilton E, Kolakowski P, Singer C, et al. Efficacy of *Lactobacillus GG* as a diarrheal preventive in travelers. J Travel Med 1997;4(1):41–3.

[62] Sazawal S, Hiremath G, Dhingra U, et al. Efficacy of probiotics in prevention of acute diarrhoea: a meta-analysis of masked, randomised, placebo-controlled trials. Lancet Infect Dis 2006;6(6):374–82.

[63] Centers for Disease Control and Prevention. Vibrio illnesses after Hurricane Katrina—multiple states, August-September 2005. MMWR Morb Mortal Wkly Rep 2005;54(37): 928–31.

[64] Centers for Disease Control and Prevention. *Vibrio vulnificus* infections associated with raw oyster consumption—Florida, 1981–1992. MMWR Morb Mortal Wkly Rep 1993;42(21): 405–7.

[65] Centers for Disease Control and Prevention. *Vibrio parahaemolyticus* infections associated with consumption of raw shellfish—three states, 2006. MMWR Morb Mortal Wkly Rep 2006;55(31):854–6.

[66] Liu JW, Lee IK, Tang HJ, et al. Prognostic factors and antibiotics in *Vibrio vulnificus* septicemia. Arch Intern Med 2006;166(19):2117–23.

[67] Tang HJ, Chang MC, Ko WC, et al. In vitro and in vivo activities of newer fluoroquinolones against *Vibrio vulnificus*. Antimicrob Agents Chemother 2002;46(11):3580–4.

[68] Borade PS, Ballary CC, Lee DK. A fishy cause of sudden near fatal hypotension. Resuscitation 2007;72(1):158–60.

[69] Centers for Disease Control and Prevention. Scombroid fish poisoning associated with tuna steaks—Louisiana and Tennessee, 2006. MMWR Morb Mortal Wkly Rep 2007;56(32):817–9.

[70] Centers for Disease Control and Prevention. Ciguatera fish poisoning—Texas, 1998, and South Carolina, 2004. MMWR Morb Mortal Wkly Rep 2006;55(34):935–7.

[71] Schnorf H, Taurarii M, Cundy T. Ciguatera fish poisoning: a double-blind randomized trial of mannitol therapy. Neurology 2002;58(6):873–80.

[72] Isbister GK, Kiernan MC. Neurotoxic marine poisoning. Lancet Neurol 2005;4(4):219–28.

[73] ProMED-mail. Paralytic Shellfish Poisoning, Human - USA (Maine). ProMED-mail 2007; 2 Aug 2007;0802.2508. Available at: http://www.promedmail.org. Accessed November 22, 2007.

[74] Gessner BD, Middaugh JP, Doucette GJ. Paralytic shellfish poisoning in Kodiak, Alaska. West J Med 1997;167(5):351–3.

[75] Kawatsu K, Hamano Y, Sugiyama A, et al. Development and application of an enzyme immunoassay based on a monoclonal antibody against gonyautoxin components of paralytic shellfish poisoning toxins. J Food Prot 2002;65(8):1304–8.

[76] Arnon SS, Schechter R, Inglesby TV, et al, Working Group on Civilian Biodefense. Botulinum toxin as a biological weapon: medical and public health management. JAMA 2001; 285(8):1059–70.

[77] Varma JK, Katsitadze G, Moiscrafishvili M, et al. Signs and symptoms predictive of death in patients with foodborne botulism—Republic of Georgia, 1980–2002. Clin Infect Dis 2004; 39(3):357–62.

[78] Centers for Disease Control and Prevention. Recognition of illness associated with the intentional release of a biologic agent. MMWR Morb Mortal Wkly Rep 2001;50(41):893–7.

[79] Centers for Disease Control and Prevention. Botulism associated with commercially canned chili sauce—Texas and Indiana, July 2007. MMWR Morb Mortal Wkly Rep 2007;56(30): 767–9.

[80] Cai S, Singh BR. Strategies to design inhibitors of *Clostridium botulinum* neurotoxins. Infect Disord Drug Targets 2007;7(1):47–57.

[81] Pier CL, Tepp WH, Bradshaw M, et al. A recombinant holo-toxoid vaccine against botulism. Infect Immun 2008;76(1):437–42.

ELSEVIER
SAUNDERS

Emerg Med Clin N Am
26 (2008) 499–516

EMERGENCY
MEDICINE
CLINICS OF
NORTH AMERICA

Travel-Related Infections

Hans R. House, MD, FACEP[a,b,*], Jesmin P. Ehlers, MD[c]

[a]*Department of Emergency Medicine, University of Iowa Hospitals and Clinics, C43 GH, 200 Hawkins Drive, Iowa City, IA 52242, USA*
[b]*Emergency Medicine Residency Program, University of Iowa Hospitals and Clinics, C43 GH, 200 Hawkins Drive, Iowa City, IA 52242, USA*
[c]*University of Iowa Carver College of Medicine, MERF, Iowa City, IA 52242, USA*

Over 50 million Americans travel internationally every year. Health problems are reported by 22% to 64% of those who travel to the developing world. Of these travelers, up to 8% seek medical care either during their travel or after returning home [1]. The duration of travel has a significant relationship to the risk of illness. Each day abroad adds a 3% to 4% risk of illness. Persons who take trips of longer than 30 days have up to an 80% risk for health complaints during or after their trip [2]. Among North American travelers, young females demonstrate the highest risk for developing an illness abroad.

Ill travelers are likely to present to emergency departments after their return, and their symptoms may be caused by common or exotic diseases. The failure to consider tropical diseases can lead to misdiagnosis and poor outcomes. This article addresses the important factors to discuss when obtaining a travel history and reviews some of the infectious diseases associated with recent travel, organized around the typical presenting symptoms. The most common symptoms for which patients seek medical care following travel include fever, diarrhea, and skin lesions.

History and risk factors

The evaluation of returning travelers should begin the same as the assessment of any other patient. Returning travelers will frequently present with illness unrelated to their recent travel; however, some unique historical

* Corresponding author. Department of Emergency Medicine, University of Iowa Hospitals and Clinics, C43 GH, 200 Hawkins Drive, Iowa City, IA 52242.
E-mail address: hans-house@uiowa.edu (H.R. House).

questions for travelers can help elucidate the likelihood of an exotic infection. It is essential to identify risk factors or medical conditions that have an impact on travel-related illnesses. A thorough travel history should be obtained in all patients with travel-related illness. The travel history should include a broad yet detailed description of various aspects of the patient's trip. Specifically, the following information should be obtained from the patient:

- Prophylactic measures taken before travel, including routine and travel-related vaccines as well as compliance with medications
- Precise dates of travel and return to home
- All destinations and the duration of stay at each destination, including whether the destinations were in industrialized versus developing countries
- Facilities where they stayed and sleeping accommodations (eg, modern hotel versus tent camping)

Discussing the reason for travel can often be helpful in evaluating a patient's exposures. Business-related travelers most often stay in modern hotels within urban areas. Adventurous travelers and those visiting family often spend significant amounts of time in more rural areas. These factors can drastically impact the exposure risk of the traveler. In addition, travelers returning to their country of origin to visit friends and relatives have an increased risk of travel-related health problems. Some specific exposures that should be questioned include the following:

- Fresh water contact
- Food intake, especially unpasteurized dairy products and potentially raw meat or fish
- Insect or tick bites or stings
- Animal contacts, including any licks, bites, or scratches
- Ill person contacts
- Barefoot exposure
- Sexual contacts
- Needle exposures
- Special activities such as diving, hiking, camping, boating, or rafting

In addition to the travel history, it is critical to obtain a thorough history of present illness and past medical conditions. If a fever has been present, identifying the pattern of the fever, including its onset and severity, can be helpful. Any associated symptoms, including sweats, rigors, chills, headache, or dermatologic symptoms, should be identified. A past medical history is helpful to identify factors that may predispose a patient to travel illness. The elderly often have multiple conditions that predispose them to infectious diseases. A history of splenectomy, immunocompromised status, or possible pregnancy are other important factors to address in the medical history [3,4].

Tropical infections presenting as undifferentiated fever

Fever is present in approximately 3% of patients after international travel [5]. It is the chief complaint in 28% of those who seek medical care after travel. The most common cause of fever in patients presenting after travel is a nonspecific viral illness, the same as in persons who have not left their home country; however, additional diseases must be considered, including malaria, dengue, typhoid, and hepatitis, among others. Certain travel destinations are associated with a higher risk of acquiring specific diseases. For example, malaria is the most likely cause of fever when a traveler returns from Sub-Saharan Africa or Oceania (Fig. 1). A detailed travel history should included the date of return to the home country and the date of the onset of symptoms. If the illness began after the patient's return and after the termination of exposure to exotic pathogens, an incubation period for the disease can be identified. This information can be useful in developing a differential list of diseases that would be consistent with the time course (Fig. 2) [5,6].

Malaria

After a viral syndrome, malaria is the most common cause of undifferentiated fever in travelers [7]. Malaria exists throughout the tropics and is especially prevalent in South Asia and Sub-Saharan Africa. The most common continent visited by returning travelers with malaria is Africa [8]. Patients who fail to adequately adhere to their chemoprophylaxis regimen are at significantly higher risk for infection [9,10].

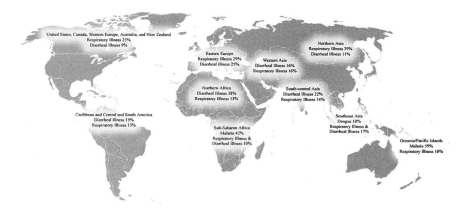

Fig. 1. Regional distribution of travelers returning ill. The percentage of travelers with fever that were diagnosed with various conditions after returning from regions across the globe is shown. Systemic febrile illness and undiagnosed febrile illness have been excluded. (*Data from* Wilson ME, Weld LH, Boggild A, et al. Fever in returned travelers: results from the GeoSentinel Surveillance Network. Clin Infect Dis 2007;44(12):1560–8.)

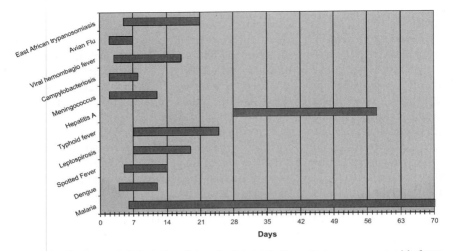

Fig. 2. Incubation period for selected travel-related infections that may present with fever. Dark bars indicate the typical incubation period. Bars that run to the end of the graph indicate possible incubation periods of prolonged timeframes. (*Data from* Ryan ET, Wilson ME, Kain KC, et al. Illness after international travel. N Engl J Med 2002;347:505–16.)

Malaria is caused by an intracellular protozoan parasite of the *Plasmodium* genus and is transmitted by the bite of the female *Anopheles* mosquito. The use of DEET-containing repellent, bed nets, and permethrin insecticide has been demonstrated to reduce the rate of *Anopheles* bites and the risk of contracting malaria [11–13]. Four *Plasmodium* species infect humans, but the most significant by far is *Plasmodium falciparum*. Due to its tendency to induce higher parasitemias (the percentage of erythrocytes infected by the parasite) and the adherence of infected cells to the endothelium, *P falciparum* accounts for the vast majority of malaria deaths.

Patients with malaria will almost always present with a chief complaint of fever, but 20% may not have the sign of fever at the time of their visit to the emergency department, reflecting the intermittent nature of the symptom. The classical cyclical fever is rarely seen. Many other symptoms may accompany malaria, including rigors, night sweats, abdominal pain, diarrhea, and even cough. The complaint of a fever in a returning traveler from a malaria-endemic region should always raise the possibility of malaria, regardless of the associated symptoms. Usual laboratory tests such as a complete blood count, chemistry, and urinalysis are nonspecific in malaria. Elevated billirubin and anemia due the intravascular destruction of erythrocytes are often seen.

Malaria is diagnosed by direct examination of thick and thin blood smears. The thick blood smear is used to identify the presence of any parasites; the thin smear is used to determine the species of the *Plasmodium* infecting the patient. Results of the thin smear are usually described as either "falciparum malaria" or "non-falciparum malaria," reflecting the importance and severity of *P falciparum* infection. Because non-falciparum infections are generally treated the same, there is little need to further speciate the sample. Multiple blood samples drawn throughout a 24-hour period may be needed to adequately rule out malaria. Serology tests for malaria are also available in some centers. These tests are not useful for natives of a malarial region, because they likely were exposed at some point in their life.

The treatment of malaria depends on the type of parasite identified. For non-falciparum species, the treatment of choice remains chloroquine. The initial dose is 600 mg base (1000 mg salt) followed by 300 mg base (500 mg salt) at 6, 24, and 48 hours after the first dose. To eradicate the hypnozoites or liver stage, chloroquine therapy should be followed by primaquine, 30 mg for 2 weeks. Patients with non-falciparum malaria should usually be admitted for treatment, but outpatient therapy can be considered for natives of a malarial region who have some baseline immunity. Because chloroquine has been known to cause a prolonged QT interval, documenting a baseline ECG before beginning therapy would be prudent. Hyperexcitability and tinnitus is expected when taking excessive doses and are an indication to decrease the dose. Is it not an appropriate drug for prolonged (more than 1 to 2 months) malaria prophylaxis because of the risk of retinopathy.

All cases of falciparum malaria must be admitted for therapy owing to the high mortality of the disease. Falciparum malaria is treated with atovaquone-proguanil (Malarone) or quinine sulfate plus doxycycline, tetracycline, or clindamycin. Severe falciparum infection, including cerebral malaria, is treated with intravenous quinidine. Since 1991, quinidine gluconate has been the only parenterally administered antimalarial drug available in the United States. It is recommended to give a loading dose of 6.25 mg base/kg (10 mg salt/kg) of quinidine gluconate infused intravenously over 1 to 2 hours followed by a continuous infusion of 0.0125 mg base/kg/min (0.02 mg salt/kg/min). At least 24 hours of quinidine infusion is recommended. Once the parasite density is less than 1% and the patient can take oral medication, the patient can complete the treatment course with oral quinine at a dosage of 10 mg salt/kg every 8 hours (for a combined treatment course of quinidine/quinine for 7 days if the disease was acquired in Southeast Asia and for 3 days if the patient has returned from Africa and South America) [14,15].

Ideally, travelers will avoid getting malaria by using adequate insect repellents and taking chemoprophylactic medications. There are essentially four choices for anti-malarial prophylaxis: chloroquine, mefloquine (Larium), atovaquone/proguanil, and doxycycline. Chloroquine is taken once per week and may only be used during travel to countries with chloroquine-sensitive areas. These countries include Central America and the Caribbean. Side effects include dizziness, insomnia, pruritis, and an exacerbation of psoriasis. Mefloquine is also taken once per week and is usually effective worldwide (areas of mefloquine-resistant malaria exist, especially in East Africa and South East Asia). Its major limitation is its tendency to cause central nervous system side effects and exacerbate psychiatric illnesses. It is contraindicated in patients suffering from major depression or a history of psychosis. Doxycycline is taken once per day and may be reliably used throughout the world. It is contraindicated in pregnancy and small children and causes photosensitivity. Atovaquone/proguanil is a relatively new agent for malaria. It is taken once per day, may be used anywhere, and is contraindicated in pregnancy, breastfeeding mothers, infants, and patients with renal impairment (creatinine clearance < 30 mL/min) [14].

Dengue

Dengue fever, a viral infection from the family Arbovirus, is transmitted by the bite of mosquitoes, most often *Aedes aegypti* and *Aedes albopictus*. The prevalence of this disease is increasing, and it has become one of the world's most common tropical diseases, especially in South America and Southeast Asia. Many popular tourist destinations, including parts of the developed world such as Hawaii, are endemic. It is now estimated that up to 16% of febrile illness in travelers returning from the tropics may be due to dengue.

The virus features a relatively short incubation period, 2 to 8 days after the initial mosquito bite, which may help distinguish it from other febrile illnesses. Initial symptoms of the disease include fever and headache. In addition, patients complain of chills, photophobia, and severe muscle, joint, and back pain. The musculoskeletal pain that often accompanies the disease has led to its nickname of "breakbone fever." Other signs of the disease may include a maculopapular or petechial rash, lymph node enlargement, and hemorrhage (usually epistaxis or gastrointestinal bleeding). There are two more serious variants of the disease: dengue hemorrhagic fever and dengue shock syndrome. Although dengue fever is a benign, self-limited disease that calls for supportive care only, fatality rates are much higher for these variants (up to 44% in dengue shock syndrome). Fortunately, these complications are rare in travelers. Diagnosis can be established by viral culture or serologic testing [16,17].

Rickettsia

Rickettsia cause several clinical syndromes, including scrub typhus and the various types of spotted fever. They are small obligate intracellular parasites of eukaryote cells that can only be grown in a cell culture. Rickettsial infections are transmitted by the bite of blood sucking arthropods, most often ticks. Activities such as camping, hiking, or traveling through grassy areas increase the risk of exposure. The clinical presentation is variable and depends on the species of organism involved. Typhus, Q fever, trench fever, ehrlichiosis, and at least 14 spotted fever syndromes are all caused by rickettsia organisms. The most common conditions seen in travelers are African tick bite fever and Mediterranean spotted fever [18].

African tick bite fever is usually a mild illness and has not been known to be fatal. Clinical symptoms typically develop 6 to 7 days after the infectious bite. Abrupt onset of fever, myalgia, regional lymphadenitis, and headache in travelers from Africa should prompt suspicion of this disease. Identification of a painless scar, an eschar, at the presumed location of the bite should confirm that suspicion. The lesion is usually black with a red halo and a necrotic center. Due to the aggressive nature of the tick vector, multiple eschars are often documented [18]. Diagnosis is most often made by the clinical history and physical examination. Patients often recover without treatment.

Mediterranean spotted fever is caused by *Rickettsia conorii* and is endemic in urban and suburban areas around the Mediterranean basin, the Middle East, India, and in parts of Sub-Saharan Africa. Because the vector for the disease is the dog tick, there is a close association with domestic dogs. Most patients will demonstrate a single inoculation eschar (in 70% of cases) and a generalized maculopapular rash (in >95% of cases). Complications are relatively common, and if left untreated, the disease carries a 2% mortality rate [18]. Treatment with tetracycline, chloramphenicol, or azithromycin is recommended in all recognized cases [19].

Leptospirosis

Leptospirosis is caused by a spirochete and is acquired by humans after contact with contaminated soil or water. Activities associated with infection include swimming or boating in contaminated fresh water as well as gardening or farming. Leptospirosis is most commonly encountered in tropical and subtropical climate regions.

Returning travelers with fever, myalgia, headache, rash, and a history of fresh water exposure should prompt suspicion for leptospirosis. The illness can also be associated with uveitis, conjunctivitis, hematuria, and aseptic meningitis. Most commonly, the diagnosis can be established by serology testing. Unfortunately, this method is often not rapid. Dark-field microscopy and subsequent culture can also aid in diagnosis. The ideal specimen to obtain for identification of the spirochete can vary by the timeline. Blood and cerebrospinal fluid are ideal within the first 10 days of disease. After the first week of illness, urine samples have a better yield. Although many cases of leptospirosis are self-limited, treatment with penicillin or tetracycline is effective and is recommended in all cases. No published studies have established the duration of treatment [20,21]. The clinical course may be complicated by renal failure, acute respiratory distress syndrome, or myocarditis. Liver failure, if present, is usually reversible.

Typhoid fever

Typhoid fever is caused by the bacterium *Salmonella typhi* and is transmitted by the fecal-oral route, most typically involving contaminated food or water. Infection after travel to highly endemic regions accounts for the majority of cases; these areas include India, the Philippines, Pakistan, Mexico, El Salvador, and Haiti. The incubation period ranges from 5 to 21 days.

As opposed to some of the other febrile illnesses discussed previously, typhoid may have a more insidious onset of symptoms. After a 5- to 21-day incubation period, typical symptoms of abdominal discomfort, constipation, fever, pulse-fever dissociation, and severe headache develop. Although the disease is caused by a salmonella infection of the Peyer's patches in the intestine, diarrhea is not a typical presenting symptom. Physical examination is often unremarkable. Typhoid vaccinations are not always effective, and the fact that a patient has been vaccinated should not rule out the diagnosis. The causative organism can be isolated from a blood culture for diagnosis. Other sites that may yield positive cultures include urine, stool, and duodenal contents. The most sensitive culture for typhoid fever is obtained from the bone marrow. The disease usually responds to treatment with fluoroquinolones for 7 to 14 days. Drug-resistant strains to other antibiotics have been reported [6,11]. If left untreated, typhoid fever can last for 3 weeks or longer and carries a mortality rate of 12% to 30%. Complications include perforation of the intestine at the Peyer's patches.

Hepatitis A

Hepatitis A is one of the most common vaccine-preventable, travel-related infections. It is caused by a virus spread by fecal-oral contact. Approximately 30% of acute hepatitis A can be attributed to travel to endemic areas. Travel to Latin America, Asia, and Africa is associated with a higher risk of infection. Specifically, poor water quality and poor sanitation are factors that contribute to the spread of hepatitis A. Vaccination is most effective when given at least 4 weeks before travel; however, because the vaccine has been shown to be effective when given in post-exposure situations, it may be protective even if given on the day of travel [22]. Over the past 20 years, hepatitis A infections have decreased significantly. Evidence suggests that children may be particularly susceptible [23]. Up to one half of travel-associated hepatitis A cases occur among children, yet the majority of international travelers are adults. North American travelers who were born and raised in developing countries are likely to have acquired immunity to hepatitis A from their childhood [24,25].

Hepatitis A virus is transmitted via a fecal-oral route, most commonly by contaminated food. Its incubation period is typically 28 to 30 days [6]. Patients typically present with fever, right upper quadrant pain, and jaundice. Additionally, they may complain of anorexia, nausea, vomiting, or malaise. Laboratory tests reveal elevations of aminotransferases, possibly into the thousands, and identification of anti–hepatitis A virus IgM antibody is diagnostic. Treatment is supportive. Most cases are self-limited, but fulminant liver failure is a rare complication.

Meningococcal meningitis

Meningococcal disease is potentially a morbid and life-threatening illness. Even with appropriate antibiotic regimens, the overall fatality rate is around 10% and is as high as 40% in cases of meningococcal sepsis [26]. In addition, approximately 15% of survivors have significant long-term complications of the illness, including hearing loss, neurologic damage, or loss of an extremity. Vaccination is available to four of the five clinically important serogroups (A, C, Y, and W-135) and should be given at least 7 to 10 days before travel. Documentation of meningococcal vaccination is required for entry into Saudi Arabia during the Haj pilgrimage [27].

Travel risk is relatively low, except for a few specific destinations. The highest documented risk for travelers is in pilgrims to Mecca and Medina in Saudi Arabia during the Haj. Annual epidemic meningococcal infections occur in the countries of the "meningitis belt," a swath of Sub-Sarahan Africa stretching from Senegal to Ethiopia. Outbreaks typically occur during the dry season, which is December through June.

The incubation period typically ranges between 2 and 10 days. Viral upper respiratory symptoms are accompanied by fever and malaise. Soon after, severe headache, nausea, vomiting, and stiff neck may follow [26,28]. Petechiae or ecchymotic lesions are the most common skin findings in this disease and may occur early in the course before systemic complications develop. Suspected cases should be treated with high-dose parenteral antibiotics such as ceftriaxone and vancomycin. Because steroids are likely to be helpful in pneumococcal meningitis, an initial dose of dexamethasone, 10 mg intravenously, should be given at the initiation of antibiotics. The steroid can be discontinued once meningococcal infection is confirmed, because it is probably not beneficial in meningococcal disease [29]. Once the gram-negative cocci has been identified in the cerebrospinal fluid, alternate therapies such as penicillin or chloramphenicol may be considered. Close contacts of patients should be offered antibiotic prophylaxis with rifampin or ciprofloxacin.

Tropical diseases presenting as diarrhea

Traveler's diarrhea

Traveler's diarrhea is the most common travel-related infection. It can be caused by a number of pathogens but most frequently is associated with enterotoxigenic *Escherichia coli* (ETEC) or *Campylobacter*. Travelers to Central America, Africa, and the Middle East are most frequently infected with ETEC, whereas travelers to Asia most often encounter *Campylobacter*. The risk of infection varies significantly based on destination but increases directly with increased exposure to local food and water [30]. Traveler's diarrhea is defined as an illness after travel featuring three or more unformed stools in 24 hours and is associated with at least one symptom of enteric disease, such as cramping, abdominal pain, nausea, vomiting, and fever. Traveler's diarrhea needs to be distinguished from dysentery, which is defined as the presence of visible blood in the stool. Dysentery may be caused by *Salmonella*, *Shigella*, and many of the same organisms that cause uncomplicated traveler's diarrhea, such as *Campylobacter*.

Patients who present with acute non-bloody diarrhea may be treated empirically with fluids, antibiotics, and antimotility agents. A single dose of ciprofloxacin, 750 mg, or azithromycin, 1 g by mouth, is effective for curing most cases. Additionally, antimotility agents such as loperamide are safe and effective at reducing the duration of symptoms [31,32]. Stool cultures for identifying causative organisms are not usually indicated because treatment with antibiotics and antimotility agents is so effective.

Although multiple prophylactic regimens are available for the prevention of traveler's diarrhea, they are not generally recommended for several reasons. First, prompt self-treatment with quinolones and antimotility agents can reduce the duration of illness to 1 day or less. Second, patients taking antibiotics for a long period of time will sustain more morbidity from side effects of the medication than from the traveler's diarrhea itself. Third, widespread antibiotic use promotes the development of resistant organisms.

Prophylactic therapy can be justified in certain situations, especially in immunocompromised patients who would face significant morbidity from bacterial enteritis. Bismuth subsalicylate (30 mL or two tablets four times a day) has been recommended in the past, but it is a difficult regimen to follow and can lead to salicylate toxicity in young patients. A newer agent, rifaximin, has been demonstrated to be effective in a placebo-controlled trial and caused only minimal change in gut flora [33]. It is probably less likely to promote resistant organisms.

For dysentery, a 3-day course of ciprofloxacin or azithromycin is recommended rather than a single dose. Randomized trials suggest that antimotility agents are safe to use even in the case of dysentery [34]. *Shigella* infections treated with antimotility agents alone are prone to develop complications such as toxic mega colon and prolonged infection; therefore, symptomatic therapy should always be combined with antibiotics when treating cases of dysentery.

Cholera

Cholera is a watery diarrheal disease that can be associated with acute dehydration. It is caused by *Vibrio cholerae,* a gram-negative rod. *V cholerae* is most frequently acquired via contaminated water or food. Although cholera can be contracted locally, foreign travel accounts for the majority of cases diagnosed in North America. Although travelers to developing countries are at risk of contracting cholera, it is estimated to occur at a rate of only 0.2 cases per 100,000 North American or European travelers. This risk is likely underestimated because, in the vast majority of instances, cholera is actually mild and may remain clinically undetected or mistaken for a more routine traveler's diarrhea.

Primary treatment for cholera is oral rehydration. In patients with severe illness, intravenous fluids and electrolyte replacement should be administered. Antibiotics usually shorten the duration of symptoms and decrease *V cholerae* excretion by half, reducing potential spread of the disease [35]. Antibiotics used in traveler's diarrhea, such as ciprofloxacin, doxycycline, and azithromycin are also effective against *V cholerae*. Localized areas of antibiotic resistance, especially to doxycycline and ciprofloxacin, are becoming more common. Cholera toxin, not the bacteria itself, mediates the disease process. Antimotility medications are not recommended and should be avoided because they carry a risk of prolonging the disease [36,37].

Tropical infections with a primarily dermatologic presentation

Cutaneous larva migrans

Cutaneous larva migrans is an epidermal eruption caused by infiltration of hookworm larvae through intact skin, usually in the feet. Infections occur most often in Africa, the Caribbean, and South-East Asia. Detailed questioning reveals a history of exposure of walking barefoot at a beach in over 95% of cases.

The incubation period for cutaneous larva migrans can vary widely, ranging from minutes to weeks. The lesions are typically described as being intensely itchy and growing a few centimeters each day. Cutaneous larva migrans appears as an erythematous tract that is typically described as serpiginous, although it may be linear. Bacterial infection of the initial lesions can subsequently occur. The most commonly affected anatomic sites include the foot, buttock, and abdomen or trunk [38].

Cutaneous larva migrans can be treated effectively with topical thiabendazole 15% for 1 to 2 weeks. Oral thiabendazole twice a day for 2 days can be used but is frequently associated with side effects such as altered mental status, gastrointestinal upset, or rash [39]. Another more recent treatment approach is a single dose of ivermectin. Cryotherapy can be attempted in pregnant patients but is often ineffective [40].

Cutaneous myiasis

Cutaneous myiasis, also called furuncular myiasis, is caused by the human botfly or the tumbu fly. It is the implantation and development of fly larvae in human skin. The larvae are transmitted to humans via a mosquito bite or by eggs hatching on the skin with subsequent penetration. The incubation period varies with the type of fly. Incubation with the botfly is usually 5 to 12 weeks and that with the tumbu fly usually 7 to 10 days. Cutaneous myiasis is typically acquired in tropical areas. The botfly is most commonly encountered in Central and South America, whereas the tumbu fly is more commonly found in Africa.

The lesions are often described as furuncle-like with discharge. The discharge can be crusting, odoriferous, purulent, or serosanguinous. Movements of the larva or bubbles can be visualized within a central punctum. The size of the lesion typically ranges from 1 to 2 cm. Patients often complain of crawling sensations within the lesion and itching. Lesions from tumbu flies are often painful. Anatomic regions typically involved with botfly bites include the head, forearms, and legs. The tumbu fly most often produces lesions on the trunk, buttocks, and thighs.

The diagnosis is clinical, and treatment consists of removal of the larva by several approaches. Manual pressure along the outside of tumbu fly lesions can express the larva. Occlusive substances applied to the lesion can cause the larva to migrate to the skin surface. Surgical excision can be employed but is often not necessary. It is important to not rupture the larva to avoid hypersensitivity or foreign body reactions to the larval antigens [19].

Leishmaniasis

Leishmania is transmitted by the bite of the sandfly. Symptoms frequently occur between 1 week and 3 months after the bite. It is caused by a tiny intracellular protozoan parasite of the genus *Leishmania*. Twenty species of organisms have been identified throughout the world, each causing a variety of clinical syndromes. Two major forms are recognized—visceral and cutaneous. Visceral leishmaniasis is rare in travelers, but cutaneous cases are occasionally seen. Over 90% of cutaneous cases occur in one of seven countries: Algeria, Iran, Iraq, Afghanistan, Saudi Arabia, Brazil, and Peru. Military personnel represent a particularly at-risk population. Several hundred cases of cutaneous leishmaniasis have been diagnosed in US soldiers returning from Iraq.

Cutaneous leishmaniasis should be suspected in a patient with a nonpainful, slowly growing ulcer over a period of weeks to months. Patients suffer a mean of 4 to 9 months from symptom onset to diagnosis. The ulcer usually ranges between 3 and 12 cm in diameter. Up to half of patients can present with multiple lesions. The border of the ulcer is violaceous and the base granular. The lesion can progress from an initial papule to a nodule and subsequently ulcerate. The lower legs and face are the typical sites affected. Diagnosis is made by skin scraping. Although some lesions may heal spontaneously, treatment consists of prolonged intravenous therapy with sodium stibogluconate, a pentavalent antimony compound [41,42].

Lyme disease

Lyme disease is caused by *Borrelia burgdorferi*, a bacterial spirochete. It is transmitted to humans through a prolonged bite of the *Ixodes* tick.

Lyme disease is prevalent in Europe, Asia, and North America. Skin lesions generally appear 3 to 30 days after the bite. An initial erythema migrans rash is present in 60% to 80% of patients. This lesion appears as an erythematous papule at the site of the bite. It typically expands over the next days to weeks with central clearing to result in the classic annular lesion. Other early manifestations of Lyme disease include malaise, myalgia, arthralgia, and generalized lymphadenopathy. In 60% of untreated patients, the disease progresses to monoarticular or oligoarticular arthritis. A smaller percentage may experience neurologic complaints, such as facial nerve palsy, or cardiac complications, most commonly atrial- ventricular block [43].

Diagnosis can be made clinically if the characteristic rash is identified; otherwise, serology is used. Treatment for early disease consists of 21 days of cefuroxime, doxycycline, or amoxicillin [44]. The key to prevention is preventing the infected tick's bite by wearing long sleeves and long pants, avoiding walks in heavily forested areas, and wearing insect repellent (preferably containing DEET). For patients who discover an attached tick in an area endemic for Lyme disease, a single 200-mg dose of doxycyline has been shown to be effective at preventing the disease [45].

Important tropical diseases rarely occurring in travelers

Yellow fever

Yellow fever is a rare disease that can occur in unvaccinated travelers. Transmitted by *Aedes* sp mosquitoes, the virus causing this hemorrhagic fever is a small (40 to 60 nm), single-stranded RNA virus of the family Flaviviridae. The disease is endemic in jungle areas in South America and Africa. From 1970 to 2002, there were nine reported cases from the United States and Europe. Immunization is the most important method of prevention, followed by prevention of mosquito bites. Immunization should ideally occur 4 weeks before travel, but the vaccine may be protective in as few as 10 days. The vaccine, a live attenuated virus, is usually well tolerated. A yellow fever–like systemic disease within 3 to 5 days (yellow fever vaccine-associated viscerotropic disease) and a post-vaccination encephalitis within 8 days (yellow fever vaccine-associated neurotropic disease) have been reported following vaccination. Patients aged more than 60 years are at higher risk for these rare complications.

Clinical presentation of yellow fever can include fever, jaundice, hemorrhage, and renal failure. Viral load is at its peak within 2 to 3 days after infection. The illness typically occurs in three phases:

1. Initial symptoms are fever, malaise, myalgia, nausea, vomiting, irritability, and dizziness. Leukopenia and elevated transaminase levels are seen for 36 to 48 hours.

2. In the latent phase, improvement of symptoms is seen for up to 48 hours with reduced fever. Some patients recover without development of jaundice.
3. In 15% of cases there is a clinical recurrence of initial symptoms with the addition of jaundice and bleeding diathesis followed by multiorgan system failure. If present, this recurrence develops 3 to 6 days after the initial symptoms begin.

Diagnosis can be confirmed by ELISA. Treatment is supportive and should involve intensive care for severe cases [46,47].

Avian flu

Millions of cases of influenza A occur every year. Since its emergence in 1997, H5N1 highly virulent avian influenza or "avian flu" has infected less than 500 people, most with an identified close contact with chickens, waterfowl, or other birds. Cases have been identified mostly in poultry farm workers or persons living with birds. Human-to-human contact, thus far, seems rare or impossible. Avian influenza typically presents with a febrile respiratory illness 2 to 5 days after exposure. The temperature of the patient is usually greater than 100.4°F and is often accompanied by leukopenia or lymphopenia. The typical initial influenza symptoms are followed by a subsequent pneumonia and worsening respiratory distress. H5-specific RNA is diagnostic when detected by polymerase chain reaction from pharyngeal or nasal swabs. Pharyngeal swabs are preferred because the virus is present in higher concentrations in the throat and lower respiratory tract [48]. Neuraminidase inhibitors such as zanamivir and oseltamivir should be started in any suspected cases. Ninety-five percent of viral isolates from South East Asia demonstrate an in vitro resistance to amantadine and rimantadine [49]. The mainstay of prevention of annual influenza in the United States, the influenza vaccine, is a subject of extensive investigation for avian flu. Although many vaccines are in clinical trials, thus far only one has been approved by the US Federal Drug Administration for use in humans [50]. It is not currently available for commercial production but will be included in the national stockpile of medications for distribution in a health care emergency.

African sleeping sickness

Sleeping sickness, also known as African trypanosomiasis, is caused by *Trypanosoma* parasites and transmitted by *Glossina* tsetse flies. This disease is fatal if untreated; death may occur from weeks to years from the time of infection depending on the type of parasite infection. The risk to travelers is low, but there are approximately one or two imported cases each year [51]. The disease is endemic in 36 countries in Sub-Saharan Africa. Prevention of the bite of the tsetse fly is key to avoiding the disease in prevalent areas.

Travelers should wear long sleeves, long pants, and DEET-containing repellent.

Recent travelers to East Africa who present with fever and cutaneous chancres should prompt suspicion of trypanosomiasis. The symptoms of this illness may mimic several other travel-related infections, including malaria and rickettsia infection. Additional symptoms may include lethargy, headache, gastrointestinal symptoms, myalgia, and delirium. The parasites can be identified in the blood or other aspirates to confirm the diagnosis. Lumbar puncture is essential to rule out central nervous system involvement, because it dictates the choice of antiparasitic therapy. In patients without central nervous system involvement, treatment with suramin is indicated. Suramin is a polysulfonated naphthylamine derivative of urea administered as a sodium salt. Due to a risk of anaphylaxis, a 200-mg test dose should be tried before administering the drug by slow infusion. The complete drug protocol, as well as the only US source of the drug, can be obtained through the Centers for Disease Control.

Patients who have positive lumbar punctures should be treated with melarsoprol, a trivalent arsenic compound [52,53]. It is commonly associated with significant toxicity. It causes vomiting, abdominal pain, hepatotoxicity, peripheral neuropathy, paraplegia, cardiac arrhythmias, and albuminuria. Arsenic encephalopathy occurs in as many as 10% of treated patients and is frequently fatal [54]. The 5% to 10% risk of mortality from the therapy is outweighed by the risk of the disease, because the mortality of central nervous system infection with African trypanosomiasis is 100%. As is true for suramin, melarsoprol is only available in the United States through the Centers for Disease Control.

Summary

Infections in travelers are a common problem presenting to the emergency department. A detailed travel history including the places visited, the activities enjoyed, and the living conditions will provide clues for the clinician regarding the risk of unusual tropical infections. Any patient returning from a malaria-endemic region with an undifferentiated fever must be ruled out for *Plasmodium* infection by the use of blood smears. The most common condition in returning travelers by far is traveler's diarrhea, which can be effectively managed with antibiotics and antimotility agents. A linear pruritic rash in a patient returning from a beach vacation to the Caribbean is most likely a sign of cutaneous larval migrans. Avian flu, yellow fever, and African sleeping sickness are dramatic but fortunately rare diseases in the returning traveler. Many of the infections acquired overseas can be prevented by vaccines, food and water precautions, and insect bite avoidance. The yellow fever vaccine is required for travel to certain regions. The risk of enteric diseases can be lessened by avoiding uncooked foods, thoroughly washing foods in clean water, and eating only peeled fruit ("boil it, cook it, peel it, or forget it"). The most severe imported diseases, including malaria, can be prevented by avoiding insect bites by wearing long sleeves and long pants, using permethrin-coated bed nets, and applying DEET-containing repellent.

References

[1] Freedman DO, Weld LH, Kozarsky PE, et al. Spectrum of disease and relation to place of exposure among ill returned travelers. N Engl J Med 2006;354(2):119–30.
[2] Hill DR. Health problems in a large cohort of Americans traveling to developing countries. J Travel Med 2000;7:259–66.
[3] Steffen R, deBernardis C, Banos A. Travel epidemiology—a global perspective. Int J Antimicrob Agents 2003;21:89–95.
[4] Leder K, Tong S, Weld L, et al. Illness in travelers visiting friends and relatives: a review of the GeoSentinel Surveillance Network. Clin Infect Dis 2006;43(9):1185–93.
[5] Wilson ME, Weld LH, Boggild A, et al. Fever in returned travelers: results from the GeoSentinel Surveillance Network. Clin Infect Dis 2007;44(12):1560–8.
[6] Ryan ET, Wilson ME, Kain KC. Illness after international travel. N Engl J Med 2002;347:505–16.
[7] Doherty JF, Grant AD, Bryceson AD. Fever as the presenting complaint of travelers returning from the tropics. QJM 1995;88(4):277–81.
[8] Askling HH, Nilsson J, Tegnell A, et al. Malaria risk in travelers. Emerg Infect Dis 2005;11(3):436–41.
[9] Jelinek T, Schulte C, Behrens R, et al. Imported falciparum malaria in Europe: sentinel surveillance data from the European Network on Surveillance of Imported Infectious Diseases. Clin Infect Dis 2002;34:572–6.
[10] Phillips-Howard PA, Radalowicz A, Mitchell J, et al. Risk of malaria in British residents returning from malarious areas. BMJ 1990;300:499–503.
[11] Lengeler C. Insecticide treated bednets and curtains for preventing malaria. In: Cochrane Infectious Diseases Group. The Cochrane Library, Issue 1. Chichester (UK): John Wiley & Sons; 2007. [search date 2003].
[12] Soto J, Medina F, Dember N, et al. Efficacy of permethrin-impregnated uniforms in the prevention of malaria and leishmaniasis in Colombian soldiers. Clin Infect Dis 1995;21:599–602.
[13] Rowland M, Downey G, Rab A, et al. DEET mosquito repellent provides personal protection against malaria: a household randomized trial in an Afghan refugee camp in Pakistan. Trop Med Int Health 2004;9:335–42.
[14] Centers for Disease Control. Treatment of malaria. Available at: www.cdc.gov. Accessed October 15, 2007.
[15] Zucker JR, Campbell CC. Malaria: principles of prevention and treatment. Infect Dis Clin North Am 1993;7(3):547–67.
[16] Jelinek T. Dengue fever in international travelers. Clin Infect Dis 2000;31:144–7.
[17] Wilder-Smith A, Schwartz E. Dengue in travelers. N Engl J Med 2005;353:924–32.
[18] Jensenius M, Fournier PE, Raoult D. Tick-borne rickettsioses in international travellers. Int J Infect Dis 2004;8(3):139–46.
[19] Lucchina LC, Wilson ME, Drake LA. Dermatology and the recently returned traveler: infectious diseases with dermatologic manifestations. Int J Dermatol 1997;36(3):167–81.
[20] Gelman SS, Gundlapalli AV, Hale D, et al. Spotting the spirochete: rapid diagnosis of leptospirosis in two returned travelers. J Travel Med 2002;9(3):165–7.
[21] Lo Re V 3rd, Gluckman SJ. Fever in the returned traveler. Am Fam Physician 2003;68(7):1343–50.

[22] Sagliocca L, Amoroso P, Adamo B, et al. Efficacy of hepatitis A vaccine in prevention of secondary hepatitis A infection. Lancet 1999;353(9159):1136–9.

[23] Gosselin C, De Serres G, Rouleau I, et al. Comparison of trip characteristics of children and adults with travel-acquired hepatitis A infection. Pediatr Infect Dis J 2006;25(12): 1184–6.

[24] Mutsch M, Spicher VM, Gut C, et al. Hepatitis A virus infections in travelers, 1988–2004. Clin Infect Dis 2006;42(4):490–7.

[25] Ciccozzi M, Tosti ME, Gallo G, et al. Risk of hepatitis A infection following travel. J Viral Hepat 2002;9:460–5.

[26] Wilder-Smith A, Memish Z. Meningococcal disease and travel. Int J Antimicrob Agents 2003;21(2):102–6.

[27] Centers for Disease Control and Prevention. Health information for international travel 2008. Atlanta (GA): US Department of Health and Human Services, Public Health Service; 2007.

[28] Memish ZA. Meningococcal disease and travel. Clin Infect Dis 2002;34:84–90.

[29] van de Beek D, de Gans J, Tunkel AR, et al. Community-acquired bacterial meningitis in adults. N Engl J Med 2006;354:44–53.

[30] Riddle MS, Sanders JW, Putnam SD, et al. Incidence, etiology, and impact of diarrhea among long-term travelers (US military and similar populations): a systematic review. Am J Trop Med Hyg 2006;74(5):891–900.

[31] Dupont HL, Jiang ZD, Belkind-Gerson J. Treatment of traveler's diarrhea: randomized trial comparing rifaximin, rifaximin plus loperamide, and loperamide alone. Clin Gastroenterol Hepatol 2007;5(4):451–6.

[32] Taylor DN, Sanchez JL, Candler W. Treatment of traveler's diarrhea: ciprofloxacin plus loperamide compared with ciprofloxacin alone. A placebo-controlled, randomized trial. Ann Intern Med 1991;114(9):731–4.

[33] DuPont HL, Jiang ZD, Okhuysen PC, et al. A randomized, double-blind, placebo-controlled trial of rifaximin to prevent traveler's diarrhea. Ann Intern Med 2005;142(10): 805–12.

[34] Murphy GS, Bodhidatta L, Echeverria P, et al. Ciprofloxacin and loperamide in the treatment of bacillary dysentery. Ann Intern Med 1993;118(8):582–6.

[35] Khan WA, Bennish ML, Seas C, et al. Randomised controlled comparison of single-dose ciprofloxacin and doxycycline for cholera caused by *Vibrio cholerae* 01 or 0139. Lancet 1996;348(9023):296–300.

[36] Steffen R, Acar J, Walker E, et al. Cholera: assessing the risk to travellers and identifying methods of protection. Travel Med Infect Dis 2003;1(2):80–8.

[37] Steinberg EB, Greene KD, Bopp CA, et al. Cholera in the United States, 1995–2000: trends at the end of the twentieth century. J Infect Dis 2001;184(6):799–802.

[38] Blackwell V, Vega-Lopez F. Cutaneous larva migrans: clinical features and management of 44 cases presenting in the returning traveller. Br J Dermatol 2001;145(3):434–7.

[39] Jelinek T, Maiwald H, Nothdurft HD, et al. Cutaneous larva migrans in travelers: synopsis of histories, symptoms, and treatment of 98 patients. Clin Infect Dis 1994;19(6):1062–6.

[40] Albanese G, Venturi C, Galbiati G. Treatment of larva migrans cutanea (creeping eruption): a comparison between albendazole and traditional therapy. Int J Dermatol 2001;40(1): 67–71.

[41] Scarisbrick JJ, Chiodini PL, Watson J, et al. Clinical features and diagnosis of 42 travellers with cutaneous leishmaniasis. Travel Med Infect Dis 2006;4(1):14–21.

[42] Antinori S, Gianelli E, Calattini S, et al. Cutaneous leishmaniasis: an increasing threat for travellers. Clin Microbiol Infect 2005;11(5):343–6.

[43] Steere AC, Schoen RT, Taylor E. The clinical evolution of Lyme arthritis. Ann Intern Med 1987;107(5):725–31.

[44] Wormser GP, Dattwyler RJ, Shapiro ED, et al. The clinical assessment, treatment, and prevention of Lyme disease, human granulocytic anaplasmosis, and babesiosis: clinical

practice guidelines by the Infectious Diseases Society of America. Clin Infect Dis 2006;43(9): 1089–134.

[45] Nadelman RB, Nowakowski J, Fish D, et al. Prophylaxis with single-dose doxycycline for the prevention of Lyme disease after an *Ixodes scapularis* tick bite. N Engl J Med 2001; 345(2):79–84.

[46] Barnett ED. Yellow fever: epidemiology and prevention. Clin Infect Dis 2007;44(6):850–6.

[47] Weir E, Haider S. Yellow fever: readily prevented but difficult to treat. CMAJ 2004;170(13): 1909–10.

[48] Juckett G. Avian influenza: preparing for a pandemic. Am Fam Physician 2006;74(5): 783–90.

[49] Cheung CL, Rayner JM, Smith GJ, et al. Distribution of amantadine-resistant H5N1 avian influenza variants in Asia. J Infect Dis 2006;193(12):1626–9.

[50] Treanor JJ, Campbell JD, Zangwill KM, et al. Safety and immunogenicity of an inactivated subvirion influenza A (H5N1) vaccine. N Engl J Med 2006;354(13):1343–51.

[51] Trypanosomiasis, African (African sleeping sickness). In: Centers for Disease Control and Prevention. Health information for international travel 2008. Atlanta (GA): US Department of Health and Human Services, Public Health Service; 2007.

[52] Oscherwitz SL. East African trypanosomiasis. J Travel Med 2003;10(2):141–3.

[53] Sinha A, Grace C, Alston WK, et al. African trypanosomiasis in two travelers from the United States. Clin Infect Dis 1999;29(4):840–4.

[54] Braakman HM, van de Molengraft FJ, Hubert WW, et al. Lethal African trypanosomiasis in a traveler: MRI and neuropathology. Neurology 2006;66(7):1094–6.

ELSEVIER
SAUNDERS

Emerg Med Clin N Am
26 (2008) 517–547

EMERGENCY
MEDICINE
CLINICS OF
NORTH AMERICA

Infectious Agents of Bioterrorism:
A Review for Emergency Physicians

Nicholas E. Kman, MD*, Richard N. Nelson, MD

*Department of Emergency Medicine, The Ohio State University Medical Center,
146 Means Hall, 1654 Upham Drive, Columbus, OH 43210-1228, USA*

In the early 1970s, much of the global community signed the Biological Weapons Convention, and the United States terminated its offensive bioweapons program. Since that time, the threat of bioterrorism had been mostly an afterthought until the terrorist attacks in September of 2001. In the time since those attacks, the world has waged a "war on terror" that includes a renewed commitment to the defense against weapons of mass destruction. Several organizations including the Centers for Disease Control (CDC), the World Health Organization (WHO), and the US Food and Drug Administration's (FDA) Center for Biologics Evaluation and Research are leading the defense effort against these weapons of mass destruction.

Bioweapons have the potential to cause mass destruction, and the world community is now working to prepare for such attacks. On July 21, 2004, the United States signed into law Project BioShield, which provides new tools to improve medical countermeasures protecting Americans against a chemical, biological, radiological, or nuclear attack. As a result of the Project BioShield legislation, the United States has already begun the process of acquiring several new medical countermeasures, including 75 million doses of a second-generation anthrax vaccine to become available for stockpiling beginning in 2008, new medical treatments for anthrax directed at neutralizing the effects of anthrax toxin, and a polyvalent botulinum antitoxin [1]. In September of 2007, the FDA announced the formulation of a second-generation smallpox vaccine [2], further illustrating the seriousness of this threat.

The medical community receives reminders of the impending threat of bioterrorism. Six years after the terrorist attacks of 2001, the WHO issued

---

* Corresponding author.
E-mail address: nicholas.kman@osumc.edu (N.E. Kman).

0733-8627/08/$ - see front matter © 2008 Elsevier Inc. All rights reserved.
doi:10.1016/j.emc.2008.01.006

a statement describing an outbreak of a virus listed as category A, the most virulent type of bioweapon [3]. Although likely natural in its origin, the outbreak of the Ebola virus in the Democratic Republic of the Congo in September of 2007 serves as a reminder that we must maintain our guard. Emergency physicians are charged with the task of maintaining a high index of suspicion for these agents because they make up the first line of defense. As emergency department volumes increase on a yearly basis, there is a high likelihood that emergency physicians will be responsible for making the diagnosis or missing the sentinel cases. Early diagnosis in the emergency department setting could prove crucial to stopping terror, panic, or a world-wide pandemic.

The CDC has classified over 30 potential biologic weapons into three broad categories lettered A through C. This article examines the most lethal or category A agents. The CDC has made these agents their highest priority because they have the highest potential to be used as weapons, are the easiest to disseminate or transmit, have potential for major public health impact and high mortality, and have potential for public panic and social disruption. Category A agents are anthrax, smallpox, plague, tularemia, the hemorrhagic fever viruses, and botulinum toxin (Table 1).

Anthrax

Background

Bacillus anthracis is an aerobic, gram-positive, spore-forming bacterium that can be found in the soil around the world. As a spore, *B anthracis* is known to be environmentally hardy. The potential of inhalational anthrax as a weapon has been known and researched for years, but the only known epidemic occurred in Sverdlovsk, Russia in 1979. In that case, there was an accidental aerosol release of 1 mg of spores (1 billion spores) from a weapons plant that resulted in 250 cases with as many as 100 deaths [4].

In September of 2001, spores were sent to several locations by US mail. Twenty-two cases resulted in five fatalities, bringing the specter of bioterror-ism and the disease anthrax to the forefront of American consciousness [4].

Epidemiology and transmission

In humans, anthrax occurs in three forms: cutaneous, gastrointestinal, and pulmonary. Anthrax is not transmitted from person to person. Cutane-ous anthrax is the most common form and results from direct contact with contaminated hides of herbivores such as sheep, goats, and cows that ingest or carry the spores through contact with contaminated soil. Approximately 2000 cases of naturally occurring cutaneous anthrax are reported worldwide each year [4].

Pulmonary or inhalational anthrax is known as wool-sorters disease in its naturally occurring state. It occurs as a result of the inhalation of spores. In

Table 1
Key characteristics of category A agents of bioterrorism

Disease	Agent	Incubation period	Transmission	Clinical symptoms and signs	Treatment
Anthrax	*Bacillus anthracis*	2–4 d	Direct contact, inhalation, or ingestion	Cutaneous eschar, fever, mediastinitis with widened mediastinum on chest radiograph	Doxycycline or ciprofloxacin plus one or two other agents (see text)
Smallpox	Smallpox virus	10–12 d	Airborne droplets and direct contact	Fever followed by vesicular rash in centrifugal distribution	Supportive treatment, consider early vaccination
Hemorrhagic fever viruses	Four families of viruses (see text)	2–21 d	Airborne droplets, bite of infected carrier, or direct contact	Virus dependent (see Table 2); fever, petechiae, bleeding, disseminated intravascular coagulation	Consider ribavirin
Plague	*Yersinia pestis*	2–4 d	Flea bite (most common), airborne droplet, and direct contact	Buboes, fever, pneumonia, acute respiratory distress syndrome, sepsis	Streptomycin or gentamicin
Botulism	*Clostridium botulinum*	12–36 h	Airborne droplet, ingestion, or contaminated wound	Descending paralysis with diplopia, dysphagia, dysarthria, and dysphonia	Supportive treatment and botulinum antitoxin
Tularemia	*Francisella tularensis*	3–5 d	Arthropod bite, airborne droplets, or ingestion	Fever, dry cough, pneumonia, pulse-temperature dissociation	Streptomycin, gentamicin, ciprofloxacin, doxycycline

Data from Refs. [4–9].

nature, these spores tend to reach the lungs from contaminated hides. In 2001, spores were delivered to unsuspecting persons through six tainted letters sent through the US Postal Service [5]. This intentional release resulted in 22 cases of anthrax, half of them pulmonary and the other half cutaneous.

Digestive, or gastrointestinal anthrax, is the least common form. The disease state occurs after the ingestion of insufficiently cooked contaminated meat.

Clinical manifestations

Like any severe life-threatening illness, early diagnosis is crucial. It has been estimated that if the time to diagnosis is delayed from 2 days to 4.8 days, the mortality would be expected to double [10]. Making the diagnosis requires attention to detail and a high clinical suspicion. There are few pathophysiologic differences between naturally occurring cases of anthrax and those caused by bioterrorism.

Cutaneous anthrax

A "malignant pustule" or cutaneous anthrax occurs on exposed areas of skin where the organism is deposited. In the cases occurring in the attacks in the United States and the release in Sverdlovsk, cases occurred from 1 to 12 days after exposure with a mean incubation period in the US cases of 5 days [4]. After the spore germinates in the skin, toxin production results in local edema. This edema subsequently develops into a black, coal-colored eschar for which anthrax is named (the Greek word for coal is *anthrakis*). The eschar is painless but often associated with extensive local edema, lymphangitis, and painful lymphadenopathy (Fig. 1). After 1 to 2 weeks, the anthrax eschar dries, loosens, and falls off.

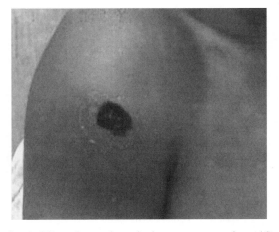

Fig. 1. Eschar on day 4 of illness in a patient who has cutaneous anthrax. (*Courtesy of* the Centers for Disease Control and Prevention [www.cdc.gov], Atlanta, GA.)

Like most of the diseases processes that present in the early stages to the emergency department, cutaneous anthrax has a wide differential diagnosis. Eschars can occur with tularemia, scrub typhus, rickettsial spotted fevers, rat bite fever, arachnid bites, vasculitidies, and ecthyma gangrenosum [4]. None of the cutaneous cases of anthrax diagnosed in 2001 were fatal, and, with appropriate treatment, this disease has a low mortality.

Gastrointestinal anthrax

Gastrointestinal anthrax results from the ingestion of bacilli from poorly cooked meat and can occur anywhere in the gastrointestinal tract. Oral-pharyngeal anthrax causes lip, oral, or esophageal ulcers and leads to lymphadenopathy, edema, and sepsis [4]. Anthrax infection of the lower gastrointestinal tract can present with nausea, vomiting, malaise, or bloody diarrhea. Infection can ultimately lead to ascites, acute abdomen, or fulminant sepsis.

Inhalational anthrax

The severe morbidity, mortality, and ease of widespread dissemination make inhalational anthrax an ideal biologic weapon. A US government analysis in 1993 estimated that the outdoor release of 100 kg of *B anthracis* upwind of Washington, DC, could produce between 130,000 and 3 million deaths [4]. Inhalational anthrax occurs when spores are inhaled and deposited on the alveolar surface where they are phagocytosed by macrophages. Surviving spores are transported to mediastinal lymph nodes where they germinate [11]. Cases occur from 2 to 43 days after exposure in humans and up to 100 days after exposure in non-human primates. Once germination occurs, rapid diagnosis is crucial. The bacteria multiply and soon produce exotoxins that quickly cause mediastinal edema and necrosis followed by bacteremia, toxemia, and sepsis, which lead to death.

The first symptoms of inhalational anthrax are nonspecific, and making the diagnosis requires a high degree of suspicion. After a typical incubation period of 1 to 6 days, patients may describe fever, dyspnea, cough, headache, chills, vomiting, weakness, or chest pain [4]. In the attacks of 2001, malaise and fever were present in all patients who had inhalational anthrax. Cough, nausea, vomiting, diaphoresis, dyspnea, chest pain, and headaches were also common in these patients. Signs that were present included fever, tachycardia, and hypoxemia.

Recent studies have attempted to aid clinicians in differentiating inhalational anthrax from community-acquired pneumonia or influenza. Nausea, vomiting, pallor/cyanosis, diaphoresis, altered mental status, a heart rate greater than 110 beats/min, a temperature greater than 100.9°F, and an increased hematocrit all seemed to predict inhalational anthrax over similar diseases [10]. Meningoencephalitis can occur with cutaneous, gastrointestinal, or inhalational anthrax. The presence of hemorrhagic meningoencephalitis should prompt a search for potential bioterrorism.

Diagnosis

The first suspicion of an anthrax illness should prompt notification of local and state health departments [12]. Routine hematologic and chemistry laboratory testing is typically not helpful, although elevated liver transaminase levels are common. Blood cultures should be performed on all suspected patients before the start of antibiotics. Cultures tend to show growth in 6 to 24 hours [11]. Aerobic blood culture growth of large, gram-positive bacilli provides preliminary identification of *Bacillus* sp. After preliminary identification, the isolate should be sent promptly to a level B or C laboratory in the Laboratory Response Network. Currently, 81 clinical laboratories in this network have diagnostic capabilities for bioterrorism pathogens [10].

A plain chest radiograph can be of great help in establishing the diagnosis. In the attacks of 2001, all ten patients had abnormal plain films of the chest. Seven had mediastinal widening, seven had infiltrates, and eight had pleural effusions. If inhalational anthrax is suspected, a chest CT scan should be obtained. As shown in Fig. 2, mediastinal widening or pleural effusions can help differentiate inhalational anthrax from community-acquired pneumonia [11]. In fact, any patient presenting to the emergency department with mediastinitis should prompt the physician to consider the diagnosis of inhalational anthrax.

Treatment

Cutaneous anthrax was previously treated with penicillin for a 7- to 10-day course. Since the bioterrorism attacks of 2001, the recommendations

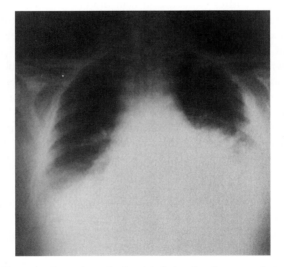

Fig. 2. Chest radiograph of a patient who has inhalational anthrax reveals typical mediastinal widening and left-sided pleural effusion. (*Courtesy of* the Centers for Disease Control and Prevention [www.cdc.gov], Atlanta, GA.)

have changed. The working group on the management of anthrax as a biologic weapon now recommends a 60-day course with oral ciprofloxacin or doxycycline [4].

Inhalational anthrax can lead to rapid sepsis or death. Early antibiotic administration is crucial, and multidrug therapy is recommended. Antibiotic therapy should include either doxycycline or ciprofloxacin plus one or two other agents. The other agents could be rifampin, vancomycin, imipenem, clindamycin, or clarithromycin. There appears to be some resistance to β-lactamase inhibitors, which are not concentrated in phagocytes and should not be used as a lone agent. Early multidrug therapy would also be effective against the frightening possibility of a genetically engineered strain of drug-resistant anthrax. Once the correct treatment is determined, it should be continued for 60 days or longer if necessary. It is wise to draw blood cultures before antibiotic administration and then tailor treatment to organism susceptibility.

In a limited casualty setting, intravenous antibiotics are indicated. In a mass casualty setting, this therapy may not be feasible, and oral antibiotics may need to be issued. Corticosteriods are recommended in all patients who have pulmonary edema, respiratory failure, and meningitis. If meningitis is suspected, ciprofloxacin with chloramphenicol, rifampin, or penicillin should be used over doxycycline to enhance cerebrospinal fluid penetration.

Public health and infection control measures

A vaccine is available in the United States for high-risk individuals. The vaccine, named anthrax vaccine absorbed (AVA), is given in a series of six inoculations over 18 months. Laboratory workers, workers who are exposed to contaminated materials or environments, and select military personnel qualify for vaccination. In July of 2004, the United States enacted Project BioShield. One of the first goals of the project is to produce 75 million doses of a second-generation anthrax vaccine to become available for stockpiling beginning in 2008. Several vaccines are currently in development, including a rapidly acting oral one-dose anthrax vaccine [10].

Postexposure prophylaxis is indicated for persons exposed to anthrax spores. Patients exposed to spores during the attacks of 2001 received a 60-day course of either ciprofloxacin or doxycycline because of the possibility of delayed germination of spores. Because inhalational anthrax has such a high morbidity and mortality, postexposure prophylaxis would most likely need to be supplemented for those who could have inhaled spores. This prophylaxis can occur in one of three ways: (1) antibiotics for 60 days accompanied by monitoring for illness and adverse events, (2) antibiotics for 100 total days (because this was the longest after exposure that spores caused illness in previous cases), or (3) a 100-day course of antimicrobial prophylaxis plus three doses of AVA vaccine given over 4 weeks [10].

Standard universal precautions should be used in the treatment of anthrax patients. Respiratory isolation is not required because person-to-person airborne transmission does not occur. If patients have draining cutaneous lesions, contact isolation precautions should be implemented. The US Environmental Protection Agency (EPA) currently recommends sodium hypochlorite solution as a sporicidal agent to decontaminate surfaces and buildings. Currently in development are biocidal gases that could kill anthrax in infected buildings and antibody-laden gels to help clean up after an anthrax attack. Two megarads of gamma radiation is known to kill the most resistant spores, and this was the decontamination method of choice after the attacks of 2001 [10].

Autonomous detection systems are currently under development to detect agents of bioweapons in the environment. These systems will eventually be able to detect biologic and chemical hazards and provide alerts that an agent is present. An autonomous detection system specifically for *B anthracis* is being deployed in hundreds of postal distribution centers across the United States. Identification of aerosolized *B anthracis* spores in an air sample can facilitate prompt on-site decontamination of workers and subsequent administration of postexposure prophylaxis to prevent inhalational anthrax [13].

Smallpox

Background

Smallpox is a large DNA virus that causes two types of disease, variola major and variola minor. At one time, smallpox was found worldwide, with a typical variola major epidemic causing fatality rates of up to 30%. Variola minor case fatality rates are typically less than 1%.

Historical evidence shows that the smallpox virus has been altering the course of human events for more than 10,000 years. Variola is thought to have evolved from African rodent poxvirus. As human population sizes grew, it became more prevalent [14]. It was first introduced to North America by the Spanish Conquistadors. Approximately one third of Native Americans died of smallpox in the decades after the Spaniards' arrival. During the French and Indian War, smallpox was first used as a biologic weapon against the Native Americans. During Pontiac's Rebellion in New England in 1763, British soldiers distributed blankets from smallpox-infected patients to the Native American population. Exposed tribe members lost half of their population because they had little immunity to this devastating virus [15].

The smallpox vaccine is the oldest of all vaccines. From India in the year 1000 BC to China in 1643, smallpox-infected materials have been used to confer immunity [14]. In 1796, Edward Jenner, with the aid of others before him, succeeded in vaccinating patients for smallpox by exposing them to cowpox or vaccinia. With an effective vaccine, the threat of smallpox as a weapon was defused. Smallpox has not been seen in the United States since 1949. In 1967, the WHO led an aggressive immunization effort that led to the eradication of smallpox 10 years later.

The threat of smallpox infection is now reborn. In 1980 at the behest of the WHO, all countries stopped immunizing. That same year, it is alleged that the Soviet Union began producing smallpox in large quantities for use in intercontinental ballistic missiles [6]. After the eradication of smallpox by global immunization, all stocks of variola virus were transferred to either the CDC in Atlanta, Georgia, or the Institutes of Virus Preparations in Moscow, Russia. There are concerns that the Russian supply of smallpox may be vulnerable to terrorist interests.

Epidemiology and transmission

Although, currently, the virus is thought to exist in only two places, it was once worldwide in its distribution. Before vaccination was practiced, almost everyone contracted a form of the disease. Unlike anthrax, smallpox is highly contagious. The virus spreads from person to person by droplets in the air and by direct contact. Contaminated clothing or bedding can spread the virus. Aerosolized smallpox virus is extremely virulent because of its low infectious dosage and the fact that individuals may be contagious during the asymptomatic late stages of incubation. Additionally, transmission of the disease can occur in healthy patients months after contact with infected corpses [16]. Epidemics in the past have led to as many as 10 to 20 second-generation cases from a single case.

The virus enters the body through oral and nasal respiratory mucosa where it travels to regional lymph nodes [17]. After several days of replication in lymphatic tissues, viremia leads to seeding of the virus in the skin and throughout the body. Almost all organs are infected to some degree. At 10 to 14 days, the incubation period ends and a rash begins. During the 7 to 10 days of rash, patients are most infectious [6]. Infectivity wanes as scabs develop, but, as previously stated, patients can remain infectious even after death.

Clinical manifestations

Smallpox infection occurs in three distinct clinical phases: incubation, prodromal illness, and fulminant infection [16]. After infection through the respiratory mucosa and multiplication in regional lymph nodes, an asymptomatic viremia develops approximately 3 to 4 days after infection. After further multiplication in the spleen, bone marrow, and lymph nodes, a secondary viremia develops on about day 8 of infection [6]. During this prodromal phase, the patient begins to show signs of a high fever, toxemia, malaise, vomiting, headache, backache, and myalgias. Two to 3 days after the onset of the prodromal illness, patients develop overt smallpox.

Slifka and Hanifin offer an excellent description of the evolution of the
rash [6]. The first lesions appear as erythematous papules and erosions in
the mouth and posterior pharynx. These lesions are followed by cutaneous
eruptions that begin as erythematous macules becoming raised and indu-
rated over the course of a few hours. In the next few days, firm, pearly,
and often umbilicated vesicles develop. During the second week of infection,
vesicles become pustular and confluent. As shown in Fig. 3, the distribution
of the rash is centrifugal, with lesions beginning on the forehead and face.
From the face, the lesions spread to the scalp, forearms, hands, back, and
upper chest. The legs and abdomen are affected last. Typically after 8 to
14 days of infection, lesions begin to dry, with thick crusting scabs leaving
deep scars.

Smallpox infection leads to severe complications. Patients can develop
panophthalmitis, blindness, keratitis, corneal ulcers, osteomyelitis, arthritis,
orchitis, and encephalitis [18]. Death most commonly occurs from bronchitis, pneumonitis, pulmonary edema, associated bacterial pneumonia, and
sepsis.

Diagnosis

Because a case of fatal smallpox has not been seen since a laboratory
worker was infected in England in 1978, clinicians must maintain a high
index of suspicion. Patients who present with a high fever, severe constitutional symptoms, and rash should be suspected to have the disease. As the
rash is observed, it will occur first on the face and then spread downward,
affecting the abdomen last. Lesions progress from vesicles to umbilicated
papules and, unlike chickenpox, are in similar stages of development. Chickenpox lesions also tend to be centripetal or denser over the trunk than the
face and extremities [6,15]. Chickenpox lesions are much more superficial
than smallpox and are also almost never seen on the palms and soles.

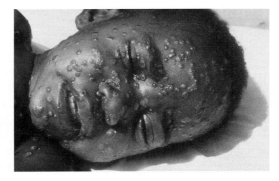

Fig. 3. Smallpox lesions on the face of a child. Lesions are more concentrated on face than
those of chickenpox and are all in similar stages of development. (*Courtesy of* the Centers
for Disease Control and Prevention [www.cdc.gov], Atlanta, GA.)

Ninety percent of smallpox cases follow the clinical path defined previously. Two other forms of smallpox are more difficult to recognize. They both bear mentioning, because it is thought that, if released intentionally, a weaponized form of smallpox may be genetically engineered to be more virulent. Hemorrhagic smallpox, or blackpox, is universally fatal and can affect anyone. It represents only 3% of cases during an outbreak. Pregnant women appear to be more susceptible to infection. The incubation period is shorter, and death occurs by the fifth or sixth day after onset of rash [6]. The rash occurs after a prodromal illness consisting of high fever, headache, back pain, and abdominal pain. The fatal rash then presents as a dark, dusky erythema that is followed by petechiae and frank hemorrhages. This illness can obviously be confused with meningococcemia or acute leukemia; therefore, diagnosis is difficult unless other cases of smallpox are observed in the same setting.

The other uncommon form of smallpox is the fatal malignant form that occurs in 5% of cases. It also occurs with an abrupt onset and severe constitutional symptoms. The rash never progresses to the pustular stage. Confluent lesions remain soft, flat, and rubbery to the touch. If the patient survives the illness, no scabbing occurs, but large amounts of epidermis peel away. This atypical presentation of smallpox would also offer diagnostic challenges unless other cases of smallpox were seen in the same setting.

Laboratory confirmation of clinical suspicion is important. After alerting local and state health officials, specimens should be collected by someone who has recently been vaccinated. Vaccination can occur on the day of specimen collection. After the specimens are harvested, they can be shipped to a high containment (biosafety level 4) laboratory. Clinicians are encouraged to contact national health officials regarding the collection and shipment of all specimens.

Smallpox infection is confirmed by electron microscopy in a biosafety level 4 laboratory where appropriate training and equipment are used. Once it is established that the epidemic is caused by smallpox, further cases can be diagnosed on clinical grounds alone.

Treatment

The only proven effective therapy for smallpox infection is supportive. The recent push for early goal-directed therapy for sepsis would benefit patients who have severe systemic symptoms. Cidofovir is a nucleoside analogue DNA polymerase inhibitor that has been studied in animal models. It might prove useful if administered within 1 or 2 days post infection but causes renal toxicity. The Working Group on Civilian Biodefense does not currently recommend it or any other drug over postexposure vaccination [6].

Public health and infection control measures

In 1972, the United States stopped its program for smallpox vaccination. The immune status of those vaccinated before 1972 is unclear. Persons who received the recommended single dose of the vaccine as children do not have lifelong immunity [6]. The CDC is in possession of a stockpile of smallpox vaccine that is reported to be sufficient to vaccinate every citizen of the United States. The current first-generation vaccine supply contains live vaccinia virus derived from calves (Dryvax; Wyeth Laboratories, Marietta, Pennsylvania) [16].

In 2002, the United States began an aggressive smallpox vaccination plan that targeted the military, government personnel, and health care workers. It was then expanded to include other first responders and, subsequently, the general public. This program was met with resistance because of concerns of safety, liability, compensation, and real smallpox risk [19]. Reported complications of this vaccine included postvaccinial encephalitis, progressive vaccinia (vaccinia gangrenosa), eczema vaccinatum, generalized vaccinia, inadvertent inoculation, and many other various rashes [6]. From the first-generation vaccine, a second-generation smallpox vaccine was recently derived.

In September of 2007, the FDA approved a second-generation smallpox vaccine. The vaccine, ACAM2000 (Acambis of Cambridge, England, and Cambridge, Massachusetts) is intended for the inoculation of people at high risk of exposure to smallpox and could be used to protect individuals and populations during a bioterrorist attack. It will be included in the CDC's Strategic National Stockpile of medical supplies [2].

According to the FDA and the manufacturer of ACAM2000, the vaccine is derived by plaque purification from the previously licensed calf lymph-produced vaccine. The new vaccine is manufactured using contemporary cell culture technology which allows manufacturers to produce large amounts while maintaining a consistent product. Over 200 million doses have been manufactured worldwide, and vaccination of the US military has already begun.

In an outbreak setting, it is recommended that all hospital employees be vaccinated. Smallpox transmission within hospitals was a serious problem before the eradication of this disease. In a limited outbreak, patients should be isolated in negative pressure rooms equipped with high-efficiency air filtration. The spread of disease from droplets, fine particle aerosol, or laundry represents such a challenge that authorities are advised to consider designating a specific hospital for a smallpox outbreak [6].

An additional approach to a large outbreak would be home isolation if specific hospitals could not be converted to care for the ill. Because primarily supportive care is used for smallpox patients, home quarantine should be used for all individuals in whom smallpox is suspected and all contacts of these cases. Isolation is important in an intentional release because the first generation of cases would spread the disease rapidly through our highly susceptible population. All individuals exposed to smallpox should be vaccinated immediately, because vaccination within 4 days of exposure has been shown to abate fatal outcome.

Once all hospital workers are vaccinated, standard precautions using gloves, gowns, and masks can be observed. All laundry and waste should be placed in biohazard containers and autoclaved before being laundered or incinerated. The rooms once occupied by infected patients should be decontaminated aggressively after their discharge. It is believed that the virus can persist for as long as 24 hours after release; therefore, care must be taken to ensure that all laundry, linen, and surfaces are thoroughly decontaminated [6].

Hemorrhagic fever viruses

Background

In September of 2007, the WHO announced the current outbreak of a category A agent of bioterrorism. At the time of this writing, Ebola hemorrhagic fever virus in the Democratic Republic of the Congo has affected 372 people, killing 166 [20]. These numbers are expected to climb. Although not thought to be related to an intentional release, this endemic outbreak serves as a stern reminder of the lethality caused by viral hemorrhagic fevers.

Several viruses that cause hemorrhagic fevers are listed by the CDC as category A agents. These viruses are Ebola, Marburg, Lassa, Junin, Machupo, Guanarito, and Sabia [21]. Viral hemorrhagic fevers are caused by RNA viruses from several families. Filoviruses (Ebola and Marburg), arenaviruses (Lassa and New World arenaviruses), bunyaviruses (Crimean-Congo hemorrhagic fever and Rift Valley fever), and flaviviruses (yellow fever, Omsk hemorrhagic fever, and Kyasanur Forest disease) are all potential agents of bioterrorism. These agents all cause fever, malaise, vomiting, bleeding diatheses, edema, and hypotension that can progress to death.

As evidenced by the nearly 50% fatality rate of the current outbreak of Ebola in Africa, these viruses pose a terrible threat if used as a bioweapon. They are widely distributed in nature, many are spread by airborne transmission, and humans are highly susceptible [22]. These viruses are also difficult to clinically distinguish from other disease processes. With such a wide differential diagnosis, making the diagnosis requires a high index of suspicion and advanced laboratory resources. Similarly, treatment, isolation, and prevention are difficult, making these agents dangerous when used as weapons.

Epidemiology and transmission

Most viral hemorrhagic fevers are spread by fine-droplet aerosol. In their endemic forms, they reside in animal hosts or arthropod vectors [7]; therefore, the viruses are confined to the geographic distribution of their hosts. Humans are infected by the bite of an infected arthropod (mosquitoes and yellow fever), via aerosol generated from infected rodent excreta, or by direct contact with infected animal carcasses, blood, or bodily secretions.

Table 2
Key clinical and epidemiologic characteristics of select hemorrhagic fever viruses

Virus	Family	Key clinical features	Vector	Person-to-person transmission	Incubation period (d)	Mortality (%)	Treatment
Ebola	Filoviridae	Sudden onset fever, weakness, muscle pain, headache, sore throat and maculopapular rash by day 5 Bleeding and disseminated intravascular coagulation common	Unknown (possibly bat)	Yes	2–21	50–90	Supportive
Marburg	Filoviridae	High fever, myalgia Nonpruritic maculopapular rash may develop Bleeding and disseminated intravascular coagulation common	Unknown (probably bat)	Yes	2–14	23–70	Supportive
Lassa fever	Arenaviridae	Early gradual fever, nausea, abdominal pain, pharyngitis, cough, conjunctivitis, cervical lymphadenopathy Late pleural and pericardial effusions Hemorrhage less common	Rodent	Yes	5–16	15–20	Ribavirin, supportive
New World arenaviruses	Arenaviridae	Gradual fever, myalgia, nausea, abdominal pain, conjunctivitis, facial flushing and generalized lymphadenopathy Possible petechiae, bleeding, and central nervous system dysfunction	Rodent	Yes	7–14	15–30	Ribavirin, supportive
Rift Valley fever	Bunyaviridae	Fever, retro-orbital headache, photophobia, jaundice, and retinitis (up to 10%) Hemorrhagic fever or encephalitis rare (>1%)	Mosquito	No	2–6	<1	Ribavirin, supportive
Yellow fever	Flaviviridae	Fever, myalgia, facial flushing, and conjunctival injection Patients either recover or experience fever, bradycardia, jaundice, renal failure, and hemorrhagic complications after short remission	Mosquito	No	3–6	20	Supportive

Modified from Borio L, Inglesby T, Peters CJ, et al. Hemorrhagic fever viruses as biological weapons: medical and public health management. JAMA 2002; 287(18):2396. Copyright © 2002, American Medical Association. All rights reserved.

occurring cases are easier to diagnose because the patient will typically have a history of travel to an endemic area. These patients may offer a history of travel to Asia, Africa, or South America. Patients may also relay a history of tick bites, mosquito bites, or exposure to an infectious source [21]. A covert bioterrorist attack would provide none of these key history items.

The Working Group on Civilian Biodefense has adapted the WHO's surveillance standards for acute viral hemorrhagic fever into guidelines on making the diagnosis [7]. The clinician should look for a temperature greater than or equal to 101°F (38.3°C) of less than 3 weeks' duration. Severe illness with no predisposing factors for hemorrhagic manifestations is typical. At least two of the following hemorrhagic symptoms should be present: hemorrhagic or purple rash, epistaxis, hematemesis, hemoptysis, blood in stools, and no other alternative diagnosis.

Once the diagnosis is suspected, laboratory confirmation can occur. Laboratory abnormalities are nonspecific and include leukopenia, anemia, thrombocytopenia, hemoconcentration, and elevated liver function tests. Coagulation abnormalities may include a prolonged bleeding time, prothrombin time, and activated partial thromboplastin time. Elevated fibrin degradation products and decreased fibrinogen may also be seen. If the diagnosis is suspected, laboratory samples need to be sent to a biosafety level 4 facility. Two capable facilities are the CDC in Atlanta, Georgia, and the US Army Medical Research Institute of Infectious Diseases in Frederick, Maryland [7]. This sample collection should be done only after suspected cases are reported immediately to local and state health departments. These health departments would then report directly to the CDC.

Treatment

Therapy for viral hemorrhagic fever is aggressive support. Fluids, electrolytes, and blood products are likely necessary in large quantities. Invasive procedures, although often necessary, should be limited secondary to the risk of needle stick infections which carry high morbidity and mortality. Currently, no antiviral drugs have been approved for the treatment of viral hemorrhagic fever by the FDA; however, ribavirin, a nucleoside analogue, has had some activity in treating viruses causing hemorrhagic fever [7].

Recent studies have shown that ribavirin is effective against arenaviruses (Lassa and New World arenaviruses) and bunyaviruses (Rift Valley fever, Crimean-Congo hemorrhagic fever, and Hantavirus). Consequently, when the viral hemorrhagic fever is identified, ribavirin is started immediately. Because diagnostic confirmation through a biosafety level 4 facility takes days, treatment is initiated as soon as possible. If infection with an arenavirus or bunyavirus is confirmed, a 10-day course of ribavirin is continued. If infection with a filovirus or flavivirus is confirmed or another diagnosis is pursued, ribavirin treatment is discontinued.

Ribavirin can be given intravenously or orally depending on disease severity, available drug, and the number of patients requiring treatment. In a contained casualty situation with a limited number of patients, the Working Group on Civilian Biodefense recommends intravenous therapy (loading dose of 30 mg/kg intravenously, followed by 16 mg/kg intravenously every 6 hours for 4 days, followed by 8 mg/kg intravenously every 8 hours for 6 days). As casualties grow, such as in a mass casualty situation, oral ribavirin can be given in the same dose recommended in chronic hepatitis C infection (2000 mg orally once, followed by 1200 mg/d orally in two divided doses for 10 days). Ribavirin is not approved for pregnant patients or children, but clinical judgment should be used as disease severity necessitates treatment. Ribavirin is also not recommended for prophylactic treatment of asymptomatic contacts [7].

Public health and infection control measures

When viral hemorrhagic fever is identified, health care personnel must work quickly to contain the disease. Most hemorrhagic fever viruses are contagious through direct contact with blood and bodily secretions. Containment of the virus must occur on several fronts. Initially, all suspected cases should be isolated from other patients and strict barrier nursing techniques implemented. Next, contacts of suspected cases should be placed under medical surveillance to ensure that the chains of transmission are broken. This surveillance includes following up any contacts of the infected patient over the incubation period to isolate them immediately if they were to become ill. Two consecutive incubation periods must elapse—a total of 42 days following the identification and isolation of the last confirmed case—before the outbreak is considered controlled [20]. If suspected contacts, including nosocomial contacts, are not symptomatic at the end of the 21-day incubation period, surveillance is discontinued. If a contact case develops a temperature of 101°F or greater and symptoms consistent with viral hemorrhagic fever, diagnostic work-up, treatment, and isolation are initiated as per the index case.

Strict barrier protective measures against nosocomial infection include hand hygiene, double gloves, impermeable gowns, N-95 masks or air-purifying respirators, negative pressure isolation rooms, leg and shoe coverings, face shields and eye protection, restricted access to all nonessential staff, dedicated disposable (or single use) medical equipment, and EPA-approved disinfectant.

When an outbreak is identified and the CDC and WHO are notified, a large multifaceted effort ensues. In the most recent Ebola outbreak, community health education was paramount [20]. Radio broadcasts reached 60% of the population. Churches, schools, military units, and markets were all informed to reduce panic and terror. Contact tracing, clinical management, infection control in health facilities, and rapid on-site laboratory diagnosis all aided in containing the number of casualties. The WHO also assists in conducting retrospective epidemiologic studies to further characterize the outbreak.

Vaccines are currently not useful in preventing the spread of viral hemorrhagic fever. Yellow fever is the only viral hemorrhagic fever with a licensed vaccine [7]. Unfortunately, even this vaccine would not be helpful in exposed patients because it takes longer than the 3- to 6-day incubation period to produce antibodies. Vaccines against Argentine hemorrhagic fever and Rift Valley fever have been developed but are not available in large quantities.

Plague

Background

Naturally occurring plague is a flea-borne zoonosis. It is caused by *Yersinia pestis*, a gram-negative coccobacillus that belongs to the Enterobacteriaceae family. Plague is known to have caused more than 200 million deaths worldwide during its numerous epidemics and three pandemics [8]. The most well-known pandemic was the second plague which started in 1346 and is known as the "Black Death." This outbreak began in Europe and eventually claimed the lives of 20 to 30 million people, or close to one third of the European population. It is thought that the use of plague as a bioweapon started during the second plague. During that time, the Tartars used catapults to launch corpses infected with plague into a Genoese city. Reportedly, the attack was successful, although it is unknown whether the disease was caused by the ballistic corpses or by infected fleas [11].

More recently, attempts have been made to weaponize *Yersinia pestis*. During World War II, members of the Japanese Army are reported to have dropped plague-infected fleas over populated areas of China. During the Cold War, the United States and Soviet Union both worked to turn plague into a biologic weapon. Although the US efforts ended in 1970 when the offensive bioweapons program was terminated, Soviet scientists were able to manufacture large quantities of weapons-grade agents [8].

Epidemiology and transmission

Naturally occurring plague exists on five continents, including Asia, Africa, North America, South America, and Europe. The CDC recorded 390 cases of plague in the United States from 1947 to 1996. The vast majority of these cases were bubonic plague, with pneumonic plague accounting for only 2% of cases [23].

The natural reservoir for plague is wild and domestic rodents, although it can also occur in prairie dogs, squirrels, rabbits, chipmunks, and domestic cats. Bacteria are usually spread to humans by the bite of a flea that previously fed on an infected rat, but humans can also become infected by coming into contact with infected tissues, bodily fluids, or respiratory droplets from infected or dead animals. This transmission can especially be seen in cats with plague pneumonia or by direct laboratory accidental inoculation [18].

Before natural human epidemics, as a harbinger of what is to come, rats frequently die in large numbers, causing the fleas to move from rats as their natural reservoir. Most persons infected by rat-borne fleas develop bubonic plague, the most common form. It is thought that infection with plague as a weapon of mass destruction would be different than this naturally occurring infection. Intentional dissemination would likely deliver *Y pestis* in an aerosolized form. A pneumonic plague would result instead of the typical bubonic plague. Symptoms would likely occur 1 to 6 days following exposure, with death quickly following the onset of symptoms. The absence of rodent deaths, cases in nonendemic locations, and the death of patients without plague risk factors would alert public health officials to the possible release of a bioweapon [8].

Clinical manifestations

In cases of naturally occurring plague, a flea bite causes direct inoculation of bacteria under the skin. The bacteria then follow the path of the cutaneous lymphatics to regional lymph nodes. In the regional lymph nodes, bacteria are phagocytosed, causing regional lymphadenopathy and abscess formation. The bacteria resist destruction and rapidly replicate. These areas of lymphadenopathy are clinically apparent as "buboes." Later, the lymph nodes become necrotic, causing the bacteria to escape with subsequent pneumonia, bacteremia, and sepsis [23].

With naturally occurring bubonic plague, patients typically develop symptoms 2 to 8 days after a flea bite. Buboes typically develop 1 day after the onset of fever, chills, and weakness. A bubo is an acutely swollen, tender lymph node that tends to develop in the groin, axilla, or cervical region (Fig. 4). Buboes range in size from 1 to 10 cm, are extremely painful, erythematous, and associated with surrounding edema and warmth [8].

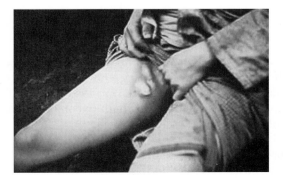

Fig. 4. Groin buboes in a patient who has plague. (*Courtesy of* the Centers for Disease Control and Prevention [www.cdc.gov], Atlanta, GA.)

The Black Death earned its name from the gangrenous lesions that developed in the digits and nose of patients with advanced disease. These lesions are a late complication of septicemic plague; therefore, they do not aid in making the diagnosis. In patients with septicemic plague, disseminated intravascular coagulation, necrosis of small vessels, and purpuric skin lesions can develop. Septicemia can arise from *Y pestis* in two ways. When sepsis develops after a flea bite with no bubo, the disease is termed *primary septicemic plague.* Although case fatality is high, only 13% of the cases of plague occurring in the United States during the last 50 years have been septicemic plague. Septicemia can also result secondary to bubonic plague. This disease is termed *secondary septicemic plague* [8].

The clinical manifestations of weaponized plague would likely be different from those observed in nature [8]. It is believed that most patients would present with primary pneumonic plague, which is very rare in nature. The symptoms would occur rapidly. In about 2 to 4 days, patients would exhibit the sudden onset of a productive cough, chills, headache, body aches, and dyspnea. They would also likely show signs of gastrointestinal illness, including nausea, vomiting, abdominal pain, and diarrhea. Two recent cases of primary pneumonic plague secondary to cat pneumonic plague exposure resulted in fatalities. Indeed, this form of plague is the most severe and rapidly fatal, usually within 24 hours of symptom onset [23].

Diagnosis

Much like all of the infectious diseases of bioterrorism, clinicians must have a high index of suspicion to make the diagnosis of plague. After an undetected terrorist attack, emergency departments in the affected area would likely see a sudden outbreak of severe pneumonia and sepsis. Interestingly, the outbreak may be similar to a terrorist attack with inhalational anthrax. Clues to the diagnosis would include a large number of previously healthy patients presenting with fever, cough, tachypnea, dyspnea, chest pain, pneumonia, and a fulminant course leading to sepsis or death. It is unlikely these patients would present with buboes [8].

After contacting the hospital epidemiologist and state and local health departments, diagnostic studies can be ordered. There are no widely available studies for plague. Chest radiographs typically show bilateral infiltrates or consolidation [8]. Blood work may not be immediately helpful in making the diagnosis. Antigen detection, IgM enzyme immunoassay, immunostaining, and polymerase chain reaction are available on a limited basis. Most hospitals would have to send specimens out of house to state laboratories, the CDC, or military laboratories, and would not have immediate confirmation. Nonspecific laboratory studies may show leukocytosis with toxic granulations, coagulation abnormalities, aminotransferase elevations, azotemia, and other evidence of multiorgan failure.

Before starting any microbial therapy, cultures should be drawn. The hospital laboratory should be notified that specimens suspicious for *Y pestis* are being sent, because these require biologic safety level 2 handling [23]. Gram stain of sputum or blood may reveal gram-negative bacilli or coccobacilli. A Wright, Giemsa, or Wayson stain may show bipolar staining [8]. Cultures of blood, sputum, or bubo aspirate should demonstrate growth in 24 to 48 hours. Cultures sent out are confirmed in specialty laboratories by immunostaining and immunoassay.

Treatment

The fatality rate of patients with pneumonic plague when treatment is delayed for greater than 24 hours is extremely high. The moment the diagnosis is suspected, the patient should be placed under droplet precautions with supportive care and antimicrobial therapy. Typically, these patients require aggressive fluid resuscitation, vasopressors, hemodynamic monitoring, and mechanical ventilation. Streptomycin is currently the drug of choice. It is given intramuscularly for a total of 10 days, or 3 days after defervescence. Gentamicin or chloramphenicol can also be used in these patients. In animal studies, fluoroquinolones are efficacious. Ciprofloxacin has shown equal efficacy as aminoglycosides and tetracyclines in animal models. Although parenteral streptomycin or gentamicin is recommended for the contained casualty setting, oral ciprofloxacin and doxycycline would be more practical in the mass casualty setting [23].

Public health and infection control measures

Symptomatic patients should be isolated with droplet precautions [8]. Gowns, gloves, and eye protection, as well as disposable surgical masks appear adequate to stop the spread of pneumonic plague. If a community is experiencing a pneumonic plague epidemic, all persons developing a temperature of 38.5°C or greater or a new cough should begin antibiotic treatment. Parenteral treatment would again be preferred, but oral treatment with doxycycline or ciprofloxacin would suffice in a mass casualty setting. The Working Group for Civilian Biodefense currently recommends a 7-day course of doxycycline for postexposure prophylaxis in exposed but asymptomatic patients [8].

Asymptomatic persons having household, hospital, or close contact with untreated pneumonic plague patients should also receive this treatment. Contacts who develop symptoms while being treated should seek prompt medical attention and begin parenteral therapy. Close contacts who refuse treatment will need to be watched carefully for the development of fever or cough during the first 7 days after exposure. They do not need to be kept in isolation but require treatment if any symptoms develop.

A vaccine for bubonic plague was available in the United States until 1999. The vaccine was not effective against primary pneumonic plague and was discontinued [8]. Current research is working toward a new vaccine that would be effective against aerosolized plague.

Botulinum toxin

Background

Clostridium botulinum is an anaerobic, gram-positive, spore-forming bacilli found globally in its natural habitat of the soil. Clostridium spores are hardy and able to survive at a wide range of temperatures. Clostridia vegetate and produce botulinum toxin in oxygen-poor, low-salt, low-sugar, and low-acidity environments [24]. Seven types of botulinum toxin employ similar mechanisms of action and have similar effects on the body. The toxin contains an enzyme that blocks acetylcholine-containing vesicles from fusing with the terminal membrane of the motor neuron. This block results in flaccid paralysis. By causing paralysis of the diaphragm and muscles of the airway, botulinum toxin causes death by asphyxiation.

Botulinum toxin is the most poisonous substance known to man. It is 100,000 times more lethal than sarin and 15,000 times more lethal than the chemical agent VX [25]. A single gram of inhaled crystalline toxin has the potential to kill over 1 million people. History has proven that the delivery of botulinum toxin is difficult, but that has not stopped several countries from working to develop the toxin as a weapon. The Soviet Union and Iraq have both tested and developed botulinum toxin as a weapon [9]. It is also believed that the terrorist nations of Iraq, Iran, North Korea, and Syria are developing botulinum toxin as a weapon [9].

Epidemiology and transmission

Botulism cannot be spread from person to person. Naturally acquired botulism is most commonly contracted by eating food that has been contaminated with spores. The spores germinate to bacilli which produce toxin that is rapidly absorbed by the gastrointestinal epithelium. The toxin is inactivated by heat (greater than or equal to 85°C for 5 minutes); therefore, it is typically transmitted by foods that are improperly heated [9]. Vegetables such as beans, peppers, carrots, or corn are most commonly implicated. In restaurants and stores, common culprits include room temperature potato salads, dips, cheese sauces, yogurts, jarred peanuts, or improperly prepared fish.

The spores cannot enter through intact skin but can infect humans by way of a contaminated wound. As a weapon, the spores would likely be aerosolized and inhaled. In the lungs, the toxin would cross the respiratory epithelium. Whether contracted from food or contaminated wounds, fewer than 200 cases are reported in the United States each year [9].

Botulism is not contagious. For that reason, it is thought that an aerosolized attack would be the most effective if botulinum spores were used as a weapon. Aerosol dissemination would result in a large number of cases sharing a similar geographic and temporal relationship. This relationship might make it easier to diagnose than some of the other agents discussed herein [24]. Although an inhalational attack would likely result in the greatest number of casualties, intentional food, water, or medication contamination are all possible.

Clinical manifestations

Whether absorbed though the respiratory epithelium, the intestinal tract, or through a contaminated wound, the results of botulinum toxin are devastating. The bloodstream carries the toxin to the peripheral cholinergic synapses where it binds irreversibly at the neuromuscular junction. The toxin blocks acetylcholine release at the neuromuscular junction, causing flaccid paralysis. The paralysis caused by all types of botulinum toxin is an acute, afebrile, symmetric, descending paralysis that always begins in the bulbar musculature [9]. The rapidity and severity of paralysis depends upon the amount of toxin absorbed and may vary from patient to patient. Because the neuromuscular blockade is irreversible, recovery can only occur when new motor axons are generated to reinnervate paralyzed muscle fibers. In adults, this process can take weeks to months. If respiratory paralysis has resulted, this time will be spent on a mechanical ventilator in an ICU.

Depending on the dose of toxin and the route through which the patient is infected, symptoms from botulinum toxin occur between 2 hours and 8 days [24]. Inhalational botulism is the most likely bioweapon-induced clinical syndrome. Health care providers could expect victims to manifest symptoms between 12 to 80 hours after attack [24]. All botulism patients typically present with vision changes, difficulty speaking, and difficulty swallowing. They will show signs of ptosis, diplopia, blurred vision, sluggishly reactive pupils, dysarthria, dysphonia, and dysphagia. Sensory changes are not seen.

Patients with botulism are afebrile and have a clear sensorium. Bulbar involvement is universal, and, as paralysis extends beyond this point, loss of head control, hypotonia, and generalized weakness are seen. Eventually, dysphagia and loss of the gag reflex make intubation and mechanical ventilation inevitable. In untreated patients, death results from airway and breathing compromise. Paralysis of the pharyngeal and upper airway muscles results in obstruction, and paralysis of the diaphragm and accessory muscles results in inadequate ventilation [9].

The Working Group on Civilian Biodefense has described a classic triad of botulism infection: (1) symmetric, descending flaccid paralysis with prominent bulbar palsies in (2) an afebrile patient with (3) a clear sensorium [9]. The bulbar palsies can be summarized as the "4 D's": diplopia, dysphagia, dysarthria, and dysphonia.

Diagnosis

Routine laboratory tests are not helpful in establishing the diagnosis of botulism, and specialized confirmatory tests take days to complete. Serum studies, cerebrospinal fluid, and imaging by either CT or MRI may be helpful in ruling out other etiologies of paralysis. Clinical acumen is the most important diagnostic tool when botulism is suspected. Once the diagnosis is clinically apparent, the hospital epidemiologist and local and state health departments should be notified. Specimen collection can then occur, with blood sent to one of the few laboratories in the United States that can confirm the diagnosis.

Because botulism is a clinical diagnosis, it is important to know the other disease processes that can mimic this condition. Guillain-Barré syndrome typically presents with an antecedent infection, paresthesias, and an ascending paralysis. Cerebrospinal fluid will eventually show an increase in protein. Patients who have myasthenia gravis present with recurrent fatigable paralysis, and a test dose of edrophonium chloride will briefly reverse symptoms. In stroke, patients will have an asymmetric paralysis, often in association with radiographic findings. Tick paralysis presents with paresthesias, ascending paralysis, and tick exposure.

Treatment

The true mainstay of treatment is supportive care with fluids, nutrition, and, often, mechanical ventilation. Patients should be monitored for their ability to maintain protection of their airway. Intensive care or step-down monitoring is typically required to monitor adequacy of gag and cough reflexes, control of secretions, oxygen saturation, vital capacity, and inspiratory force [9].

Supportive care can be supplemented with passive immunization with equine or human antitoxin [9]. Botulism toxin binds irreversibly; therefore, antitoxin cannot reverse effects that have already occurred but can help stop disease progression. For maximum effect, the clinician must administer the antitoxin as soon as botulism is suspected. The antitoxin is given early so it has enough time to neutralize circulating toxin before it irreversibly binds to the presynaptic neuromuscular terminal. Antitoxin is generally not recommended if a patient's exposure is greater than 72 hours before administration [9].

The available form of antitoxin in the United States is a trivalent (against types A, B, and E), equine-derived antitoxin [24]. It is effective against the three most common forms of the toxin and is available only through state health departments and the CDC. The US Army maintains a supply of hexavalent (A-G) antitoxin that is only available with their permission and support. A single vial of antitoxin diluted 1:10 in normal saline is effective when administered over 30 to 60 minutes. Because this substance is equine derived, preparations need to be taken against the risk of anaphylaxis and allergic reaction [24]. Skin testing should be done before the antitoxin is administered.

Public health and infection control measures

Because botulism is difficult and costly to treat once illness occurs, avoidance of contamination is paramount. Proper food preparation, storage, and consumption can easily eliminate most cases of food-borne botulism. Heating food to an internal temperature of 85°C for at least 5 minutes will detoxify contaminated food or drink. Surveillance for contaminated foods is important, because most of the 10 to 30 outbreaks that are reported annually in the United States are associated with inadequately processed, home-canned foods. In commercially produced foods, if infection is suspected, the FDA will perform a class I recall, their highest priority recall.

All cases of botulism should be regarded as public health emergencies, and the appropriate authorities should be notified. Although botulism concerning for bioterrorism would likely occur in unusual locales, with large numbers of victims, or with atypical presentations, any case should prompt epidemiologic investigation.

Medical personnel caring for patients with suspected botulism can use standard precautions. After exposure to botulinum toxin, clothing and skin should be washed with soap and water. Contaminated objects should be cleaned with 0.1% hypochlorite bleach solution. The use of antitoxin for postexposure prophylaxis is limited by its scarcity and its high potential for allergy.

Tularemia

Background

Tularemia is a bacterial zoonosis caused by *Francisella tularensis*. *F tularensis* is extremely virulent, with as few as ten organisms causing infection. The bacterium was first isolated less than a century ago. It is an extremely hardy, aerobic, intracellular, gram-negative coccobacillus that can survive for weeks in water, soil, animal carcasses, hides, frozen meat, and hay or straw [26].

Tularemia, like the other category A agents discussed herein, was maintained in the US arsenal until stockpile destruction in 1970. It was weaponized by freeze drying bacteria-laden slurry and milling it into a fine powder for aerosolized attack. The former Soviet Union also maintained stocks of weaponized tularemia but is never known to have used it in an attack. Japanese germ warfare research units also studied this agent, among others, from 1932 to 1945 [27]. A WHO report from 1969 revealed that aerosol dispersal of 50 kg of *F tularensis* in an area inhabited by 5 million people would result in 19,000 deaths and 250,000 persons with severe illness [26]. In the

United States, the reported lethality rate was 3.6% to 33% in the preantibiotic era [28].

Epidemiology and transmission

Tularemia is naturally transmitted from an arthropod bite. It is not transmitted from person to person. Contact with blood or tissues of infected
animals, ingestion of contaminated water or meat, or inhalation of aerosols
or soil can also cause disease. Aerosols that are produced by lawn mowing,
laboratory cultures, or, potentially, bioterrorists can all cause infection.
Most cases occur in rural areas where the animals that serve as natural reservoirs live.

In the United States, cottontail rabbits and jack rabbits are the most
common reservoirs for the vector. East of the Mississippi, the disease is
generally contracted through contact with infected animals. This contact
primarily occurs during the winter hunting season. Squirrels, beavers, musk-
rats, meadow voles, cats, and rodents have also been linked to the disease.
Bites from any of these animals have been known to transmit infection.
These reservoirs harbor ticks, mosquitoes, deer flies, and fleas which are
the arthropod vectors of tularemia. West of the Mississippi, tick-borne tularemia dominates and is more common in the summer. In the United States,
ticks are responsible for 75% of cases [26].

Tularemia occurs primarily in the United States, Europe, and Asia. Most
American infections occur in the south-central and western states. The majority of the cases occur in late spring and summer when arthropod bites are
more common. Much like plague, large quantities of dead animal hosts can
herald impending human outbreaks. Persons who perform activities such as
hunting, trapping, butchering, farming, or laboratory work are at increased
risk for infection [27].

Inhalational tularemia is extremely rare in the United States. Although
any case of tularemia is reportable to the CDC, inhalational tularemia
infections would be especially concerning. The Working Group for Civilian
Biodefense believes that an aerosolized attack would be the most likely
method used by terrorists because it has the highest potential for adverse
consequences [27].

Clinical manifestations

Infection with *F tularensis* typically occurs 3 to 5 days after exposure
(range, 1–21 days). Patients present with an abrupt onset of fever, chills,
headache, coryza, sore throat, myalgia, arthralgia, and fatigue. A pulse-
temperature dissociation in which the pulse is slower than expected for
the degree of fever has been seen in as many as 42% of patients [27]. The
severity, type of symptoms, and time to onset often depend on the route
of exposure, dose, and virulence of organism. Depending on the route of

infection, patients can present with one of six clinical syndromes: ulcero-glandular, glandular, oculoglandular, oropharyngeal, typhoidal, and pneu-monic [28]. These syndromes are not always distinct, and patients may present with any combination of overlapping features [11]. In addition to these syndromes, tularemia may spread hematogenously to cause meningi-tis, pericarditis, pneumonia, hepatitis, peritonitis, endocarditis, ataxia, oste-omyelitis, sepsis, rhabdomyolitis, and acute renal failure.

Ulceroglandular tularemia is the most common natural presentation of the disease. It occurs in 75% to 85% of presentations and arises from handling a contaminated carcass or following an arthropod bite. At the inoculation site, a tender or pruritic papule develops 2 to 5 days after expo-sure. The papule enlarges, typically turning into a tender ulcer which may be covered by an eschar. Associated regional lymph nodes may become en-larged and tender within several days of papule appearance. Bacteremia may occur as infected lymph nodes become fluctuant and drain [26,27].

Glandular (5%–10% of cases) and oculoglandular (1%–2% of cases) tu-laremia are less common. Glandular tularemia is characterized by fever and tender lymphadenopathy with no evidence of cutaneous involvement. Ocu-loglandular tularemia occurs after inoculation of the eye with contaminated fingers or with accidental inoculation with infected matter. Patients com-monly exhibit painful purulent unilateral conjunctivitis with cervical and preauricular lymphadenopathy [26].

Oropharyngeal tularemia is acquired by drinking contaminated water, eating contaminated food or undercooked meat, and, less commonly, by inhaling infectious droplets. Patients present with pharyngitis, tonsillitis, or stomatitis with cervical adenopathy. They may also manifest gastrointes-tinal symptoms of abdominal pain, nausea, vomiting, diarrhea, intestinal ul-cerations, gastrointestinal bleeding, and mesenteric lymphadenopathy [26].

Tularemia pneumonia can present much like other atypical pneumonias. Lung infection can occur from inhaling contaminated aerosols or can be sec-ondary to hematogenous spread. Symptoms include fever and nonproduc-tive cough, dyspnea, and pleuritic chest pain. Although rare in nature, this would be a likely clinical syndrome after a bioterrorist attack.

Typhoidal tularemia is rare in the United States but is potentially severe. Inoculation may occur by any means. Patients exhibit systemic symptoms without evidence of skin, mucosal, or lymphatic involvement. Unless recog-nized early in the clinical course, systemic inflammatory response syndrome, sepsis, disseminated intravascular coagulation, acute respiratory distress syndrome, and multisystem organ failure can occur [27].

Diagnosis

Much like the other category A agents of bioterrorism, making the diagnosis of tularemia depends on a high index of suspicion. Patients pre-senting to the emergency department with any of the clinical manifestations described previously should raise the concern for tularemia. Specifically, clusters of acute, severe respiratory illness with unusual epidemiologic features should prompt clinicians to alert hospital, local, and state epidemiologists.

Laboratory findings in tularemia are nonspecific. Leukocytosis and mildly elevated transaminases may be seen, but, otherwise, the complete blood count will likely be normal. If pulmonary involvement occurs, chest radiographs may show multifocal segmental or lobar infiltrates. Mediastinal lymphadenopathy, cavitary lesions, and pleural effusions may also be present [26].

Serologic testing and cultures may help confirm the diagnosis, but treatment should not be delayed pending these results. Serologic evidence of tularemia is established with detection of antibody response to a micro-agglutination test or enzyme-linked immunosorbent assay. A serum micro-agglutination test is diagnostic with a fourfold rise in convalescent titer or presumed positive with a single titer greater than 1:160. Growth of *F tularensis* in culture is the definitive means of confirming the diagnosis. Cultures can be grown from pharyngeal washings, sputum specimens, and, occasionally, from the blood. Antigen detection assays, polymerase chain reaction, enzyme-linked immunoassays, immunoblotting, and electrophoresis are available in research and reference laboratories to more quickly determine the diagnosis [27].

Treatment

Treatment of tularemia has traditionally been performed with aminoglycosides. Today, experience with fluoroquinolones has shifted this pattern [28]. The Working Group on Civilian Biodefense has recommended several treatment regimens for tularemia [27]. In isolated or contained cases, streptomycin is preferred at a dose of 1 g intramuscularly twice daily for 10 days. As an alternative, gentamicin can be used, 5 mg/kg intravenously or intramuscularly every day for 10 days. In a mass casualty event, ciprofloxacin is recommended, 500 mg orally twice daily for 10 days. As an alternative, doxycycline can be used, 100 mg orally twice daily for 10 to 14 days. In children, the same medical regimens can be used because the risks of tularemia far outweigh the risk of medication-related side effects. For pregnant patients, oral ciprofloxacin is considered the preferred treatment option [27].

Public health and infection control measures

Avoidance of exposure is the key to preventing tularemia infection. Although there is no human-to-human spread, animal handlers should take extra precautions in endemic areas or when handling sick animals. In known endemic areas, ticks, mosquitoes, and deer flies should be avoided or promptly removed. A protective mask should be used when performing activities that create dust, such as landscaping or construction [28].

Whether by covert terrorist attack or laboratory exposure, postexposure prophylaxis is recommended for tularemia contacts [28]. If it can be given within 24 hours of exposure, a 14-day course of ciprofloxacin or doxycycline is effective treatment. If the release of tularemia occurs covertly and the diagnosis is not made until casualties present with symptoms, suspected contacts should conduct a fever watch. If symptoms arise within 14 days of presumed exposure, standard treatment regimens would apply [27]. Because human-to-human transmission does not occur, persons who are not exposed to initial aerosol or contaminate do not need prophylaxis. The vaccine is not recommended for postexposure prophylaxis.

The Working Group on Civilian Biodefense recommends the use of the live vaccine only for laboratory workers exposed to *F tularensis* [27]. The vaccine is derived from avirulent *F tularensis* biovar *palaearctica* (type B) and only produces partial protection. Vaccine-induced protection could be overwhelmed by high doses of tularemia.

In the natural setting, *F tularensis* is hardy and can survive for extended periods in a cool moist environment. In the setting of a bioterrorist release of tularemia aerosol, it is unclear how long aerosol would survive. In this event, exposed parties should decontaminate skin and clothing with soap and water. Decontamination of exposed surfaces and objects can occur with 10% bleach solution followed in 10 minutes by 70% alcohol solution. Standard levels of chlorine in municipal water sources should protect against water-borne infection [26].

Summary

The terrorist attacks of September 11, 2001, and the anthrax scare that followed changed our lives forever. We now find ourselves engaged in a war against terror. In this ongoing battle, nuclear, radiologic, chemical, and biologic weapons present an ominous threat. Emergency physicians stand on the front lines in the war against bioterror. If ever unleashed on mankind, the agents of bioterrorism are sure to end up in emergency departments across the United States. It is the duty and responsibility of emergency physicians to be prepared to meet this challenge. Using knowledge, vigilance, preparation, and suspicion, this challenge can be met, preventing needless casualties.

References

[1] The Office of the Press Secretary. Project bioshield. Available at: www.whitehouse.gov/infocus/bioshield. Accessed October 18, 2007.
[2] Food and Drug Administration. FDA approves a second-generation small pox vaccine. FDA News Released September 1, 2007.
[3] Centers for Disease Control. Biological and chemical terrorism: strategic plan for preparedness and response. MMWR Recomm Rep 2000;49(RR04):1–14.

[4] Inglesby TV, O'Toole T, Henderson DA, et al. Anthrax as a biological weapon, 2002: updated recommendations for management. JAMA 2002;287:2236–52.

[5] Shannon M. Management of infectious agents of bioterrorism. Clinical Pediatric Emergency Medicine 2004;5:63–71.

[6] Henderson DA, Inglesby TV, Bartlett JG. Smallpox as a biological weapon: medical and public health management. JAMA 1999;281(22):2127–37.

[7] Borio L, Inglesby T, Peters CJ, et al. Hemorrhagic fever viruses as biological weapons: medical and public health management. JAMA 2002;287(18):2391–405.

[8] Inglesby TV, Dennis DT, Henderson DA, et al. Plague as a biological weapon. JAMA 2000; 283:2281–90.

[9] Arnon SS, Schechter R, Inglesby TV. Botulinum toxin as a biological weapon. JAMA 2001; 285:1059–81.

[10] Kyriacou DN, Adamski A, Khardori N. Anthrax: from antiquity and obscurity to a front-runner in bioterrorism. Infect Dis Clin North Am 2006;20:227–51.

[11] Daya M, Nakamura Y. Pulmonary disease from biological agents: anthrax, plague, Q fever, and tularemia. Crit Care Clin 2005;21:747–63.

[12] Centers for Disease Control. Nationally notifiable infectious diseases: United States, 2007 revised. Available at: www.cdc.gov/epo/dphsi/phs/infdis2007r.htm. Accessed December 21, 2007.

[13] Meehan PJ, Rosenstein NE, Gillen M, et al. Responding to detection of aerosolized *Bacillus anthracis* by autonomous detection systems in the workplace. MMWR Recomm Rep 2004; 53(Early Release):1–11.

[14] Cleri DJ, Porwancher RB, Ricketti AJ, et al. Smallpox as a bioterrorist weapon: myth or menace? Infect Dis Clin North Am 2006;20:329–57.

[15] Hendrickson RG, Hedges JR. Introduction: what critical care practitioners should know about terrorism agents. Crit Care Clin 2005;21:641–52.

[16] Nafziger SD. Smallpox. Crit Care Clin 2005;21:739–46.

[17] Slifka MK, Hanifin JM. Smallpox: the basics. Dermatol Clin 2004;22:263–74.

[18] Bossi P, Garin D, Guihot A, et al. Bioterrorism: management of major biological agents. Cell Mol Life Sci 2006;63:2196–212.

[19] Saks MA, Karras D. Emergency medicine and the public's health: emerging infectious diseases. Emerg Med Clin North Am 2006;24:1019–33.

[20] World Health Organization News release: Ebola hemorrhagic fever in the Democratic Republic of the Congo. 2007. Available at: www.who.int/csr/don. Accessed October 3, 2007[Updates 1–4].

[21] Pigott DC. Hemorrhagic fever viruses. Crit Care Clin 2005;21:765–83.

[22] Cleri DJ, Ricketti AJ, Porwancher RB, et al. Viral hemorrhagic fevers: current status of endemic disease and strategies for control. Infect Dis Clin North Am 2006;20:359–93.

[23] Koirala J. Plague: disease, management, and recognition of act of terrorism. Infect Dis Clin North Am 2006;20:273–87.

[24] Villar RG, Elliott SP, Davenport KM. Botulism: the many faces of botulinum toxin and its potential for bioterrorism. Infect Dis Clin North Am 2006;20:313–27.

[25] Osterbauer PJ, Dobbs MR. Neurobiological weapons. Neurol Clin 2005;23:599–621.

[26] Cronquist SD. Tularemia: the disease and the weapon. Dermatol Clin 2004;22:313–20.

[27] Dennis DT, Inglesby TV, Henderson DA. Tularemia as a biological weapon. JAMA 2001; 285:2763–73.

[28] Eliasson H, Broman T, Forsman M, et al. Tularemia: current epidemiology and disease management. Infect Dis Clin North Am 2006;20:289–311.

ELSEVIER
SAUNDERS

Emerg Med Clin N Am
26 (2008) 549–570

EMERGENCY
MEDICINE
CLINICS OF
NORTH AMERICA

Influenza and Pneumococcal Vaccinations in the Emergency Department

Daniel R. Martin, MD[a,*], Mark E. Brauner, DO[a],
Joseph F. Plouffe, MD[b]

[a]Department of Emergency Medicine, The Ohio State University Medical Center,
410 West 10th Avenue, Columbus, OH 43210, USA
[b]5205 Canterbury Drive, Sarasota, FL 34243, USA

The most recent data suggest that nationwide, emergency department (ED) visits continue to increase, with estimates from 2005 of 115.3 million visits [1] and recent preliminary data from 2006 of just more than 119 million visits (Centers for Disease Control and Prevention [CDC], personal communications, 2006). Several studies have shown that this population is underimmunized. It is currently recommended that patients older than 50 years of age should be immunized annually against influenza and those older than 65 years of age should be immunized once against pneumococcus [2], and both are recommended for patients younger than these ages with several chronic diseases. Clearly, the percentage of the population older than 55 to 65 years of age continues to increase, as does the contribution of this population in EDs. Because the ED population is underimmunized and less likely to receive regular physician care and more likely to be of lower socioeconomic status, the ED provides an excellent opportunity to facilitate the attainment of the objective of vaccinating 90% of eligible patients against influenza and pneumococcal disease. The precise strategy of how to initiate this process and which patients should be immunized and the evidence for such a program in the ED are discussed.

* Corresponding author.
E-mail address: martin.23@osu.edu (D.R. Martin).

0733-8627/08/$ - see front matter © 2008 Elsevier Inc. All rights reserved.
doi:10.1016/j.emc.2008.02.004   *emed.theclinics.com*

Tetanus immunizations in the emergency department

Although it is generally recommended that immunizations be administered by patients' private physicians, immunizations against organisms, such as tetanus, hepatitis, and rabies, have been administered in the ED for years. One analysis using the National Hospital Ambulatory Medical Care Survey from 1992 to 2000 showed that EDs gave 27,738,000 vaccines and 93% were against tetanus [3]. One recent study performed at five university-affiliated EDs (1999–2000) reported a seroconversion rate of 90.2% [4]. Although it is not clear precisely when tetanus immunization in the ED began, it is clear that this is common practice and standard of care for patients who have wounds. In fact, tetanus immunizations have been administered in the ED since the 1970s and the beginning of organized emergency medicine as a specialty. The CDC reported an annual incidence of 0.16 cases per million population, or an average of 43 cases per year [5]. Although uncommon in developed countries, such as the United States, tetanus remains a much larger problem in developing countries, with some estimates of 1 million cases worldwide each year [6]. The World Health Organization (WHO) estimated that there were 309,000 deaths from tetanus in 2000, and 200,000 of these were estimated to have occurred from neonatal tetanus [7]. These reports clearly show a reduced incidence in developed countries and a much lower case fatality rate in patients who have up-to-date tetanus toxoid immunization status. From these large numbers of tetanus immunizations given in EDs and in primary care physicians' offices, one can conclude that our current emphasis on preventing tetanus has been successful to a large extent. Despite the gravity and impact of influenza and pneumococcal diseases in EDs and the relatively rare cases of tetanus, however, the former vaccines remain underused in EDs.

Influenza and pneumococcal immunizations in the emergency department

Immunizations against influenza and pneumococcal disease have been widely believed to be underused in Americans 65 years of age and older [8], and this has occurred despite the fact that influenza is believed to cause more than 100,000 excess hospitalizations and 20,000 deaths per year [9]. Because hospitalized patients are at particularly high risk for these diseases and many have been hospitalized in the previous 3 to 5 years, the Advisory Committee on Immunization Practices (ACIP) has recommended immunizing eligible hospitalized adults against influenza and pneumococcal diseases as a strategy to increase the rate of vaccination [9,10]. The process of immunizing hospitalized patients against influenza and pneumococcal diseases has been recommended by the Centers for Medicare and Medicaid Service (CMS) as a method to improve the quality of care given to Medicare beneficiaries [11]. In fact, these vaccinations have been recommended since the 1980s [12,13]. This practice continues to be recommended today and was part of the combined recommendations by the American Thoracic Society (ATS) and Infectious Diseases Society of American (IDSA) in their most recent guidelines for the treatment of community-acquired pneumonia [2]. Clearly, the administration of influenza and pneumococcal vaccinations to eligible patients has been demonstrated to reduce morbidity and mortality and to save costs [14–19]. Also, administration of these immunizations to hospitalized patients has become a crucial method to improve these vaccination rates.

From these studies, it follows that vaccination programs based in EDs represent important additional methods of vaccinating eligible patients. Furthermore, of the 119 million patients seen in US EDs, only a relatively small proportion are admitted, and those treated and sent home represent an excellent opportunity to administer influenza and pneumococcal vaccinations, especially because many have no primary care physician. Initially, reports from patients in the ED showed that only approximately 20% of eligible patients in the ED had even heard of pneumococcal immunization and only 8.6% had been immunized [20,21]. Patients who could identify a primary care provider or a clinic at which they were followed were much more likely to have received pneumococcal and influenza vaccinations. Of the eligible patients in the ED, approximately 60% said they would receive the vaccine in the ED. Subsequent reports continued to verify low immunization rates among eligible patients in the ED, with 75% to 82% of eligible patients in the ED reporting that they had not received pneumococcal vaccinations and 57% to 63% reporting that they had not received influenza vaccinations [22,23]. More than 50% of patients who had not received previous vaccinations consented to receive the vaccinations in the ED. Similar results were obtained in studies based at four EDs in Canada, and most emergency physicians surveyed were willing to prescribe vaccinations for influenza [24]. A similar study in an inner city county hospital population found that only 3% of high-risk patients had received previous pneumococcal vaccinations [25]. From these studies, it is evident that patients in the ED represent a patient population that is largely underimmunized against pneumococcal disease and influenza; furthermore, more than half of these patients are willing to receive these immunizations in the ED.

From a disease prevention standpoint, many of those patients eventually diagnosed with pneumococcal bacteremia had been previously seen in an ED, often more than once [26]. In one study of patients who had pneumococcal bacteremia, of those with risk factors, nearly 90% had been seen in an ED during the previous 5 years, whereas only approximately half (49.7%) had been on an inpatient medicine ward and only approximately a third (30.6%) had been seen in a general medicine clinic setting [27]. Not only did both studies report that administration of these vaccines in the ED would be cost-effective, but the latter also suggested that a vaccination program in the ED has greater potential to reach more high-risk patients than the general medicine inpatient wards or the general medicine clinic setting.

Arguments for using EDs for administration of influenza and pneumococcal vaccinations have been numerous. According to the National Ambulatory Medical Care Survey, ED visits in our country have increased from 90.3 to 113.9 million visits in 2003 to just more than 119 million visits in 2006 (CDC, personal communications, 2006). The population represented by those older than 65 years of age has increased by 26%, and, similarly, representation of many socioeconomically disadvantaged populations has also increased in the ED. The missed opportunities for immunization of high-risk patients loom larger than ever.

Influenza and pneumococcal disease have more direct effects on EDs, creating more urgent needs for administering influenza and pneumococcal vaccines. Influenza outbreaks were associated with a significant increase in elder (65 years of age and older) persons' use of the ED for influenza-related infections and upper respiratory infections [28]. In this study, the investigators reported that for every 10 new cases of influenza in the community, there was a 1.5% increase in the proportion of elderly patients in the ED who presented with influenza-related infections and upper respiratory infections. During periods in which the CDC declared "widespread influenza activity," there was generally noted to be a marked increased in resource use [29]. The resources considered included increased admission rate, increased ED length of stay for admitted and discharged patients, increased ED saturation time, and increased numbers of patients who left the ED without being seen. Influenza outbreaks were also associated with increased ambulance diversion [30]. For every 100 cases of influenza per week, ambulance diversion increased by 2.5 hour per week. Other reports demonstrated a substantial increase in ED visits during influenza outbreaks, especially for patients who had respiratory illnesses, such as influenza, pneumonia, and exacerbations of chronic lung diseases [31]. These data suggest that, clearly, pneumococcal and influenza infections contribute to all the complications associated with ED overcrowding.

Several organizations also recommend strategies for administration of immunizations in EDs. The CDC and ACIP have recommended initiating influenza and pneumococcal immunizations in the ED for years. In 1998, at the American College of Emergency Physicians (ACEP) annual council meeting, a resolution was passed asking the ACEP to address this issue and endorse the immunization of high-risk populations in our EDs [32]. Subsequent ACEP policy statements to address this issue were made in 2000 and 2002. The 2000 policy statement recommended that health care workers be immunized and that high-risk patients be identified and appropriately referred [33]. It was recommended that EDs should consider administering vaccinations in the elderly if no other resources are available, especially if there is a widespread outbreak or epidemic. The 2002 ACEP Policy statement simply stated that the ACEP supports the immunization of high-risk patients in the ED against pneumococcal disease and influenza [34].

Not only has administration of pneumococcal and influenza vaccinations been demonstrated to be cost-effective, but Medicare Part B pays or reimburses for administration of these vaccines at a rate beyond the inpatient diagnosis-related group payment for hospitalized patients [35]. The reimbursement for these vaccines has been made even easier, because billing can be accomplished through roster billing, wherein hospitals or health care providers need only submit a list of patient names and Medicare numbers [36].

Pediatric influenza and pneumococcal immunizations in the emergency department

Unlike adults, children are not generally underimmunized in the United States. Childhood immunization rates are currently at record levels and approaching CDC and ACIP *Healthy People 2010* goals [37]. Pneumococcal and, to a much greater extent, influenza immunization rates continue to lag behind more traditional childhood immunizations, however. Surprisingly, influenza vaccination is not currently part of the baseline series of vaccinations so effectively administered by US health care providers [38]. Although rates of pneumococcal immunizations have increased since 2005, and the literature has demonstrated a decrease in pneumococcal disease [39,40], influenza immunization rates remain low.

In 2006, the ACIP expanded its recommendations for routine influenza vaccination of healthy children from the age of 6 months to 5 years [41]. In 2007, using data from several sentinel sites, the CDC found that approximately 30% of children aged 6 to 23 months and approximately 20% of children aged 2 to 5 years were appropriately vaccinated. The study also reported high geographic and socioeconomic variability not associated with other childhood immunization programs [42]. In children younger than 2 years of age, those with comorbidities, and those in undeveloped countries, influenza and pneumococcal infections can cause significant childhood mortality and morbidity secondary to severe pneumonia, meningitis, and bacteremia [43]. Influenza and pneumococcal infections are often concomitant and are, to a large extent, vaccine preventable [44].

There is also a significant socioeconomic burden on the community associated with pediatric influenza because of missed school, work absenteeism, more doctors' appointments, increased antibiotic use, and other influenza-related costs in children with verified influenza versus other respiratory infections [45]. Influenza-infected children also shed virus for longer periods than do adults, and are therefore considered to be more infectious to the general population [46]. Pediatric populations visiting EDs are underimmunized compared with the general pediatric population [47], and more than 75% of frequent pediatric ED users have chronic underlying disease [48]. Despite the evidence for ED-based influenza and pneumococcal immunization programs for pediatric patients and the demonstrated effectiveness of these programs, controversy exists because of the desire by some pediatric and family physicians to keep pediatric immunizations part of primary care [49–52].

Other potential benefits of influenza and pneumococcal immunizations in the emergency department

The influenza vaccine has been reported to decrease mortality and morbidity in persons with cardiovascular disease (CVD) and to prevent asthma exacerbations in children. The evidence is compelling in regard to CVD, but the balance of evidence suggests that influenza vaccination may instead be linked to increased rates of asthma exacerbation in children.

In persons older than 65 years of age with CVD, influenza vaccination has been reported to result in a 60% reduction in death from all causes. This includes death from myocardial infarction (MI), cerebrovascular accident (CVA), and congestive heart failure (CHF) exacerbations. Strong evidence for CVD protection comes from the Flu Vaccination in Acute Coronary Syndromes (FLUVACS) trial. This prospective randomized study showed a relative risk reduction of a composite end point (cardiovascular death, nonfatal MI, or severe ischemia) to be 0.59% (95% confidence interval [CI]: 0.30 to 0.86; 11% [nonimmunized] versus 23% [immunized]) [53]. There are other well-designed studies that refute any reduction in the risk for MI specifically [54]. Severe pneumonia has consistently been associated with increased rates of CVA and exacerbation of CHF symptoms and is thought to accelerate atherosclerotic processes. Strong convincing evidence for a direct cause-and-effect relation between severe respiratory infection and CVA has not been statistically established, however. In 2006, the American Heart Association (AHA) and the American College of Cardiology (ACC) recommended influenza vaccination as a secondary prevention measure in adults and children with known CVD. There is no evidence to suggest that influenza vaccination is harmful to persons with CVD.

Influenza vaccination has been evaluated in children for reduction of acute asthma exacerbation. There have been four major studies: three were retrospective cohort studies, and one was a prospective placebo-controlled trial [55]. Two of three cohort studies showed an increase in the number of acute exacerbations. One cohort study by Smits and colleagues [56] did show protective effect in children younger than 6 years of age. The prospective trial did not show benefit and did show a nonsignificant trend toward harm in children with asthma. Although the results of the cohort studies were negative, the studies were subject to considerable bias and may not reflect real-world clinical conditions. Despite a lack of clear evidence, the US Department of Health and Human Services (DHHS) advocates routine influenza immunization for children younger than 6 years of age with all clinical subtypes of asthma [57,58].

Influenza

The influenza virus is one of the most common infectious diseases worldwide. It is estimated that between 20 and 50 million people died worldwide from the H1N1 type influenza pandemic that occurred in 1918 to 1919. There were approximately 670,000 deaths in the United States [58]. Influenza has untold effects on the economy, health care system, and human suffering.

Epidemics generally occur in the winter months and often affect millions of people each year in the United States. Influenza occurs year round in the tropics. The frequency and severity depend on the virulence of the virus subtype [59]. The CDC estimates that 20,000 deaths occur annually in the United States as a result of influenza infection. Adults older than 50 years of age, those with chronic medical conditions, and children younger than 2 years of age are at higher risk for severe complications, namely, pneumonia [42].

Influenza is an acute febrile illness that can be challenging to diagnose secondary to a highly variable presentation. Many patients present early, before significant prostration, with signs and symptoms consistent with a common upper respiratory infection. Alternatively, many patients at highest risk for severe disease also have comorbidities that can obfuscate the clinical picture. One symptom that does seem to predict influenza independently is disproportionate prostration [60]. Death is usually associated with severe secondary bacterial pneumonia caused by *Streptococcus pneumoniae*, *Haemophilus influenzae*, or *Staphylococcus aureus*.

The virus is highly contagious and is spread by large droplets and small-particle aerosols from the respiratory tract of infected individuals. Adult patients are generally infected 1 to 2 days before symptom presentation and are contagious because of viral shedding for approximately 1 day before and 5 to 10 days after presentation [61]. School- aged children (especially 5–9 years old) typically shed for longer periods and represent a major source of infection in the community, especially to the elderly, who are at greatest risk for severe infection [46].

Influenza is a zoonotic infection caused by a single-stranded RNA virus with three major subtypes (A, B, and C), which are classified within the family Orthomyxoviridae. Major virulence factors are the surface proteins hemagglutinin and neuraminidase, and are thus targets for pharmacotherapeutic treatments. Influenza type A is the most pathogenic and causes the greatest human disease burden. The most common influenza A subtypes are H1N1 and H3N2. The trivalent inactive vaccine (TIV), which is developed annually and is used worldwide, contains A strains from H1N1, H3N2, and one influenza B strain.

Pandemics occur when the influenza virus acquires a new genetic code for hemagglutinin or neuraminidase proteins. The encoding of hemagglutinin and neuraminidase by separate RNA molecules facilitates the reassortment of these genes in animals simultaneously infected by two different subtypes. Theoretically, reassortment can occur in human beings with dual infections. The abrupt genetic change is called antigenic shift. Until these new proteins are identified and incorporated into vaccines, there can be no large-scale immunity. New virus configurations may confer severe virulence with increased infectivity and profound mortality and morbidity [62].

Epidemics occur when there are missense mutations in the hemagglutinin and, to a lesser extent, the neuraminidase genes, altering the epitope so that the virus is not recognized by circulating acquired antibodies. The gradual accumulation of new epitopes on the hemagglutinin and neuraminidase proteins is called antigenic drift. In the immunocompetent host, influenza infection elicits a strong immune response against only the specific strain that caused it. Within a brief period, antigenic drift makes one susceptible to a new viral variant. Mass immunization with influenza vaccines has proven to be helpful in reducing the size and severity of new epidemics [63].

The WHO Global Influenza Surveillance Network was established in 1952. The network consists of several hundred organizations that collectively perform regional primary virus isolation and preliminary antigenic characterization. New strains are isolated and evaluated for high-level antigenic and genetic analysis. The pooled data, along with expert consensus, form the basis for WHO recommendations on the formulation of influenza vaccines. Different vaccine formulations are developed for the Northern and Southern Hemispheres [64].

Influenza vaccines

The influenza vaccine should ideally be administered in September through November and especially in high-risk groups. This schedule provides adequate time for immunogenic response before the influenza virus arrives in the community (United States). Because peak influenza season in the United States is January through March, immunizations should continue as long as vaccine is available [42].

There are two basic types of influenza vaccines: inactive and live-attenuated virus vaccines. The first to be developed and the most commonly used vaccine currently consists of one of three subtypes of inactive virus (killed viruses): (1) whole-virus vaccines, (2) inactivated virus particles (split-virus vaccines), or (3) purified hemagglutinin protein vaccines. All inactive vaccine formulations contain A strains from H1N1, H3N2, and one influenza B strain, and are thus called TIVs. All inactive virus vaccines are formulated for intramuscular delivery [65].

The second type and, arguably, the most effective vaccine consists of live-attenuated virus and an intranasal delivery system. Both types of vaccines incorporate antigens from the three major viral strains predicted to be in circulation. The live-attenuated virus vaccines are developed to replicate well in the cool physiologic environment found in the upper respiratory system and poorly in the warmer lower respiratory system [42]. The intranasal live-attenuated vaccine formulation is often referred to as a cold-adapted influenza vaccine (CAIV-T).

The influenza vaccine is produced by a small number of manufacturers [42]. The viral antigens are grown in fertilized chicken eggs. In North America, the vaccine is produced by only six manufacturers and is dispensed predominantly in individual-dose vials or intranasal devices. Some newer single-dose vials obviate the need for the use of a mercury-containing compound (thimerosal) traditionally used for preservation and antibiosis in multidose vials. It has been shown by the CDC, with the support of several studies, that there is no correlation between thimerosal and neurologic sequelae, including autism. Despite the CDC position, the US Food and Drug Administration has recently called for the elimination of thimerosal from all formulations [66]. Egg-based vaccines are contraindicated in people with severe allergies to egg protein and those with a history of Guillain-Barré syndrome [67].

Egg-based vaccine production has many limitations when it comes to ramping up for a surge in response to an influenza pandemic. Egg-based production requires having millions of 11-day-old chicken eggs available continuously. This is a dubious process, considering that a major current public health concern (especially in Asia) is avian influenza, which exhibits high lethality in chickens. Despite the current limitations of egg-based production, expert consensus advocates leveraging the egg-based manufacturing infrastructure for pandemic vaccine production while simultaneously and aggressively exploring strategies to improve vaccine immunogenicity, evaluating vaccine adjuvants, and developing larger capacity cell culture–based live-attenuated virus vaccine production and methods to induce durable immunity [68].

Most commercially available viral vaccines (except for influenza) are manufactured using cell culture technology. Cell culture–based production uses bioreactors, which grow viruses in a closed environment utilizing a readily available growth medium. Cell culture–based production is insensitive to having millions of precisely aged chicken eggs, and production could potentially be expanded faster to meet surge capacity. Many governmental organizations, including the DHHS, are promoting and investing worldwide in cell culture–based influenza vaccination production [69].

Both types of vaccines have been well studied. There is, however, considerably more data using the inactivated virus vaccines. Studies have been performed in animal models and prospective human clinical trials, and several meta-analyses have been reported [15,70]. Testing the efficiency of the vaccine is straightforward. Healthy adults are given the vaccine and then infected with live virus. Antibody production is also measured as an indicator of efficiency.

Both types of vaccines are efficient at producing an immunogenic response. The intranasal live-attenuated virus produces circulating antibodies and a large number of immunoglobulin A (IgA) antibodies in the respiratory mucosa. Mucosal immunity is theoretically more helpful for preventing influenza infection through the respiratory tract [71]. Ethical considerations obviate the ability to test vaccine efficiency in the patient populations at greatest risk for severe disease as a result of the concerns for inducing influenza infections in these patients.

Reporting effectiveness of influenza vaccination with certainty is impossible. There are no prospective clinical trials in the populations at greatest risk. There is a predominance of meta-analyses in the literature, and some questionable statistical methods have driven public health policy [72–74]. The level of evidence supporting influenza vaccine effectiveness falls short of standards that have been adopted in many other clinical specialties. This being said, public health concerns with endemic influenza, ethical considerations regarding trial design, a rapidly aging population, and the potential magnitude of a severe influenza pandemic do not allow for passive public health policy. Influenza vaccination effectiveness in the literature is controversial and is cited in the context of the best supporting evidence.

In clinical practice, effectiveness is measured in a vaccinated individual as the practical reduction in risk for mortality and morbidity. Data on the effectiveness of influenza vaccination can be delineated into four age groups: (1) immunocompetent adults, (2) the elderly (>65 years of age), (3) children (5–18 years of age), and (4) children younger than 2 years of age.

In the immunocompetent adult, influenza vaccines are highly effective against the viral strains found in the vaccine. There is only a marginal effect on the rate of infection and no effect on the rate of hospitalization, however. This is partially attributable to the large number of mild disease-causing influenza strains and other respiratory viruses found in the community.

Similarly, in children, efficiency is high, but effectiveness is only high in children older than 6 years of age. There is poor effectiveness in children younger than 2 years of age, as demonstrated by a clear increase in mortality and morbidity in this age group [75]. One important phase 3 study in children aged 6 to 59 months showed a risk reduction of 55% in laboratory-confirmed influenza cases [76]. Another systematic review showed that in children younger than 16 years of age, there was a risk reduction of 79% to 80% in laboratory-confirmed influenza and a reduction in clinical illness of 34% to 38% [77].

In the elderly, the efficiency is high and the effectiveness is complex and, in part, socially dependent; vaccination does not alter the rate of infection, but it does decrease the frequency of pneumonia, severe infection, and rate of hospitalization and death from pneumonia. The risk reduction is reported to be 70% to 90%. Reduction in hospitalization is 25% to 39%, and there is a 39% to 75% reduction in death [78]. The effectiveness also seems to be higher in institutionalized elderly persons versus those from the community at large. Among nursing home residents, influenza vaccination can reduce hospitalizations (all causes) by approximately 50%, the risk for pneumonia by approximately 60%, and the risk for death (all causes) by 68% [79] (Box 1, Table 1).

In terms of safety, TIVs and CAIV-Ts are considered safe. The TIV subtypes do exhibit different rates of reactogenicity, however. Whole-virus vaccines exhibit a 15% to 20% rate of local reaction (whole-virus vaccines are not available in the United States). The local reaction is predominantly in young children and is self-limited, rarely lasting longer than 1 to 2 days.

Box 1. Persons for whom annual influenza vaccination is recommended

- All persons, including school-aged children, who want to reduce the risk for becoming ill with influenza or of transmitting influenza to others
- All children aged 6 to 59 months (ie, 6 months to 5 years)
- All persons aged 50 years or older
- Children and adolescents (aged 6 months to 18 years) receiving long-term aspirin therapy who therefore might be at risk for experiencing Reye syndrome after influenza virus infection
- Women who are pregnant during the influenza season
- Adults and children who have chronic pulmonary (including asthma), cardiovascular (except hypertension), renal, hepatic, hematologic, or metabolic disorders (including diabetes mellitus)
- Adults and children who have immunosuppression (caused by medications or HIV)
- Adults and children who have any condition (eg, cognitive dysfunction, spinal cord injuries, seizure disorders, other neuromuscular disorders) that can compromise respiratory function or that can increase the risk for aspiration
- Residents of nursing homes and other chronic care facilities
- Health care personnel
- Healthy household contacts (including children) and caregivers of children aged younger than 5 years and adults aged 50 years or older, with special emphasis on vaccinating contacts of children aged younger than 6 months
- Healthy household contacts (including children) and caregivers of persons with medical conditions that put them at higher risk for severe complications from influenza

---

Adapted from Prevention and control of influenza—recommendations of the Advisory Committee on Immunization Practices (ACIP). MMWR Morb Mortal Wkly Rep 2007;56(RR06):2.

Table 1
Approved influenza vaccines for different age groups—United States

Vaccine	Generic name	Manufacturer	Preparation	Age group	No. doses	Route
TIV	Influenza vaccine	Sanofi Pasteur	0.25-mL prefilled syringe	6–35 months	1 or 2[a]	Intramuscular
			0.5-mL prefilled syringe	36 months and older	1 or 2[a]	Intramuscular
			0.5-mL vial	36 months and older	1 or 2[a]	Intramuscular
			5.0-mL multidose vial	6 months and older	1 or 2[a]	Intramuscular
TIV	Influenza vaccine	Novartis vaccine	5.0-mL multidose vial	4 years and older	1 or 2[a]	Intramuscular
TIV	Influenza vaccine	GlaxoSmith Kline	0.5-mL prefilled syringe	18 years and older	1	Intramuscular
TIV	Influenza vaccine	GlaxoSmith Kline	5.0-mL multidose vial	18 years and older	1	Intramuscular
LAIV	Influenza nasal vaccine, live	MedImmune	0.2-mL sprayer	5–49 years	1 or 2[b]	Intranasal

Abbreviations: LAIV, live attenuated influenza virus vaccine; TIV, trivalent inactivated influenza virus vaccine.

[a] Two doses administered at least 1 month apart are recommended for children aged 6 months to 8 years who are receiving TIV for the first time, and those who only received one dose in their first year of vaccination should receive two doses in the following year.

[b] Two doses administered at least 6 weeks apart are recommended for children aged 5–8 years who are receiving LAIV for the first time, and those who received only 1 dose in their first year of vaccination should receive 2 doses the following year.

Adapted from CDC 2007 to 2008 influenza prevention and control recommendations.

Minor systemic reactions, including, fever, malaise, myalgias, cellulites, and serum sickness, occur in less than 3% of vaccine recipients. The reactions are transient and generally occur within 6 to 12 hours of vaccination [42]. As one would expect, split-virus vaccines and subunit vaccines exhibit substantially less systemic reactogenicity. The reduced reactogenicity is found in all age groups [80]. There are certain TIV formulations (namely, the 1979 Northern Hemisphere formulation) that have been associated with a slight but nonsignificant increase in the risk for Guillain-Barré syndrome [81]. The most common side effects from CAIV-Ts are rhinorrhea, fever, myalgias, and mild abdominal pain. The illness pattern is self-limited and is not associated with systemic allergic reactions. Influenza vaccines have been found to be safe in pediatric and adult patients who have HIV [82].

Antiviral therapy and chemoprophylaxis against influenza

Comprehensive influenza vaccination is clearly the best primary preventative measure against influenza infection. Based on several ED studies mentioned previously [20–27], we know that many patients in the ED are not being properly immunized. To this end, antiviral drugs can be used clinically to attenuate influenza symptoms and, to a lesser extent, to prevent influenza infection in individuals at high risk who may have not been immunized before the detection of influenza in their community [83].

There are currently two approved antiviral medicines recommended for use in the United States: oseltamivir and zanamivir. They are chemically related antiviral compounds that target neuraminidase and have excellent activity against influenza A and B viruses. Antiviral therapy must be started within 24 to 48 hours after the onset of symptoms. Antiviral therapy can attenuate illness severity and shorten the duration of illness by 24 to 36 hours [84]. Antiviral therapy for influenza may also prevent serious influenza-related complications, but the data supporting this are incomplete [85]. Antiviral medications are reported to be 70% to 90% effective in preventing influenza and are useful adjuncts to vaccination in certain populations [86,87]. Antiviral medicines are also effective at preventing disease in those using them as chemoprophylaxis with household members with confirmed influenza [88]. Amantadine and rimantadine are no longer recommended by the CDC.

Oseltamivir is approved for the treatment of individuals 1 year of age or older. Zanamivir is approved for the treatment of individuals 7 years of age or older. The recommended duration of treatment with oseltamivir or zanamivir is 5 days. Oseltamivir is licensed for use as chemoprophylaxis in people 1 year of age or older. Zanamivir is licensed for use as chemoprophylaxis in people 5 years of age or older. To be effective as prophylaxis, antiviral therapy must delivered for the duration of exposure to individuals with influenza or until immunity after vaccination develops. It generally takes 2 weeks to develop acquired antibodies in adults, and it can take significantly longer in children depending on age and health status. The supply and cost of antiviral therapy significantly limit their utility in epidemics and pandemic situations and underscore the role of vaccination as the primary preventive measure against influenza.

Pneumococcal disease

Pneumococcal disease is a leading cause of serious illness, hospitalization, and death in children and adults worldwide. Pneumococcal disease causes upper and lower respiratory tract infections and invasive systemic disease. Pneumococcus is an encapsulated gram-positive bacterial organism. The disease process is primarily a result of massive bacterial replication because it has few significant virulence factors. Encapsulation does allow the bacterial organism to avoid phagocytosis, amplifying its ability to replicate and stimulate a complex inflammatory cascade.

In the United States, pneumococcal disease is responsible for causing most cases of community-acquired bacterial pneumonia ($>$ 500,000 cases a year), bacteremia ($>$ 50,000 cases a year), and meningitis ($>$ 3000 cases a year)

[89]. Pneumococcus also causes otitis media (>7 million cases a year) and sinusitis [90]. The incidence of invasive pneumococcal disease is significantly higher in the developing world than in industrialized nations [91]. There are manifold pneumococcal types (>90); the 10 most common types account for approximately 62% of invasive disease worldwide [92].

Pneumococcal disease is more common in winter months and when respiratory viruses, such as influenza, are prevalent. Endemic pneumococcal disease is not common but can occur in institutionalized patient populations and in school children. In the United States, most deaths from pneumococcal disease occur in the elderly, although in developing countries, child mortality is still high. In 2000, a new pneumococcal conjugate vaccine (PCV) was introduced in the United States for routine childhood immunization and has dramatically reduced the incidence of severe pneumococcal disease in children [93]. During the same time, rates of childhood immunization have also dramatically increased. Pediatric pneumococcal immunization in the United States is currently approximately 87% [37]. Because PCV interrupts person-to-person transmission, the incidence of severe pneumococcal disease in older children and adults has also declined [93]. Pneumococcal vaccination is recommended by all major clinical advisory groups including the CDC, AICP, ACEP, and Cochrane Database of Systematic Reviews [94].

Pneumococcal disease is a febrile illness in most forms of pneumococcal infection and may account for the only symptoms in pediatric patients who have bacteremia. Patients who have pneumococcal pneumonia typically have cough, dyspnea, or pleuritic chest pain and may have shaking chills. Fever and sputum production may be absent in elderly persons with pneumococcal pneumonia. Pneumococcal meningitis, otitis media, or sinus infections may present with signs consistent with other bacterial or viral infections.

Two vaccines are currently available in the United States to prevent pneumococcal disease: (1) the pneumococcal conjugate vaccine 7 (PCV7) and (2) the pneumococcal polysaccharide vaccine 23 (PPV23). Both vaccines are effective at inducing antibodies to pneumococcal capsular proteins and are effective at preventing invasive disease [95]. The PCV7 prevents some pneumonia and otitis media and sinusitis in children [96].

The PCV7 is part of the routine infant immunization schedule in the United States and is recommended for all children younger than 2 years of age and for children 2 to 4 years of age who have certain underlying conditions [10]. Pediatric pneumococcal rates are high (<87%). The PPV23 is part of the routine adult immunization schedule, but many adults are under-immunized [8]. In 2003, only 64% of adults 65 years of age or older had received the vaccine [97].

Pneumococcal vaccines

A single dose of PPV23 should be given to persons 65 years of age or older or to persons 2 to 64 years of age with high-risk comorbidities.

Children 2 to 4 years of age with indications for PPV23 should receive PPV23 at least 2 months after receiving doses of PCV7. Persons with an indication for PCV7 but with an uncertain vaccination history should receive one dose. A second dose of vaccine should be used for the following groups: (1) persons 65 years of age or older who received the vaccine at least 5 years before and were younger than 65 years of age at the time of initial vaccination; (2) persons with sickle cell disease, asplenia, renal disease, hematologic disease, malignancy, or HIV/AIDS; and (3) children younger than 10 years of age, in whom the second dose may be given 3 years or more after the first dose (Box 2) [98].

Severe reactions are rare with pneumococcal vaccination (PCV7 and PPV23). Adverse effects are mild and generally consist of transient localized reactions, such as erythema, swelling, and tenderness. Mild reactions occur in 10% to 23% of infants after PCV7 vaccination. In 1% to 9% of cases, larger regional areas of erythema and swelling may occur. Low-grade fever can occur in up to 24% of children after PCV7 vaccination. For PPV23 vaccination, mild transient local side effects occur in approximately 50% of patients and are more common after subsequent vaccinations. Systemic symptoms, including myalgias and fever, are rare after PPV23 vaccination [99].

Implementation of immunization programs in the emergency department

Although the possible administration of influenza and pneumococcal immunization in the ED has been considered for more than 20 years, with the earliest report occurring in 1987 by Polis and colleagues [20], and many subsequent reports and organizations have recommended that these vaccines be administered in the ED, widespread use continues to be lacking. In a recent CDC publication that included the ACIP recommendations, it was reported that influenza immunizations have been administered successfully in outpatient facilities, managed care organizations, assisted living facilities, correctional facilities, pharmacies, and adult workplaces [42].

Administration of influenza vaccines in pharmacy-based supermarket chains was described by Weitzel and colleagues [100]; currently, these programs exist in several department store and supermarket chains. When surveyed, vaccinations in nontraditional setting, such as stores, community centers, and the workplace, were more likely for young healthy adults [101]. In another report, emergency medical services (EMS) personal immunized 2075 adults in a variety of locations, including EMS stations, churches, senior citizen complexes, and private residences [102]. In the recently published ACIP recommendations [43], standing orders to offer influenza vaccines to all hospitalized persons in acute care hospitals was recommended. The long-term care facilities have used standing orders programs for these vaccines, and it is recommended that such programs be conducted under the supervision of licensed practitioners so that patients can be

Box 2. Persons for whom pneumococcal vaccination is recommended

Immunocompetent persons (give vaccine if earlier vaccination status is unknown)

- All persons aged 65 years or older (strength of recommendation A). Revaccinate if the patient received the vaccine 5 years or longer ago when they were younger than the age of 65 years.
- All persons aged 2 to 64 years with chronic CVD, chronic pulmonary disease, or diabetes mellitus (strength of recommendation A)
- All persons aged 2 to 64 years with functional or anatomic asplenia (including patients who have sickle cell disease) (strength of recommendation A). Revaccinate if the patient is younger than 10 years of age, with a single revaccination 5 years or longer after the previous dose. If the patient is 10 years of age or younger, consider revaccination 3 years after the previous dose.
- All persons aged 2 to 64 years with alcoholism, chronic liver disease, or cerebrospinal fluid leak (strength of recommendation B)
- All persons aged 2 to 64 years living in special environments or social settings (including Alaskan Natives and certain American Indian populations) (strength of recommendation C)

Immunocompromised persons and

- Persons aged 2 years of age or older, including those with HIV infection, leukemia, lymphoma, Hodgkin's disease, multiple myeloma, generalized malignancy, chronic renal failure, or nephritic syndrome; those receiving immunosuppressive chemotherapy (including corticosteroids); and those who have received an organ or bone marrow transplant (strength of recommendation C). Revaccinate with a single dose if 5 years or more have elapsed since the first dose. If patient is 10 years of age or younger, consider revaccination 3 years after the previous dose.

From CDC. Prevention of pneumococcal disease: recommendations of the Advisory Committee on Immunization Practices (ACIP). MMWR Morb Mortal Wkly Rep 1997;46(RR-8):12.

Box 3. Reasons for administering influenza vaccinations in the emergency department

1. Patient volumes in the ED are increasing, and vaccination rates are low in this population [1,22–25].
2. Several studies have demonstrated that eligible patients in the ED can be successfully vaccinated in the ED [21–25].
3. ED vaccination programs can help with racial, ethnic, and socioeconomic disparities.
4. Influenza infections adversely affect ED throughput, ED diversion, and ED use [28,30,31].
5. Numerous professional organizations, such as the CDC, ACIP, and ACEP, have recommended that the ED administer these vaccines [35,42].
6. Influenza and pneumococcal vaccines are reimbursable by third-party payers, and Part B Medicare is also available [42].
7. ED vaccination programs are cost-effective [27].
8. Emergency medicine needs to keep up with other inpatient services and other locations in which these vaccines are administered [42,101]. If supermarket chains can do this, why cannot EDs [100]?
9. ED vaccinations have been successful for tetanus [3].
10. Yes, this is primary care in the ED, but this is what we do.

---

appropriately screened, vaccines appropriately administered, and adverse events monitored. Although it is generally recommended that outpatient facilities, such as physicians' offices and a list of other specialty clinics, administer these immunizations, it was also recommended by the ACIP that outpatient facilities providing episodic acute care, such as EDs and walk-in care clinics, also administer these vaccines.

Payment for influenza and pneumococcal vaccines is available under Medicare Part B, and roster billing can be used. In EDs, there are many impediments to administering vaccines. Increasing patient volumes and overcrowding make it more difficult for ED personnel to take the time to screen for eligible patients. In many of the reported ED-based studies, additional nurses or research personnel were used for this purpose. Standing orders have been recommended, but ED personnel still are required for screening. The implementation of computerized order entry for admitted patients with mandatory immunization screening has helped to increase the rates of immunization for eligible hospitalized patients. As computerized chart documentation and order entry become more popular in the ED, such programs, coupled with standing orders, may help to increase administration rates of these vaccines. As with any medication or immunization administered in the ED, efforts to monitor safety and to inform patients' physicians should ideally become part of the program as well.

During a recent lecture by the primary author, a "top 10" list was provided regarding the rationale for implementing an ED-based influenza administration program. The 10 reasons are listed here in no particular order of importance (Box 3).

References

[1] Nawar EW, Niska RW, Jianmin X. re Statistics National Hospital Ambulatory Medical Care Survey: 2005 Emergency Department summary. Available at: http://www.cdc.gov/nchs/data/ad/ad386.pdf. Accessed February 4, 2008.

[2] Mandell LA, Wunderink RG, Anzueto A, et al. Infectious Diseases Society of America/American Thoracic Society consensus guidelines on the management of community-acquired pneumonia in adults. Clin Infect Dis 2007;44:S27–72.

[3] Pallin DJ, Muennig PA, Emond JA, et al. Vaccination practices in U.S. emergency departments. Vaccine 2005;23:1048–52.

[4] Talan DA, Abrahamian FM, Moran GJ, et al. Tetanus immunity and physician compliance with tetanus prophylaxis practices among ED patients presenting with wounds. Ann Emerg Med 2004;43:305–14.

[5] Pascual FB, McGinley EL, Zanardi LR, et al. Tetanus surveillance US 1998–2000. MMWR Surveill Summ 2003;52:1–8.

[6] Thwaites CL, Farrar JJ. Preventing and treating tetanus. BMJ 2003;326:117–8.

[7] Vandelaer J, Birmingham M, Gasse FL, et al. Tetanus in developing countries: an update on the maternal and neonatal tetanus elimination initiative. Vaccine 2003;21:3442–5.

[8] Center for Disease Control and Prevention (CDC). Influenza and pneumococcal vaccination levels among persons aged >65 years—United States, 1999. MMWR Morb Mortal Wkly Rep 2001;50:532–7.

[9] Bridges CB, Fukuda K, Cox NJ, et al. Advisory Committee on Immunization Practices. Prevention and control of influenza: recommendations of the Advisory Committee on Immunization Practice (ACIP). MMWR Morb Mortal Wkly Rep 2001;50(RR-4):1–44.

[10] CDC. Prevention of pneumococcal disease: recommendations of the Advisory Committee on Immunization Practices (ACIP). MMWR Morb Mortal Wkly Rep 1997;46(RR-8): 1–24.

[11] Bratzler DW, Houck PM, Jiang H, et al. Failure to vaccinate Medicare inpatients. Arch Intern Med 2002;162:2349–56.

[12] Association for Practitioners of Infection Control. Position paper: immunizations. Am J Infect Control 1992;20:131–2.

[13] Fedson DS. Adult immunization. Summary of the National Vaccine Advisory Committee. JAMA 1994;272:1133–7.

[14] Fisman DN, Abrutyn E, Spaude KA, et al. Prior pneumococcal vaccination is associated with reduced death, complications, and length of stay among hospitalized adults with community acquired pneumonia. Clin Infect Dis 2006;42:1093–101.

[15] Gross PA, Hermogenes AW, Sacks HS, et al. The efficacy of influenza vaccine in elderly persons: a meta-analysis and review of the literature. Ann Intern Med 1995;123:518–27.

[16] Nichol KL, Baken L, Nelson A. Relation between influenza vaccination and outpatient visits, hospitalizations, and mortality in elderly persons with chronic lung disease. Ann Intern Med 1999;130:397–403.

[17] McDonald CJ, Hui SL, Tiemey WM. Effects of computer reminders for influenza vaccination on morbidity during influenza epidemics. MD Comput 1992;9:304–12.

[18] Nichol KL, Margolis KL, Wuorenma J, et al. The efficacy and cost effectiveness of vaccination against influenza among elderly persons living in the community. N Engl J Med 1994;331:778–84.

[19] Sisk JE, Moskowitz AJ, Whang W, et al. Cost-effectiveness of vaccination against pneumococcal bacteremia among elderly people. JAMA 1997;278:1333–9.

[20] Polis MA, Smith JP, Sainer D, et al. Prospects for an emergency department-based adult immunization program. Arch Intern Med 1987;147:1999–2001.

[21] Polis MA, Davey VJ, Collins ED, et al. The emergency department as part of a successful strategy for increasing adult immunization. Ann Emerg Med 1988;17:1016–8.

[22] Rodriguez RM, Baraff LJ. Emergency department immunization of the elderly with pneumococcal and influenza vaccines. Ann Emerg Med 1993;22:1729–32.

[23] Wrenn K, Zeldin M, Miller O. Influenza and pneumococcal vaccination in the ED: is it feasible? J Gen Intern Med 1994;9:425–9.

[24] Kapur AK, Tenenbein M. Vaccination of ED patients at high risk for influenza. Acad Emerg Med 2000;7:354–8.

[25] Slobodkin D, Zielske PG, Kitlas JL, et al. Demonstration of the feasibility of ED immunization against influenza and pneumococcus. Ann Emerg Med 1998;32:537–43.

[26] Stack SJ, Martin DR, Plouffe JF. An emergency department-based pneumococcal vaccination program could save money and lives. Ann Emerg Med 1999;33:299–303.

[27] Hussain S, Slobodkin D, Weinstein RA. Pneumococcal vaccination: analysis of opportunities in an inner city hospital. Arch Intern Med 2002;162:1961–5.

[28] Schull MJ, Mamdani MM, Fang J. Influenza and ED utilization by elders. Acad Emerg Med 2005;12:338–44.

[29] Silka PA, Geiderman JM, Goldberg JB, et al. Demand on ED resources during periods of widespread influenza activity. Am J Emerg Med 2003;21:534–9.

[30] Schull MJ, Mamdani MM, Fang J. Community influenza and emergency department ambulance diversion. Ann Emerg Med 2004;44:61–7.

[31] Menec VH, Black C, MacWilliam L, et al. The impact of influenza-associated respiratory illnesses on hospitalizations, physician visits, ER visits and mortality. Can J Public Health 2003;94:59–63.

[32] American College of Emergency Physicians Council (ACEP). Resolution 18, influenza and pneumococcal immunizations. Available at: http://www.acep.org/Content.aspx?id=23216.

[33] ACEP. Immunization of adult patients. Available at: http://www.acep.org/practres.aspx?id=29516. Accessed December 1, 2007.

[34] ACEP. Immunizations in the ED. Available at: http://www.acep.org/practres.aspx?id=29522. Accessed December 1, 2007.

[35] Butler JC, Shapiro ED, Carlone GM. Pneumococcal vaccines: history, current status and future directions. Am J Med 1999;107(1A):69S–76S.

[36] Centers for Medicare and Medicaid Services. 2001 Fact sheet for Medicare influenza/pneumococcal vaccination benefits. Available at: http://cms.hhs.gov/preventiveservices/2.asp#1. Accessed April 8, 2002.

[37] CDC. Healthy People 2010 database. Available at: http://wonder.cdc.gov/data2010/. Accessed January 22, 2008.

[38] Center for Disease Control and Prevention. Recommended childhood immunization schedule—United States. JAMA 1998;279:495–6.

[39] CDC. National Immunization Survey 2005 Report. Available at: http://www.cdc.gov/vaccines/stats-surv/nis/data/tables_2005.htm. Accessed January 22, 2008.

[40] CDC. National Immunization Survey 2006 Report. Available at: http://www.cdc.gov/vaccines/stats-surv/nis/data/tables_2006.htm. Accessed January 22, 2008.

[41] Kroger AT, Atkinson WL, Marcuse EK, et al. Advisory Committee on Immunization Practices (ACIP), Centers for Disease Control and Prevention. General recommendations on immunization: recommendations of the Advisory Committee on Immunization Practices (ACIP). MMWR Morb Mortal Wkly Rep 2006;55(RR15):1–48.

[42] Fiore AE, Shay DK, Haber P, et al. Advisory Committee on Immunization Practices (ACIP) Centers for Disease Control an Prevention (CDC). Prevention and control of influenza—recommendations of the Advisory Committee on Immunization Practices (ACIP). MMWR Morb Mortal Wkly Rep 2007;56(RR06):1–54.
[43] Morens DM. Influenza-related mortality: considerations for practice and public health. JAMA 2003;289:227–9.
[44] Brundage JF. Interactions between influenza and bacterial respiratory pathogens: implications for pandemic preparedness. Lancet Infect Dis 2006;6:303–12.
[45] Neuzil KM, Mellen BG, Wright PF, et al. The effect of influenza on hospitalizations, outpatient visits, and courses of antibiotics in children. N Engl J Med 2000;342:225–31.
[46] Monto AS, Sullivan KM. Acute respiratory illness in the community: frequency of illness and the agents involved. Epidemiol Infect 1993;110:145–60.
[47] Lutwick S. Pediatric vaccine compliance. Pediatr Clin North Am 2000;47:427–34.
[48] Esposito S, Marchisio P, Droghetti R, et al. Influenza vaccination coverage among children with high-risk medical conditions. Vaccine 2006;24:5251–5.
[49] Atkinson W, Hamborsky J. CDC epidemiology and prevention of vaccine-preventable diseases. 10th edition. Washington, DC: Public Health Foundation; 2007.
[50] National Vaccine Advisory Committee. Standards for child and adolescent immunization practices: National Vaccine Advisory Committee. Pediatrics 2003;112:958–63.
[51] Pappano D, Humiston S, Goepp J. Efficacy of a pediatric ED based influenza vaccination program. Arch Pediatr Adolesc Med 2004;158:1077–83.
[52] Humiston SG, Lerner EB, Hepworth E, et al. Parent opinions about universal influenza vaccination for infants and toddlers. Arch Pediatr Adolesc Med 2005;159:108–12.
[53] Gurfinkel EP, Leon de la Fuente R, Mendiz O, et al. Flu Vaccination in Acute Coronary Syndromes and Planned Percutaneous Coronary Interventions (FLUVACS) study. Eur Heart J 2004;25:25–31.
[54] Jackson LA, Yu O, Heckbert SR, et al. Influenza vaccination is not associated with a reduction in the risk of recurrent coronary events. Am J Epidemiol 2002;156:634–40.
[55] Cates CJ, Jefferson TO, Bara AI, et al. Vaccines for preventing influenza in people with asthma (Cochrane Review). Cochrane Database Syst Rev 2000;(4):CD000364.
[56] Smits AJ, Hak E, Stallman WA, et al. Clinical effectiveness of conventional influenza vaccination in asthmatic children. Epidemiol Infect 2002;128:205–11.
[57] National Asthma Education and Prevention Program. Expert panel report 2: guidelines for the diagnosis and management of asthma. Bethesda (MD): 146 US Department of Health and Human Services, Public Health Service, National Institutes of Health, National Heart, Lung and Blood Institute; 1997.
[58] Taubenberger JK, Morens DM. 1918 influenza: the mother of all pandemics. Emerg Infect Dis 2006. Available at: http://www.cdc.gov/ncidod/EID/vol12no01/05-0979.htm. Accessed January 22, 2008.
[59] Cox NJ, Fukuda K. Influenza. Infect Dis Clin North Am 1998;12:27–38.
[60] Monmany J, Rabella N, Margall N, et al. Unmasking influenza virus infection in patients attended to in the ED. Infection 2004;32:89–97.
[61] Long CE, Hall CB, Cunningham CK, et al. Influenza surveillance in community-dwelling elderly compared with children. Arch Fam Med 1997;6:459–65.
[62] Cunha B. Influenza: historical aspects of epidemics and pandemics. Infect Dis Clin North Am 2004;18:141–55.
[63] Simonsen L, Taylor RJ, Viboud C, et al. Mortality benefits of influenza vaccination in elderly people: an ongoing controversy. Lancet Infect Dis 2007;7:658–66.
[64] The World Health Organization (WHO). Global Influenza Surveillance Network. Available at: http://www.who.int/csr/disease/influenza/influenzanetwork/en/index.html. Accessed January 22, 2008.
[65] Reid KC, Grizarrd TA, Poland GA. Adult immunizations: recommendations for practice. Mayo Clin Proc 1999;74:377–84.

[66] Ball LK, Ball R, Pratt RD. An assessment of thimerosal use in childhood vaccines. Pediatrics 2001;107(5):1147–54.

[67] Juurlink DN, Stukel TA, Kwong J, et al. Guillain-Barré syndrome after influenza vaccination in adults; a population-based study. Arch Intern Med 2006;166:2217–21.

[68] United States Government Accountability Office (GAO). GAO Report to the Committee on Oversight and Government Reform, House of Representatives: INFLUENZA VACCINE issues related to production, distribution, and public health messages, October 2007. Available at: http://www.gao.gov/new.items/d0827.pdf. Accessed January 22, 2008.

[69] Homeland Security Council. The White House: National Strategy for Pandemic Influenza Implementation Plan One Year Summary, July 17, 2007. Available at: http://www.whitehouse.gov/homeland/pandemic-influenza-oneyear.html. Accessed January 22, 2008.

[70] Negri E, Colombo C, Giordano L, et al. Influenza vaccine in healthy children: a meta-analysis. Vaccine 2005;23:2851–61.

[71] Belshe R, Mendelman P. Safety and efficacy of live attenuated, cold-adapted, influenza vaccine-trivalent. Immunol Allergy Clin North Am 2003;23:745–67.

[72] Witte K, Allen M. A meta-analysis of fear appeals: implications for effective public health campaigns. Health Educ Behav 2000;27:591–615.

[73] Hak E, Hoes AW, Nordin J, et al. Benefits of influenza vaccine in US elderly—appreciating issues of confounding bias and precision. Int J Epidemiol 2006;35:800–2.

[74] Jackson LA, Jackson ML, Nelson JC, et al. Evidence of bias in estimates of influenza vaccine effectiveness in seniors. Int J Epidemiol 2006;35:337–44.

[75] Nichol KL. Benefits of influenza vaccination among healthy and high-risk persons across the age spectrum. International Congress Series 2004;1263:48–50.

[76] Zangwill KM, Belshe RB. Safety and efficacy of trivalent inactivated influenza vaccine in young children: a summary of the new era of routine vaccination. Pediatr Infect Dis J 2004;23:189–97.

[77] Neuzil KM, Dupont WD, Wright PF, et al. Efficacy of inactivated and cold-adapted vaccines against influenza A infection, 1985 to 1990: the pediatric experience. Pediatr Infect Dis J 2001;20:733–40.

[78] Nichol KL, Nordin JD, Nelson NB, et al. Effectiveness of influenza vaccine in the community-dwelling elderly. N Engl J Med 2007;357:1373–81.

[79] Nichol KL, Nordin J, Mullooly J, et al. Influenza vaccination and reduction in hospitalizations for cardiac disease and stroke among the elderly. N Engl J Med 2003;348:1322–32.

[80] Gillim-Ross L, Subbarao K. Emerging respiratory viruses: challenges and vaccine strategies. Clin Microbiol Rev 2006;19:614–36.

[81] Giovanetti F. Travel medicine interventions and neurological disease. Travel Med Infect Dis 2007;5:7–17.

[82] Zanetti AR, Amendola A, Besana S, et al. Safety and immunogenicity of influenza vaccination in individuals infected with HIV. Vaccine 2002;20(Suppl 5):B29–32.

[83] Medimmune Vaccines Incorporated. FluMist [package insert]. Gaithersburg (MD): Medimmune Vaccines, Inc.; 2007. Available at: http://www.flumist.com/pdf/flumist-prescribing-information.pdf. Accessed January 22, 2008.

[84] Schmidt AC. Antiviral therapy for influenza: a clinical and economic comparative review. Drugs 2004;64:2031–46.

[85] Kaiser L, Wat C, Mills T, et al. Impact of oseltamivir treatment on influenza-related lower respiratory tract complications and hospitalizations. Arch Intern Med 2003;163:1667–72.

[86] Monto AS, Fleming DM, Henry D, et al. Efficacy and safety of the neuraminidase inhibitor zanamivir in the treatment of influenza A and B virus infections. J Infect Dis 1999;180:254–61.

[87] Hayden FG, Atmar RL, Schilling M, et al. Use of the selective oral neuraminidase inhibitor oseltamivir to prevent influenza. N Engl J Med 1999;341:1336–43.

[88] Hayden FG, Gubareva LV, Monto AS, et al. Inhaled zanamivir for the prevention of influenza in families. Zanamivir Family Study Group. N Engl J Med 2000;343:1282–9.

[89] Robinson KA, Baughman W, Rothrock G. Epidemiology of invasive Streptococcus pneumoniae infections in the United States, 1995–1998. Opportunities for prevention in the conjugate vaccine era. JAMA 2001;285:1729–35.

[90] CDC. Preventing pneumococcal disease among infants and young children. MMWR Morb Mortal Wkly Rep 2000;49:1–35.

[91] World Health Organization. Pneumococcal vaccines. Wkly Epidemiol Rec 2003;14:110–9.

[92] CDC. Active Bacterial Core Surveillance (ABCs)/Emerging Infections Program (EIP) Network, 2000. Available at: http://www.cdc.gov/ncidod/dbmd/abcs/survreports/spneu98.pdf. Accessed January 22, 2008.

[93] Whitney CG, Farley MM, Hadler J. Decline in invasive pneumococcal disease after the introduction of protein-polysaccharide conjugate vaccine. N Engl J Med 2003;348:1737–46.

[94] Lucero MG, Dulalia VE, Parreno RN, et al. Pneumococcal conjugate vaccines for preventing vaccine-type invasive pneumococcal disease and pneumonia with consolidation on x-ray in children under two years of age. Cochrane Database Syst Rev 2004;(4):CD004977.

[95] Fedson DS. The clinical effectiveness of pneumococcal vaccination: a brief review. Vaccine 1999;17(Suppl 1):S85–90.

[96] Eskola J, Kilpi T, Palmu A, et al. Efficacy of a pneumococcal conjugate vaccine against acute otitis media. N Engl J Med 2001;344:403–9.

[97] National Center for Health Statistics. Early release of selected estimates based on data from the January-September National Health Interview Survey (NHIS) [monograph on the Internet]. Atlanta (GA): Centers for Disease Control and Prevention; 2003. Available at: http://www.cdc.gov/nchs/about/major/nhis/released200303.htm#5. Accessed January 22, 2008.

[98] CDC. Pneumococcal polysaccharide vaccine—what you need to know. Available at: http://www.cdc.gov/vaccines/pubs/vis/downloads/vis-ppv.pdf. Accessed January 22, 2008.

[99] Fedson DS, Musher DM. Pneumococcal vaccine. In: Plotkin SA, Mortimer EA Jr, editors. Vaccines. 2nd edition. Philadelphia: WB Saunders; 1994. p. 517–63.

[100] Weitzel KW, Goode JV. Implementation of a pharmacy-based immunization program in a supermarket chain. J Am Pharm Assoc (Wash) 2000;40:252–6.

[101] Singleton JA, Poel AJ, Lu PJ, et al. Where adults reported receiving influenza vaccination in the United States. Am J Infect Control 2005;33:563–70.

[102] Mosesso VN Jr, Packer CR, McMahon J, et al. Influenza immunization by EMS agencies: the MEDICVAX Project. Prehosp Emerg Care 2003;7:74–8.

ELSEVIER
SAUNDERS

Emerg Med Clin N Am
26 (2008) 571–595

EMERGENCY
MEDICINE
CLINICS OF
NORTH AMERICA

Hyperbaric Oxygen: Applications in Infectious Disease

Colin G. Kaide, MD, FACEP, FAAEM*,
Sorabh Khandelwal, MD

*Department of Emergency Medicine, The Ohio State University Medical Center,
0136 Means Hall, 1654 Upham Drive, Columbus, OH 43240, USA*

The first hyperbaric chamber was built in 1662 by a British clergyman named Nathaniel Henshaw. It was compressed manually with a bellows using room air and likely did not reach pressures that had any clinical significance. From that time until 1955 various hyperbaric apparatus have been used with varying (limited) success to treat certain conditions. There was little if any science or understanding behind the application of hyperbarics during this period. In 1955, Churchill-Davidson and colleagues used hyperbaric oxygen (HBO) to try to augment the effects of radiation therapy for patients who had cancer, which began the era of the scientific use of HBO in clinical medicine.

Over its long history, HBO has been used for many purposes, ranging from "anti-aging treatments" and boosting the athletic ability of competitors to treatment of chronic neurologic conditions. For many of these applications, the scientific foundations were weak and the research backing their use was questionable.

The Undersea and Hyperbaric Medicine Society (UHMS) was founded in 1967 (originally as the Undersea Medical Society) to help promote the exchange of data and research within the commercial and military dive medicine communities. Later, the clinical practice of hyperbaric medicine came under the auspices of the UHMS. It now acts as the primary scientific body for hyperbaric medicine. In 1976 the UHMS developed the multispecialty Hyperbaric Oxygen Therapy Committee to oversee the development of an evidence-guided list of indications for the use of HBO. There are currently

* Corresponding author.
  E-mail address: colin.kaide@osumc.edu (C.G. Kaide).

0733-8627/08/$ - see front matter © 2008 Elsevier Inc. All rights reserved.
doi:10.1016/j.emc.2008.01.005   *emed.theclinics.com*

13 indications for HBO for which there is in vitro and in vivo evidence to support its use (Box 1) [1]. Some of these conditions involve infectious processes.

In this article we discuss the use of HBO as an adjunct to aggressive medical and surgical management of infectious processes.

Hyperbaric physiology

HBO therapy is the application of pressures greater than 1 atmosphere absolute (ATA) to an environment of 100% oxygen, which results in the increase in the partial pressure of oxygen, proportional to the increase in pressure. When a patient is placed into a hyperbaric chamber, the oxygen is delivered by the lungs to the entire body. This systemic delivery of oxygen should not be confused with topical oxygen therapy, in which a specific body part is subjected to oxygen under pressure with the oxygen delivered locally to an open wound.

Under normobaric conditions, we live at 1 ATA of pressure measured at sea level. That is to say that a person at sea level has downward pressure exerted on his body equal to the weight of the atmosphere above him. In medial applications, it is customary to measure atmospheric pressure in millimeters of mercury (mm Hg). A pressure of 760 mm Hg is equal to 1 ATA, 14.7 psi, 760 torr, or 33 ft of seawater.

At the depth of 33 ft of seawater, a diver is exposed to 2 ATA: 1 ATA from the atmosphere above the water and 1 ATA from the pressure exerted by the 33 ft (10 m) of seawater. Henry's law specifies that the partial pressure

---

Box 1. Indications for hyperbaric oxygen therapy

Air/gas embolism
Decompression sickness
Carbon monoxide poisoning
Crush injury, compartment syndrome, and other acute ischemias
Exceptional blood loss anemia
Delayed radiation injury (osteo and soft tissue)
Skin grafts and flaps
Thermal burns
Enhancement of healing in selected problem wounds
Necrotizing soft tissue infections
Clostridial myositis and myonecrosis (gas gangrene)
Osteomyelitis (refractory), includes malignant otitis externa
Intracranial abscesses

Data from Feldmeier JJ, editor. Hyperbaric oxygen 2003: indications and results: the Hyperbaric Oxygen Therapy Committee Report. Kensington (MD): Undersea and Hyperbaric Medical Society; 2003.

of a gas dissolved in a liquid is proportional to the pressure exerted on that gas. At 2 ATA a diver breathing 21% oxygen would develop a Po_2 of 320 mm Hg, twice the Po_2 at 1 ATA. Although the percentage of oxygen at 2 ATA is still 21%, the diver is breathing in twice as many molecules of oxygen per breath, which is equivalent to breathing 42% oxygen at 1 ATA. Conversely, if that individual were to travel to a higher elevation, such as 8000 ft (2440 m), the pressure exerted by the atmosphere would be equal to 75% of the pressure at sea level. The Po_2 would be 120 (0.75 × 160) and the resultant effective fraction of inspired oxygen would be 15.75%.

There are two gas laws that explain the effects of HBO: Boyle's law and Henry's law. Boyle's law describes the change in volume of a gas as a function of pressure and Henry's law states that the concentration of a gas dissolved in a liquid is proportional to the partial pressure of that gas above the solution. HBO capitalizes on Henry's law by significantly increasing the ambient Po_2 causing a dramatic increase in the amount of dissolved oxygen carried by the blood. As the partial pressure of oxygen reaches 100 mm Hg, hemoglobin becomes fully saturated. Under normobaric conditions, the dissolved oxygen is negligible, representing only 0.3 mL of oxygen per 100 mL of blood (called volume percent—vol%), compared with 20 vol% carried by hemoglobin. Under hyperbaric conditions, however, the Pao_2 at 2.5 ATA (a typical HBO treatment pressure) approaches 2000 mm Hg. This pressure is high enough to generate 5.4 vol% of dissolved oxygen, which can sustain basal metabolic functions in the complete absence of any hemoglobin. Hyperoxygenated plasma can transport oxygen to areas that are inaccessible to red cells, delivering oxygen to relatively hypoxic tissues in proportion to the oxygen tension of the plasma (Box 2).

Mechanisms of antimicrobial effect of hyperbaric oxygen therapy

As the result of the hyperoxic environment generated by HBO, some physiologic and biochemical changes occur, which promote an additional antimicrobial effect that can enhance or modulate standard therapy. Some effects of the hyperoxic environment as they pertain to infectious diseases include the following:

Suppression of clostridial alpha toxin production in gas gangrene (discussed later in this article) [2].

Box 2. Oxygen content calculation

The oxygen content of the blood is determined by the combination of the oxygen carried by hemoglobin plus the oxygen dissolved in the blood.

Oxygen Content = 1.34 (HgB) (% Saturation) + PO_2 (.003)

Enhancement of leukocyte-killing activity. Granulocytes kill microorganisms by oxygen-independent and oxygen-dependent mechanisms. The oxygen-independent system alone is inadequate to eradicate all of the wound pathogens, as evidenced by a decrease in microorganism killing in hypoxic environments [3,4]. The oxygen-dependent system consumes large amounts of molecular oxygen to produce an "oxidative burst" after phagocytosis of offending pathogens. The burst consists of oxygen radicals, such as hydroxyl radicals, peroxides, and superoxide. The production of these substances increases in a fashion directly proportional to the amount of available oxygen [5]. Further, it has been shown that this process is significantly retarded in a hypoxic environment.

Bacterial growth suppression in hyperoxic tissues. Healthy normoxic wounds with adequate perfusion are highly resistant to infection [6]. In multiple animal models, it has been clearly demonstrated that bacterial growth in hypoxic, poorly perfused tissues increases. In tissues where the oxygen tension fell below 30 mm Hg, an established bacterial infection quickly destroyed the tissue. In a controlled environment, the elevation of oxygen tension in inoculated tissue caused a resistance to infection that was slightly better than in the comparison group that received antibiotics alone. Moreover, there seemed to be a synergistic effect between a hyperoxic environment plus antibiotics [7].

Enhancement of antibiotic effects. Certain antibiotics show improved efficacy when delivered in a hyperoxic environment. The activity of aminoglycosides and the antimetabolite agents trimethoprim, sulfamethoxazole, and sulfasoxazole all show an increase in effectiveness in high oxygen tensions [8,9]. Additionally, agents such as vancomycin and the fluoroquinolones show decreased activity in a hypoxic milieu [10,11]. The effectiveness of these agents returns to normal when normoxia is restored.

Improvement in tissue repair. Poorly vascularized, ischemic tissue shows a significantly decreased healing response and increased susceptibility to infection [12]. The presence of necrotic tissue and infection in the open wound further slows the healing process. When exposed to HBO following standard treatment protocols, clearing of the infection and wound closure are significantly improved. HBO has little effect on wound closure in adequately vascularized, normoxic tissues. Enhancement of osteoclastic and osteoblastic activity also occurs, which enhances the clearing of bone infections and promotes healing in osteomyelitis.

Effects on anaerobic bacteria. Anaerobic bacteria lack the ability to defend adequately against free radicals and other toxic oxygen species. The enhancement of production of these endogenous antimicrobial agents by granulocytes is the primary mechanism by which HBO can be bacteriocidal to anaerobic organisms.

Necrotizing soft tissue infections

Necrotizing fasciitis (NF) is a rapidly progressive, life-threatening, deep-seated soft tissue infection that causes necrosis of the fascia and subcutaneous tissues. Bacterial endotoxins, exotoxins, and protease enzymes degrade fat and the extracellular matrix, resulting in rapid and extensive tissue damage and severe systemic toxicity [13]. Although NF is a relatively uncommon infection with 500 to 1500 cases reported in the United States annually, it incurs a mortality of 20% to 40% [14,15]. Those who survive NF usually have significant morbidity, frequently undergoing multiple surgical débridements and possibly even amputation.

NF can occur in two distinct populations of patients. Type I NF occurs in individuals who have a history of peripheral vascular disease, immune compromise, diabetes, or surgery, and is a polymicrobial disease. Typically, the inciting factor is a wound (eg, trauma to the skin, a decubitus ulcer, postoperative wound, animal or insect bite, or insulin injection site). Type I NF flora can be composed of both aerobic and anaerobic bacteria with common isolates including *Staphylococcus aureus*, *Escherichia coli*, *Bacteroides fragilis*, and various species of *Streptococci*, *Enterococci*, *Peptostreptococcus*, *Prevotella*, *Porphyromonas*, and *Clostridium* [16]. A particular form of NF called Fournier gangrene is also a polymicrobial infection, usually composed of enteric organisms. It attacks the perineal region and anterior abdominal wall. In males, the penis and scrotum are also affected.

Type II NF accounts for about 10% to 15% of cases [15,17]. It is the monomicrobial form and is caused by Group A *Streptococcus* (*Streptococcus pyogenes*). Recently, however, cases caused by community-associated, methicillin-resistant *S aureus* (MRSA) as the sole organism have been reported [18]. Type II NF can develop spontaneously in apparently healthy people who have minimal or no prior trauma and in the absence of a known causative factor or portal of entry for bacteria [19,20]. In some patients, predisposing factors, such as skin trauma and blunt injury, can sometimes be found.

Rationale and evidence for hyperbaric oxygen therapy

The primary modalities for treatment of NF are aggressive, early surgical débridement along with broad-spectrum antibiotic therapy directed at presumed causative agents. Surgical treatment includes the excision of necrotic fascia, compromised skin, and subcutaneous tissue. Frequently, multiple débridements are necessary within the first 24-hour period [21]. Although antibiotic therapy is essential in the treatment of NF, it is secondary in importance to surgical débridement [21]. The use of HBO in NF plays a complimentary and adjunctive role and should never substitute for the primary interventions [14,22]. Although there are no large randomized controlled studies that clearly demonstrate the effectiveness of HBO in NF, clinical experience and multiple small clinical reports suggest that HBO can play a valuable role in the overall management plan for many patients suffering from this devastating disease [21].

Of the clinical series supporting the use of HBO in NF, the most compelling were published by Mader (1988), Riseman (1990), and Escobar (2005) [23–25]. Mader [24] reported on 22 patients who had NF involving the scrotum and perineum (Fournier gangrene). He noted a reduction in mortality from 67% to 25% when HBO was added to standard treatment.

Riseman and colleagues [25] reported on 17 patients who had NF who received HBO plus standard therapy compared with 12 patients who received standard therapy alone. The HBO group was described as more seriously ill on admission. The reduction in mortality from 66% to 23% in the HBO group, along with a decrease in the number of necessary débridements, prompted the authors to strongly advocate that HBO be added to standard therapy in institutions where it is available. The authors went as far as to say that withholding HBO will cause unnecessary deaths and is therefore unethical.

The most recent study by Escobar and colleagues (2005) [23] retrospectively evaluated 42 patients who had NF in various body locations. These patients had significant comorbidities, including diabetes mellitus, chronic renal failure, intravenous drug abuse, peripheral vascular disease, and malignancy. They used a standard regimen for HBO, which was added to aggressive surgical débridement, antibiotic therapy, and critical care. Their patient population incurred a mortality of 11.9%, compared with the national average mortality rate of 34%. There were no amputations in the HBO-treated group compared with the reported rate of 50% nationally. Their study further refuted two common criticisms of HBO: delaying surgical intervention and creation of HBO-induced complications. They demonstrated no delays to operative intervention or interference in standard care. There were no clinically relevant complications related to the HBO.

To date there has only been one study that suggested a potential harm associated with HBO in NF. In 1977, Tehrani and Ledingham [26] reported an 88% mortality in 14 patients who received HBO along with conservative surgical treatment. In this study, however, the first 8 patients received HBO plus only incision and drainage as the primary surgical intervention as opposed to aggressive surgical debridement. Seven of the patients died. In the final 6 patients, a more aggressive surgical débridement along with HBO lead to a 33% mortality. This outcome argues more against the dangers of conservative surgical intervention than it does regarding the adjunctive HBO. See Table 1 for a summary of studies of HBO in NF.

Management with hyperbaric oxygen

Box 3 outlines the treatment protocol for necrotizing fasciitis.

Table 1
Summary of studies on hyperbaric oxygen treatment in necrotizing fasciitis

Author	Year	Study conclusions
Tehrani et al [26]	1977	Conservative surgery combined with HBO therapy was associated with high mortality (88%)
Eltorai et al [98]	1986	100% survival
Gozal et al [99]	1986	Mortality rate of 12.5%
Riseman et al [25]	1990	Significant decrease in mortality and the number of débridements in the HBO-treated group
Brown et al [100]	1994	A nonsignificant decrease in mortality with HBO therapy; no difference in length of hospitalization or number of débridements
Shupak et al [101]	1995	No significant difference in mortality or number of débridements
Korhonen et al [102]	1998	Mortality rate of 9% in patients who had Fournier gangrene
Escobar et al [23]	2005	11.9% mortality in HBO group with no amputations; 34% mortality in historical controls with 50% amputation rate

Summary for necrotizing fasciitis

Based on data accumulated from the trials done to date, it is reasonable to recommend HBO as adjunctive to aggressive surgical débridement. There seems to be a decrease in mortality and number of débridements required in patients who receive HBO. It is important to understand that HBO can never substitute for aggressive débridement and definitive operative management of NF should not be delayed awaiting HBO treatment. If a substantial time delay in going to the operating room (OR) is encountered, HBO

Box 3. Hyperbaric oxygen treatment protocol for necrotizing fasciitis

Pressure: HBO treatments started at 2.0–2.5 ATA

Duration: 90–120 minutes

Frequency: Treatment is initially done twice daily until the patient's condition is stabilized; then treatments can be changed to once daily.

Treatments: Treatments can continue until clinical improvement is maximized.

Use review: The continued use of HBO should be reviewed after 30 treatments.

Data from Feldmeier JJ, editor. Hyperbaric oxygen 2003: indications and results: the Hyperbaric Oxygen Therapy Committee Report. Kensington (MD): Undersea and Hyperbaric Medical Society; 2003.

may be initiated before surgery only if the treatment does not further delay débridement. When patients are at hospitals that do not have HBO available, surgical management should take precedence and transfer to an HBO center can be done postoperatively after the patient is stabilized if it is clinically indicated.

Gas gangrene

Gas gangrene is a rapidly progressive, invasive clostridial infection of previously healthy muscle tissue. It is also known as clostridial myonecrosis. It produces massive local tissue destruction along with severe systemic symptoms. It is a relatively rare disease with 1000 to 3000 cases per year in the United States [27].

Gas gangrene is caused by various species of *Clostridium*. These are Gram-positive, spore-forming, anaerobic rods normally found in soil and the human and animal gastrointestinal tract. The most common species implicated in gas gangrene is *Clostridium perfringens* (80%–90%) [28]. This organism is the causative agent in traumatic and postsurgical cases. Direct inoculation of a traumatic wound with *C perfringens* in a hypoxic wound environment with a compromised blood supply is the perfect milieu for growth. Many traumatic wounds are contaminated with *Clostridium* spores, but only a small percentage actually develop gas gangrene. It seems that both inoculation with the organism and a relatively hypoxic tissue environment are necessary for the clinical disease process to develop. Although it is an anaerobe, *C perfringens* can grow in a restricted fashion in oxygen tensions up to 70 mm Hg.

Clostridium septicum, which is more aerotolerant, is most commonly implicated in cases of spontaneous gas gangrene [28]. This infection usually occurs when bacteria enter from the gut by way of breaks in the gastric mucosa in patients who have colon cancer. Hematogenous spread causes infection in muscle tissue. Other *Clostridia* species make up a minority of cases and include *bifermentans*, *fallax*, *histolyticum*, and a few others.

The clinical syndrome of infection with *C perfringens* begins with pain at the infection site that seems out of proportion to the size of the wounded area. Local tissue destruction results in bleb and bullae formation. Rapid extension of the wound almost seems to happen in real time, at rates up to 15 cm/h [29]. When present, gas can sometimes be seen on radiographs and felt in the tissue as crepitus [28]. In at least 50% of cases, however, gas is not demonstrable, either on radiographs or clinically. Owing to variability, the detection of gas should not be used to make or break the diagnosis of clostridial infection. A "sickly sweet" odor can be detected from the wound drainage. Systemic symptoms include a low-grade fever, disproportionate tachycardia (140–160), and cognitive symptoms ranging from a flat affect to severe anxiety. Hypotension is a late finding and heralds impending circulatory collapse and death.

Clostridium spreads rapidly in the tissue not so much as a function of bacterial replication but rather by the elaboration of many exotoxins [30]. These various toxins break down connective tissue, lyse blood components, and cause necrosis of muscle tissue. Systemic effects are also seen, including shock, myocardial depression, capillary leaking, renal failure, and death. The most clinically important of the toxins seems to be alpha toxin. Alpha toxin is a phospholipase C that acts along with less important toxins to degrade cell membranes and produce a liquefactive necrosis. Further, it can promote local vasoconstriction and platelet aggregation leading to occlusion of small vessels. This process can help to create an environment of tissue hypoxia and contribute to the spread of the bacteria. Studies looking at *Clostridium* that contained a mutant, nonfunctional form of alpha toxin showed that the bacteria lost all virulence and did not produce the characteristic muscle necrosis and tissue destruction [31]. Reintroduction of the gene with a normal form of alpha toxin restored the bacteria's virulence and destructive properties. Finally, alpha toxin, acting with other toxins (primarily theta toxin) causes a powerful myocardial depressant effect.

Rationale and evidence for hyperbaric oxygen therapy

Alpha toxin is rapidly cleared from the body within 2 hours of production. For the bacteria to continue to spread, continuous elaboration of alpha toxin is required. At a tissue Po_2 of 250 mm Hg, alpha toxin production by *Clostridium* completely ceases [2]. This level of tissue oxygen is easily produced in hyperbaric conditions at 3 ATA. Because dead tissue cannot be salvaged and normal tissue is not yet affected, the target for therapy is to stop the alpha toxin in the infected but salvageable tissue in between. The faster this is accomplished, the more tissue can be spared; to borrow a concept from the world of heart attacks, "time is muscle." Unstable patients who may be too sick to go to the OR for formal débridement may be made stable enough hemodynamically to tolerate aggressive OR procedures immediately after the first HBO treatment. The authors of this chapter have observed this phenomenon in at least five patients in the last 5 years (Colin G. Kaide, MD, FACEP, FAAEM and Sorabh Khandelwal, MD, unpublished data, 2002–2007).

In addition to inhibiting the production of alpha toxin, HBO also has an anti-anaerobic organism effect and suppresses the growth of clostridia [32]. This effect has been shown in vitro and in vivo. Many subsequent basic science and animal studies clearly demonstrated inhibition of alpha toxin formation, inhibition of the growth of clostridia, and a potential bactericidal effect of HBO delivered at a pressure of 3 ATA [28].

Since the 1960s, HBO therapy has been used for the treatment of gas gangrene. Early animal study protocols showed that HBO alone was not sufficient to eradicate clostridial infections. When HBO was used in combination with antibiotics and aggressive debridement, mortality was significantly improved over surgery and antibiotics taken together or separately [33].

To date there have been no randomized controlled trials (RCTs) in humans to compare the addition of HBO to standard therapy for gas gangrene. Based on a review of results published through 1984, Peirce [34] concluded that HBO should be a standard addition to antibiotics and surgical débridement and further stated that an RCT to compare these modalities would be unethical. In 1977, Heimbach and colleagues [35] reported on the substantial decrease in mortality seen with the use of HBO in the cumulative series of more than 1200 patients from 117 reports in the world's literature. Bakker [36] added an additional 600 patients for which HBO demonstrated a clear reduction in mortality and morbidity when used in conjunction with surgery and antibiotic therapy. A review in the *New England Journal of Medicine* in 1996 concluded that despite the lack of RCTs the evidence supports HBO as an adjunctive therapy with the following benefits: improved demarcation of viable and dead tissue allowing for more judicious débridement, decreased amputation rate, and a substantial improvement in systemic symptoms [37].

Management with hyperbaric oxygen therapy

Unlike necrotizing fasciitis, HBO should be started before surgical débridement when possible, especially in unstable, systemically ill patients. Those who are too sick to tolerate formal operative procedures could have initial fasciotomies performed at the bedside, followed by immediate HBO treatment. Definitive operative management should then be performed with HBO interposed between débridements. Treatment should be continued until definitive improvement is seen. Transfer to an HBO facility is recommended when possible. The conditions of the patient, proximity to an HBO center, and the comfort level of the practitioners should be factored into the decision as to whether to transfer a patient immediately or to do so after initial operative management (Box 4).

Box 4. Hyperbaric oxygen treatment protocol for gas gangrene

Pressure: HBO treatments started at 3 ATA
Duration: 90 minutes
Frequency: Treatment is initially done three times in the first 24 hours then twice daily for the next 2–5 days.
Treatments: If the patient remains toxic, the treatment profile needs to be extended.
Use review: The continued use of HBO should be reviewed after 10 treatments.

Data from Feldmeier JJ, editor. Hyperbaric oxygen 2003: indications and results: the Hyperbaric Oxygen Therapy Committee Report. Kensington (MD): Undersea and Hyperbaric Medical Society; 2003.

Summary for gas gangrene

Despite the lack of an RCT comparing HBO to standard therapy, the sheer number of published results, which all are consistent in their findings, allow for the strong recommendation that HBO therapy be an integral part of the management of clostridial gas gangrene. Good evidence shows that HBO acts to halt alpha toxin production, substantially decreases the reproduction of clostridium, and augments the killing of the organism. Morbidity and mortality are decreased along with the extent of débridements and the number of limb amputations required.

Chronic refractory osteomyelitis

Osteomyelitis is an infectious process of the bone accompanied by inflammatory mediated bony destruction. Osteomyelitis can be further broken down into acute and chronic subtypes. Acute osteomyelitis develops over days or weeks, whereas chronic osteomyelitis is defined as a longstanding infection that evolves over months or even years. The chronic form is characterized by the persistence of microorganisms, low-grade inflammation, and the presence of necrotic bone and fistulous tracts [38]. Refractory osteomyelitis is a chronic osteomyelitis that persists or recurs after appropriate interventions have been performed. It is also termed refractory when an acute osteomyelitis does not respond to accepted management interventions, including antibiotics and surgery [39]. The functional definition most commonly applied to hyperbaric candidates includes failure to respond to a 4- to 6-week course of appropriate parenteral antibiotics [40].

Rationale and evidence for hyperbaric oxygen therapy

There are several mechanisms that may explain the effects of HBO in chronic refractory osteomyelitis. They all stem from the increase in oxygen tension that is produced during HBO treatments. Oxygen tension in infected bone is decreased. Breathing 100% oxygen in hyperbaric conditions can normalize and even produce supraphysiologic tissue oxygen tensions in infected bone [41,42].

When oxygen tensions fall below 30 to 40 mm Hg, leukocyte-mediated killing of aerobic Gram-positive and Gram-negative organisms is impaired [43]. Several animal models have demonstrated the benefit of HBO in animal models of chronic *S aureus* and *Pseudomonas aeruginosa* osteomyelitis [44]. By increasing tissue oxygen levels, HBO has also been also shown to have a direct suppressive effect on anaerobic organisms [45,46]. As described earlier, HBO augments the efficacy of several classes of antibiotics, such as aminoglycosides and cephalosporins. This effect may be because of enhancement of antibiotic transport across bacterial cell walls because transport is oxygen dependent and does not occur if oxygen tensions are less than 20 to 30 mm Hg [47]. HBO may also play a role in osteogenesis by promoting fibroblast activity, which allows for collagen synthesis necessary for healing [40], and by enhancing osteoclast activity. An increase in osteoclastic activity improves the overall quality of débridement and reduced the chances that local infection will recur [44]. Finally, in the acute phase, HBO combats factors that lower tissue oxygen tension by reducing tissue edema, decreasing elevated compartmental pressures, and limiting the effects of inflammation. In the long term, HBO promotes new collagen formation and angiogenesis. This neovascularization reduces the likelihood of recurrent infection and thus limits further bone destruction [44].

There are no controlled, prospective, randomized trials on the use of HBO in chronic refractory osteomyelitis. Although this type of trial is preferred, it would be difficult to accomplish, given the relative infrequency of the illness and the varied patient and disease characteristics.

Initial evidence for the use of HBO in chronic refractory osteomyelitis first appeared in a paper published in the Lancet in 1965 [48]. There have been numerous studies since then that have argued in favor of HBO. Morrey followed 40 patients for an average of 23 months after HBO for refractory cases of osteomyelitis and noted an 85% remission rate [49]. Davis and colleagues [50] similarly reported successful results with 38 patients demonstrating an 89% remission rate. Bingham and Hart [51] reported on their series of 70 patients treated with HBO and demonstrated improvement in all patients with 63% of them remaining disease free. Depenbusch [52] reported on 50 patients who had success rates around 70%. More recently there have been several additional articles that have reported the long-term success with HBO. Chen and colleagues [53] demonstrated an 86% remission rate in 15 patients who had an average follow-up period of 17.2 months. Aitasalo and colleagues [54] demonstrated a 79% remission rate in 33 patients who had a median follow-up period of 34 months. Maynor and colleagues [55] demonstrated resolution of wound drainage in 86% at a 24-month follow-up, 80% at 60 months, and 63% at 84 months. Only one retrospective study found no benefit with HBO [56]. After a closer review of the data, it seems that treatment failures were attributable to patients' noncompliance with surgery rather than whether the patient received HBO.

Management with hyperbaric oxygen therapy

The Cierney-Mader classification system of osteomyelitis is a useful way of characterizing which patients may benefit from HBO (Fig. 1) [57,58]. The Cierney-Mader classification system stages osteomyelitis by severity and incorporates systemic and local factors that may have an effect on immune surveillance, metabolism, and local vascularity. Using this classification, adjunctive HBO may be useful for the most difficult cases of refractory osteomyelitis, including those in stage 3 or 4, accompanied by the systemic and local factors mentioned previously [59]. Some have proposed including HBO on any patient who has recurrence of osteomyelitis after appropriate

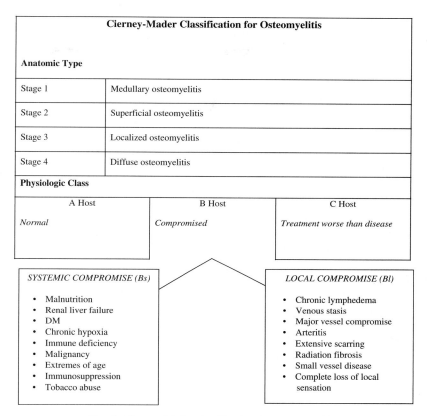

Fig. 1. Cierney-Mader classification for osteomyelitis.

surgical and medical management regardless of coexistent compromising factors (Box 5).

Summary for osteomyelitis

Successful treatment of chronic refractory osteomyelitis does not depend on HBO alone. It requires a multidisciplinary approach that includes aggressive débridement, good local wound care, and appropriate antibiotic use. It is also critical to maximize off-loading if the ulcer is located on a pressure point. Additional systemic factors that contribute to successful treatment include maximizing nutritional intake (especially protein) and controlling serum glucose levels.

The evidence supports the use of HBO in chronic refractory osteomyelitis given the ample animal data and in vitro experimental studies along with a large body of clinical experience. Because of the absence of RCTs, HBO receives a class-II evidence-based indication based on the AHA 1999 Guidelines [60].

Box 5. Hyperbaric oxygen treatment protocol for chronic refractory osteomyelitis

Pressure: HBO treatments at 2.0–2.5 ATA
Duration: 90–120 minutes
Frequency: Treatment is done once daily
Treatments: Treatments on average range from 15–40 per
    infectious episode
Use review: The continued use of HBO should be reviewed after
    40 treatments

    More frequent treatments or treatments greater than 3 ATA may actually hinder bone repair.
    Data from Feldmeier JJ, editor. Hyperbaric oxygen 2003: indications and results: the Hyperbaric Oxygen Therapy Committee Report. Kensington (MD): Undersea and Hyperbaric Medical Society; 2003.

The addition of HBO as an adjunctive therapy significantly increases the upfront cost of treatment. In complicated cases of refractory osteomyelitis, however, the long-term expenses associated with prolonged hospitalization, long courses of antimicrobial therapy, and additional surgery actually offset the differences, frequently making HBO cost effective.

Zygomycosis (mucormycosis) fungal disease

Mucormycosis is a term used to define infections caused by molds of the order Mucorales, under the class Zygomycetes. Zygomycosis is a term used to describe any invasive infection caused by the class Zygomycetes, which includes Mucorales and Entomophthorales. Although both orders are capable of causing significant disease, fungi belonging to the order Mucorales are angiotropic, cause tissue infarction, and are associated with disseminated and frequently fatal infections, especially when associated with various immunosuppressive conditions, such as poorly controlled diabetes mellitus, neutropenia, malignancies, transplants, burns, chronic renal failure, and the use of immunosuppressive and deferoxamine therapy [61,62]. Mucormycosis most commonly causes rhinocerebral syndromes. Less common presentations include pulmonary, cutaneous, gastrointestinal, and disseminated infections. Definitive diagnosis almost always requires histopathologic evidence of fungal invasion of tissue. Management traditionally has depended on timely diagnosis, aggressive surgical débridement, and rapid administration of antifungal therapy.

Rationale and evidence for hyperbaric oxygen therapy

Most of the clinical series of HBO use in fungal infections involve mucormycosis. The rationale for its use most likely lies in augmentation of the bactericidal action of the polymorphonuclear leukocytes [3,41,63]. Other potential mechanisms of action include enhancement of macrophage function and synergism with amphotericin B through the correction of lactic acidosis [64,65]. Additional contributing factors include fibroblast activation, neovascularization, and the increase in oxygen tension in infected tissues to normal or supraphysiologic levels [65].

Although there are no randomized clinical trials on the use of HBO in mucormycosis, the data coming from published reports/series are compelling. Price and Stevens [66] reported a successful outcome on a case of fulminant rhinocerebral mucormycosis using HBO after all other therapy failed. Ferguson and colleagues [67] retrospectively looked at 12 patients who had rhinocerebral mucormycosis and found that 4 of 6 not receiving HBO died and only 2 of 6 receiving HBO died, with one of these patients actually showing improvement in the disease process. Couch and colleagues [68] reported successful outcomes on two cases of rhinocerebral mucormycosis with brain tumor abscesses not responding to standard care. Survival with a diagnosis of bilateral cerebro-rhino-orbital mucormycosis is uncommon with surgical and medical management alone. De La Paz and colleagues [69], however, reported a successful outcome in a case of a 66-year-old man who had this disease using adjunctive HBO. Yohai and colleagues [70] reviewed 145 patients (139 from the literature and 6 from his own institution) looking at survival factors. They found a favorable effect of HBO on the prognosis of mucormycosis. More recently, Segal and colleagues [71] looked at 14 patients who had invasive fungal infections by Mucorales or *Aspergillus* spp over a 12-year period. These cases showed a 50% survival with a treatment regimen consisting of surgery, antibiotics, and HBO. Simmons and colleagues [72] report a case of a an 8-year-old girl who had type 1 diabetes who survived rhinocerebral mucormycosis complicated by internal carotid artery and cavernous sinus thromboses using HBO as part of her treatment regimen. John and colleagues [62] reviewed 28 cases, many of which are mentioned above, in which zygomycosis was treated with HBO, and concluded that HBO is a promising treatment modality but does not make any firm conclusions given that most of the evidence is from case reports/series.

Management with hyperbaric oxygen therapy

Box 6 outlines the protocol for treating mucormycosis with hyperbaric oxygen therapy.

Summary for mucormycosis

Given that it is unlikely that any randomized study will be performed on this disease process, the clinical evidence strongly supports using HBO in the management of the highly fatal rhinocerebral mucormycosis.

Box 6. Hyperbaric oxygen treatment protocol for mucormycosis

Pressure: HBO treatments at 2.0–2.5 ATA
Duration: 90–120 minutes
Frequency: Treatment is done one to two times daily
Treatments: Treatments should continue to a minimum of 40
   with up to 80 having been used in previous reports

Data from Feldmeier JJ, editor. Hyperbaric oxygen 2003: indications and results: the Hyperbaric Oxygen Therapy Committee Report. Kensington (MD): Undersea and Hyperbaric Medical Society; 2003.

Diabetic foot ulcerations

Although diabetes affects only 3% of the population, foot ulcers in patients who have diabetes contribute to more than half of all lower extremity amputations performed in the United States [73]. Diabetic foot ulcers occur in 1.9% of adults annually [74] resulting in amputation rates of 15% to 20% within 5 years [75]. The physiology behind ulcer development in the diabetic foot has been reviewed extensively and is beyond the scope of this reading [76]. Universally accepted care for diabetic foot ulcers includes (a) optimized nutritional support and glycemic control; (b) appropriate off-loading; (c) débridement of nonviable tissue; (d) provision of a moist, clean environment for support of granulation tissue and epithelialization; (e) surgical remedy of vascular insufficiency; and (f) infection control [77–79]. Infection, overcolonization, and osteomyelitis are frequent complications in diabetic foot ulcers.

Rationale and evidence for hyperbaric oxygen therapy

The rationale for HBO therapy in diabetic foot ulcerations is multifactorial [80–82]. Effects stem primarily from optimization of the oxygen concentration and the oxygen gradient from wound edge to the hypoxic center, which stimulates neovascularization and fibroblast replication with subsequent collagen deposition. Phagocyte activity and leukocyte-mediated killing are enhanced. Finally, under hyperbaric conditions there is an upregulation of vascular endothelial growth factor and platelet-derived growth factor.

There is much debate about whether HBO is effective as an adjunct in the treatment of diabetic foot ulceration [83,84]. Evidenced-based guidelines (Infectious Disease Society of America, US Public Health Service grade B-I) favor the use of HBO in ulcers not responsive to conventional therapy and surgery [79]. A systematic review undertaken by Roeckl-Wiedman and colleagues [85] also found that HBO therapy confers a significant reduction in the risk for major amputation with an number needed to treat of 4. Although there was a trend toward greater ulcer healing, there was no statistically significant difference in wound area reduction or need for minor amputation.

In 2001 Centers for Medicare & Medicaid Services (CMS), after reviewing a technology assessment report by the New England Medical Center and other reviews, made a positive determination on the use of HBO therapy in diabetic foot ulcers.

Management with hyperbaric oxygen therapy

Box 7 shows the treatment protocol for diabetic foot ulcers. The CMS criteria [86] for the use of HBO in diabetic foot ulcers are:

Patient has type 1 or 2 diabetes and has a lower extremity wound that is attributable to diabetes

Patient has a wound classified as Wagner grade III or higher (Table 2) [87,88].

Patient has failed an adequate course of standard wound therapy (defined as 30 days of standard treatment, including assessment and correction of vascular abnormalities, optimization of nutritional status, and glucose control, débridement, moist wound healing, off-loading, and infection control).

Summary for diabetic foot ulcers

The UHMS Hyperbaric Oxygen Therapy Committee report summarizes individual studies in this area and concludes that HBO for diabetic foot ulcers meets the requirements for AHA class I (definitely recommend) based on level I evidence [1]. The use of HBO not only leads to more expeditious wound healing but it also results in a decrease in the rate of major amputations.

Intracranial abscess

Intracranial abscess (ICA) encompasses cerebral abscess, subdural empyema, and epidural empyema. Although many factors, such as early and

---

Box 7. Hyperbaric oxygen treatment protocol for diabetic foot ulcers

Pressure: HBO treatments at 2.0–2.5 ATA
Duration: 90–120 minutes
Frequency: Treatment is done one to two times daily
Treatments: Use review is required each 30 days of treatment.

Data from Feldmeier JJ, editor. Hyperbaric oxygen 2003: indications and results: the Hyperbaric Oxygen Therapy Committee Report. Kensington (MD): Undersea and Hyperbaric Medical Society; 2003.

Table 2
Wagner grading system for diabetic foot ulcers

Grade	Clinical description
0	Intact skin
1	Superficial without penetration into deeper layers
2	Deeper, reaching tendon, bone, or joint capsule
3	Deeper, with abscess, osteomyelitis, or tendonitis extending to those structures
4	Gangrene of some portion of the toe or forefoot
5	Gangrene involving the entire foot or enough of the foot that local procedures are not an option

Data from Feldmeier JJ, editor. Hyperbaric oxygen 2003: indications and results: the Hyperbaric Oxygen Therapy Committee Report. Kensington (MD): Undersea and Hyperbaric Medical Society; 2003; with permission.

more accurate diagnosis, better surgical techniques, and more accurate antibiotic coverage, have led to decreases in mortality over time, ICA continues to show mortality rates of around 20% [89].

Rationale and evidence for hyperbaric oxygen therapy

The rationale for using HBO in ICA includes inhibition of anaerobic organisms that make up the flora [45,46], reduction in perifocal brain edema [90–92], and enhancement of leukocyte-mediated killing of bacteria [43]. Additional benefit is seen in cases with concomitant skull osteomyelitis, which is frequently present in cases of rhinogenic and otogenic intracranial abscesses [93].

Randomized studies of this disease are unlikely and treatment recommendations for HBO are based on case reports and case series. These are infrequent in the literature. Lampl and Frey [93] summarized data available through 1998 (publications, conference proceedings, and unpublished sources) and found a total of 48 patients treated with HBO incurring a 2% mortality. Two recent articles addressing adjunctive HBO for intracranial abscess were also positive. Kutlay and colleagues [94] reported on their experiences from 1999 to 2004 on 13 patients who had bacterial brain abscesses treated with stereotactic aspiration combined with HBO and antibiotics. They found that adjunctive HBO can reduce the need for reoperations, duration of antibiotic therapy, and overall costs. Kurschel and colleagues [95] reported on the successful use of adjunct HBO therapy in five children treated between 1995 and 2002, stating that adjunct HBO can result in reduction in the duration of antibiotic use, directly affecting the length of hospitalization.

Management with hyperbaric oxygen therapy

Although some patients who have ICA may do well with a more conservative therapeutic approach, there are certain conditions and complications that warrant a more aggressive strategy (Box 8). Adjunctive HBO therapy should be considered if any of the following are present [89]:

Multiple abscesses
Abscesses in a deep or dominant location
A compromised host
Situations in which surgery is contraindicated
Inadequate or no response to standard surgical and antibiotic treatment

Summary for intracranial abscess

Admittedly, the limited number of patients who have ICA treated with HBO makes it difficult to draw any definitive conclusions, but the low mortality seen thus far is encouraging and strongly supports the consideration of adjunct HBO therapy in this group of illnesses.

Malignant otitis externa

Malignant otitis externa (MOE) is an uncommon but potentially life-threatening infection in immunocompromised patients and elderly people who have diabetes. *P aeruginosa* is the causative organism in 98% of cases and the remaining 2% are caused by *S aureus, Proteus mirabilis, Klebsiella oxytoca, Pseudomonas cepacia, Staphylococcus epidermidis*, and rarely *Aspergillus fumigatus* [64]. Complications of MOE include osteomyelitis of the base of the skull, involvement of the temporomandibular joint, cranial nerve palsies, and central nervous system complications, which are the most common cause of death. These complications include meningitis, intracranial abscess, and cerebral venous sinus thrombosis. Management

---

Box 8. Hyperbaric oxygen treatment protocol for intracranial abscess

Pressure: HBO treatments started at 2.0–2.5 ATA
Duration: 60–90 minutes
Frequency: Daily or twice daily depending on clinical condition
Treatments: The total number of treatments is variable, depending on clinical response. In the largest series of patients who had ICA who were treated with HBO, the average number of treatments was 13.
Use review: The continued use of HBO should be reviewed after 20 treatments.

Data from Feldmeier JJ, editor. Hyperbaric oxygen 2003: indications and results: the Hyperbaric Oxygen Therapy Committee Report. Kensington (MD): Undersea and Hyperbaric Medical Society; 2003.

traditionally has relied on aggressive use of antibiotics and surgical débridement if possible. HBO should be considered in recurrent cases and in patients who have advanced MOE in whom the disease process seems refractory to antibiotics [44]. Rationale for its use stems from its effectiveness in normalizing oxygen tension in infected tissue. This process is necessary for leukocyte-mediated killing of bacteria, neovascularization, and augmentation of osteoclastic and osteoblastic activity. Davis and colleagues [96] reported on 17 patients who had MOE who received adjunctive treatment with HBO. All 17 patients responded well to HBO, as defined by 90% or greater return of cranial nerve function and an infection-free interval of 1 year. More importantly, 9 patients who had advanced disease failing antibiotics and surgery responded to HBO. Narozny and colleagues [97] reported on their experiences using adjunctive HBO for MOE and believed that it was a valuable and beneficial modality. Similar to chronic refractory osteomyelitis, HBO treatments should be performed at 2 to 2.5 ATA for 90 to 120 minutes per treatment.

Contraindications to and side effects of hyperbaric oxygen therapy

There are only two absolute contraindications to HBO treatment. Untreated pneumothorax presents a problem in that transfer or diffusion of additional oxygen into the space outside of the lung subsequently expands on a decrease in the pressure as the patient returns to the normobaric state, with the potential to cause tension physiology. The concurrent use of cisplatin and HBO can delay wound healing. Concurrent use of bleomycin or a history of bleomycin use at any time in the past along with HBO has been associated with significant lung injury from interstitial pneumonitis. HBO seems to enhance the cardiac toxicity of doxorubicin and is contraindicated until well after the doxorubicin is stopped.

Relative contraindications and their potential problems are listed in Table 3. Side effects of HBO include middle ear and sinus barotrauma,

Table 3
Relative contraindications to hyperbaric oxygen therapy

Upper respiratory infections Chronic sinusitis Stapes implant	These problems contribute to difficulty equalizing the pressure in the middle ear
Chronic obstructive pulmonary disease with CO_2 retention	Theoretically, high levels of oxygen may interfere with hypoxic drive in CO_2
Seizure disorder High fever	High levels of oxygen can cause oxygen toxicity seizures in approximately 1 in 4000 patients. Fever slightly increases the risk for seizure[a]
History of thoracic surgery History of spontaneous pneumothorax Pulmonary lesions on chest radiograph	Increases the risk for pneumothorax

[a] Seizures are usually self-limited and of little clinical consequence.

claustrophobia, oxygen-induced seizure, tension pneumothorax, maturation of existing cataracts, and progressive myopia that resolves within a few weeks after treatments stop.

Summary

HBO is clearly not a panacea. It has some specific, generally accepted applications in infectious diseases that are often additive or adjunctive to regular medical therapy. Admittedly, there is a paucity of RCTs for HBO. With the low incidence of the diseases discussed above, however, the randomization of patients would be difficult. In our opinion, withholding HBO because of the lack of randomized trials in the face of a huge body of clinical experience and in vitro studies, especially in these devastating disease processes, would be bordering on unethical.

References

[1] Feldmeier JJ, editor. Hyperbaric oxygen 2003: indications and results: the Hyperbaric Oxygen Therapy Committee Report. Kensington (MD): Undersea and Hyperbaric Medical Society; 2003. p. 2.
[2] VanUnnik A. Inhibition of toxin production in Clostridium perfringens in vitro by hyperbaric oxygen. Antonie Leeuwenhoek Microbiology 1965;31:181–6.
[3] Hohn D, et al. Effect of oxygen tension on microbicidal function of leukocytes in wounds and in vitro. Surg Forum 1976;27:18–20.
[4] Hunt T, et al. The effect of differing ambient oxygen tensions on wound infection. Ann Surg 1975;181:35–9.
[5] Babior B. Oxygen-dependent microbial killing by phagocytes. N Engl J Med 1978;298: 659–68.
[6] Jonsson K, Hunt TK. Oxygen as an isolated variable influences resistance to infection. Ann Surg 1988;208(6):783–7.
[7] Knighton D, Halliday B, Hunt TH. Oxygen as an antibiotic: a comparison of inspired oxygen concentration and antibiotic administration on in vivo bacterial clearance. Arch Surg 1986;121:191–5.
[8] Park M, et al. Hyperoxia prolongs the aminoglycoside-induced post antibiotic effect in Pseudomonas aeruginosa. Antimicrob Agents Chemother 1991;35:691–5.
[9] Gottlieb SF, et al. Synergistic action of increased oxygen tensions and PABA-folic acid antagonists on bacterial growth. Aerosp Med 1974;45(8):829–33.
[10] Norden CW, Shaffer M. Treatment of experimental chronic osteomyelitis due to staphylococcus aureus with vancomycin and rifampin. J Infect Dis 1983;147(2):352–7.
[11] Smith J, Lewin C. Chemistry and mechanisms of action of the quinolone antibacterials. In: Andriole V, editor. The quinolones. New York: Acad Press; 1988. p. 23–82.
[12] Kivisaari J, Niinikoski J. Effects of hyperbaric oxygenation and prolonged hypoxia on the healing of open wounds. Acta Chir Scand 1975;141:14–9.
[13] Mandell GL, et al. Mandell, Douglas, and Bennett's principles and practice of infectious diseases. New York: Churchill-Livingston; 2005.
[14] Jallali WS, Butler PE. Hyperbaric oxygen as adjuvant therapy in the management of necrotizing fasciitis. Am J Surg 2005;189(4):462–6.
[15] Levine EG, Manders SM. Life-threatening necrotizing fasciitis. Clin Dermatol 2005;23(2): 144–7.

[16] Brook I, Frazier E. Clinical and microbiological features of necrotizing fasciitis. J Clin Microbiol 1995;33(9):2382–7.
[17] Hasham S, et al. Necrotising fasciitis. BMJ 2005;330(7495):830–3.
[18] Miller LG, et al. Necrotizing fasciitis caused by community-associated methicillin-resistant Staphylococcus aureus in Los Angeles. N Engl J Med 2005;352(14):1445–53.
[19] Childers BJ, et al. Necrotizing fasciitis: a fourteen-year retrospective study of 163 consecutive patients. Am Surg 2002;68(2):109–16.
[20] McHenry CR, et al. Idiopathic necrotizing fasciitis: recognition, incidence, and outcome of therapy. Am Surg 1994;60(7):490–4.
[21] Bakker D. Selected aerobic and anaerobic soft tissue infections. In: Kindwall E, Whelan H, editors. Hyperbaric medicine practice. Flagstaff (AZ): Best Pub. Co.; 2004. p. 575–601.
[22] Jallali N. Necrotising fasciitis: its aetiology, diagnosis and management. J Wound Care 2003;12:297–300.
[23] Escobar SJ, et al. Adjuvant hyperbaric oxygen therapy (HBO2) for treatment of necrotizing fasciitis reduces mortality and amputation rate. Undersea Hyperb Med 2005;32(6):437–43.
[24] Mader J. Mixed anaerobic and aerobic soft tissue infections. In: Davis J, Hunt T, editors. Problem wounds: the role of oxygen. New York: Elsevier; 1988. p. 153–72.
[25] Riseman JA, et al. Hyperbaric oxygen therapy for necrotizing fasciitis reduces mortality and the need for débridements. Surgery 1990;108(5):847–50.
[26] Tehrani M, Ledingham M. Necrotising fasciitis. Postgrad Med J 1977;53:237–42.
[27] Hart G, Lamb R, Strauss M. Gas gangrene. J Trauma 1983;23(11):991–1000.
[28] Heimbach R. Gas gangrene. In: Kindwall E, Whelan H, editors. Hyperbaric medicine practice. Flagstaff (AZ): Best Pub. Co.; 2004. p. 549–65.
[29] Bakker D. Clostridial myonecrosis (gas gangrene). In: Feldmeier J, editor. Hyperbaric Oxygen Therapy Committee Report 2003. Dunkirk (France): Undersea and Hyperbaric Medical Society; 2003. p. 19–25.
[30] Titball RW. Gas gangrene: an open and closed case. Microbiology 2005;151(Pt 9):2821–8.
[31] Awad MM, et al. Virulence studies on chromosomal alpha-toxin and theta-toxin mutants constructed by allelic exchange provide genetic evidence for the essential role of alpha-toxin in Clostridium perfringens-mediated gas gangrene. Mol Microbiol 1995;15(2):191–202.
[32] Demello F, et al. The effects of hyperbaric oxygen on the germination and toxin production of Clostridium perfringens spores. In: Proceedings of the fourth international congress on hyperbaric medicine. Baltimore (MD): Williams & Wilkins.
[33] Demello FJ, Haglin JJ, Hitchcock CR. Comparative study of experimental Clostridium perfringens infection in dogs treated with antibiotics, surgery, and hyperbaric oxygen. Surgery 1973;73(6):936–41.
[34] Peirce EI. Gas gangrene: a critique of therapy. Surg Rounds 1984;7:17–25.
[35] Heimbach R, et al. Current therapy of gas gangrene. In: Davis J, Hunt T, editors. Hyperbaric oxygen therapy. Bethesda (MD): Undersea Medical Society, Inc; 1977. p. 153.
[36] Bakker D. Clostridial myonecrosis. In: Bakker D, Cramer F, editors. Hyperbaric surgery. Flagstaff (AZ): Best Publ.; 2002. p. 283–316.
[37] Tibbles PM, Edelsberg JS. Hyperbaric-oxygen therapy. N Engl J Med 1996;334(25):1642–8.
[38] Lew DP, Waldvogel FA. Osteomyelitis. Lancet 2004;364(9431):369–79.
[39] Strauss M. Chronic refractory osteomyelitis: review and role of hyperbaric oxygen. Hyperbaric Oxygen Review 1980;1:231–56.
[40] Mader JT, et al. Antimicrobial treatment of chronic osteomyelitis. Clin Orthop Relat Res 1999;360:47–65.
[41] Mader JT, et al. A mechanism for the amelioration by hyperbaric oxygen of experimental staphylococcal osteomyelitis in rabbits. J Infect Dis 1980;142(6):915–22.
[42] Niinikoski J, Hunt TK. Oxygen tensions in healing bone. Surg Gynecol Obstet 1972;134(5):746–50.

[43] Hohn D. Oxygen and leukocyte microbial killing. In: Davis J, Hunt T, editors. Hyperbaric oxygen therapy. Bethesda (MD): Undersea and Hyperbaric Medical Society; 1977. p. 101–10.

[44] Hart BB. Refractory osteomyelitis. In: Feldmeier JJ, editor. Hyperbaric oxygen 2003: indications and results: the Hyperbaric Oxygen Therapy Committee Report. Kensington (MD): Undersea and Hyperbaric Medical Society; 2003. p. 79–85.

[45] Slack WK. Hyperbaric oxygen therapy in anaerobic infections. Med Times 1978;106(10): 15d(82)–16d(82), 21d(82).

[46] Park MK, Myers RA, Marzella L. Oxygen tensions and infections: modulation of microbial growth, activity of antimicrobial agents, and immunologic responses. Clin Infect Dis 1992; 14(3):720–40.

[47] Verklin RM Jr, Mandell GL. Alteration of effectiveness of antibiotics by anaerobiosis. J Lab Clin Med 1977;89(1):65–71.

[48] Slack WK, Thomas DA, Perrins D. Hyperbaric oxygenation chronic osteomyelitis. Lancet 1965;1:1093–4.

[49] Morrey BF, et al. Hyperbaric oxygen and chronic osteomyelitis. Clin Orthop Relat Res 1979;(144):121–7.

[50] Davis JC, et al. Chronic non-hematogenous osteomyelitis treated with adjuvant hyperbaric oxygen. J Bone Joint Surg Am 1986;68(8):1210–7.

[51] Bingham EL, Hart GB. Hyperbaric oxygen treatment of refractory osteomyelitis. Postgrad Med 1977;61(6):70–6.

[52] Depenbusch FL, Thompson RE, Hart GB. Use of hyperbaric oxygen in the treatment of refractory osteomyelitis: a preliminary report. J Trauma 1972;12(9):807–12.

[53] Chen CY, et al. Chronic refractory tibia osteomyelitis treated with adjuvant hyperbaric oxygen: a preliminary report. Changgeng Yi Xue Za Zhi 1998;21(2):165–71.

[54] Aitasalo K, et al. A modified protocol to treat early osteoradionecrosis of the mandible. Undersea Hyperb Med 1995;22(2):161–70.

[55] Maynor ML, et al. Chronic osteomyelitis of the tibia: treatment with hyperbaric oxygen and autogenous microsurgical muscle transplantation. J South Orthop Assoc 1998;7(1): 43–57.

[56] Esterhai JL Jr, et al. Adjunctive hyperbaric oxygen therapy in the treatment of chronic refractory osteomyelitis. J Trauma 1987;27(7):763–8.

[57] Cierny G, Mader J, Pennick J. A clinical staging system for adult osteomyelitis. Contemp Orthop 1985;10:17–37.

[58] Mader J, Davis J. General concept of osteomyelitis. In: Mandell G, Bennet J, Dolin R, editors. Principles and practice of infectious disease. New York: Churchill Livingston; 1995.

[59] Strauss MB, Bryant B. Hyperbaric oxygen. Orthopedics 2002;25(3):303–10.

[60] Strauss M. The role of hyperbaric oxygen in the surgical management of chronic refractory osteomyelitis. In: Bakker DJ, Cramer FS, editors. Hyperbaric surgery. Flagstaff (AZ): Best Publishing; 2002. p. 59.

[61] Kontoyiannis DP, Lewis RE. Invasive zygomycosis: update on pathogenesis, clinical manifestations, and management. Infect Dis Clin North Am 2006;20(3):581–607, vi.

[62] John BV, Chamilos G, Kontoyiannis DP. Hyperbaric oxygen as an adjunctive treatment for zygomycosis. Clin Microbiol Infect 2005;11(7):515–7.

[63] Mandell GL. Bactericidal activity of aerobic and anaerobic polymorphonuclear neutrophils. Infect Immun 1974;9(2):337–41.

[64] Gupta S, et al. Infections in diabetes mellitus and hyperglycemia. Infect Dis Clin North Am 2007;21(3):617–38, vii.

[65] Farmer J, Kindwall E. Use of adjunctive hyperbaric oxygen in the management of fungal disease. In: Feldmeier J, editor. Hyperbaric oxygen 2003: indications and results: the Hyperbaric Oxygen Therapy Committee Report. Dunkirk (France): Undersea and Hyperbaric Medical Society; 2004. p. 656–61.

[66] Price JC, Stevens DL. Hyperbaric oxygen in the treatment of rhinocerebral mucormycosis. Laryngoscope 1980;90(5 Pt 1):737–47.

[67] Ferguson BJ, et al. Adjunctive hyperbaric oxygen for treatment of rhinocerebral mucormycosis. Rev Infect Dis 1988;10(3):551–9.

[68] Couch L, Theilen F, Mader JT. Rhinocerebral mucormycosis with cerebral extension successfully treated with adjunctive hyperbaric oxygen therapy. Arch Otolaryngol Head Neck Surg 1988;114(7):791–4.

[69] De La Paz MA, et al. Adjunctive hyperbaric oxygen in the treatment of bilateral cerebro-rhino-orbital mucormycosis. Am J Ophthalmol 1992;114(2):208–11.

[70] Yohai RA, et al. Survival factors in rhino-orbital-cerebral mucormycosis. Surv Ophthalmol 1994;39(1):3–22.

[71] Segal E, Menhusen MJ, Shawn S. Hyperbaric oxygen in the treatment of invasive fungal infections: a single-center experience. Isr Med Assoc J 2007;9(5):355–7.

[72] Simmons JH, et al. Rhinocerebral mucormycosis complicated by internal carotid artery thrombosis in a pediatric patient with type 1 diabetes mellitus: a case report and review of the literature. Pediatr Diabetes 2005;6(4):234–8.

[73] Reiber GE, Smith DG. Lower extremity foot ulcers and amputations in diabetes. In: National Diabetes Data Group, National Institutes of Health, National Institute of Diabetes and Digestive and Kidney Diseases, editors. Diabetes in America. p. 409–28.

[74] Ramsey SD, et al. Incidence, outcomes, and cost of foot ulcers in patients with diabetes. Diabetes Care 1999;22(3):382–7.

[75] Moulik PK, Mtonga R, Gill GV. Amputation and mortality in new-onset diabetic foot ulcers stratified by etiology. Diabetes Care 2003;26(2):491–4.

[76] Falanga V. Wound healing and its impairment in the diabetic foot. Lancet 2005;366(9498): 1736–43.

[77] Consensus Development Conference on Diabetic Foot Wound Care: 7–8 April 1999, Boston, Massachusetts. American Diabetes Association. Diabetes Care 1999;22(8):1354–60.

[78] O'Meara S, et al. Systematic reviews of wound care management: (3) antimicrobial agents for chronic wounds; (4) diabetic foot ulceration. Health Technol Assess 2000;4(21):1–237.

[79] Lipsky BA, et al. Diagnosis and treatment of diabetic foot infections. Clin Infect Dis 2004; 39(7):885–910.

[80] Hunt TK, Pai MP. The effect of varying ambient oxygen tensions on wound metabolism and collagen synthesis. Surg Gynecol Obstet 1972;135(4):561–7.

[81] Knighton DR, Silver IA, Hunt TK. Regulation of wound-healing angiogenesis-effect of oxygen gradients and inspired oxygen concentration. Surgery 1981;90(2):262–70.

[82] Zhao LL, et al. Effect of hyperbaric oxygen and growth factors on rabbit ear ischemic ulcers. Arch Surg 1994;129(10):1043–9.

[83] Berendt AR. Counterpoint: hyperbaric oxygen for diabetic foot wounds is not effective. Clin Infect Dis 2006;43(2):193–8.

[84] Barnes RC. Point: hyperbaric oxygen is beneficial for diabetic foot wounds. Clin Infect Dis 2006;43(2):188–92.

[85] Roeckl-Wiedmann I, Bennett M, Kranke P. Systematic review of hyperbaric oxygen in the management of chronic wounds. Br J Surg 2005;92(1):24–32.

[86] Shuren J, et al. Coverage decision memorandum for hyperbaric oxygen therapy in the treatment of hypoxic wounds and diabetic wounds of the lower extremities. 2002.

[87] Wagner FW Jr. The dysvascular foot: a system for diagnosis and treatment. Foot Ankle 1981;2(2):64–122.

[88] Smith RG. Validation of Wagner's classification: a literature review. Ostomy Wound Manage 2003;49(1):54–62.

[89] Feldmeier JJ. chairman and editor. Chapter reviewed by Irving JacobyIntracranial abscess. In: Feldmeier JJ, editor. Hyperbaric oxygen 2003: indications and results: the Hyperbaric Oxygen Therapy Committee Report. Kensington (MD): Undersea and Hyperbaric Medical Society; 2003. p. 63–5, 63–7.

[90] Mogami H, et al. Clinical application of hyperbaric oxygenation in the treatment of acute cerebral damage. J Neurosurg 1969;31(6):636–43.

[91] Moody RA, et al. Therapeutic value of oxygen at normal and hyperbaric pressure in experimental head injury. J Neurosurg 1970;32(1):51–4.

[92] Pierce ECI, Jacobson JH II. Cerebral edema. In: Davis JC, Hunt TK, editors. Hyperbaric oxygen therapy. Bethesda (MD): Undersea Medical Society; 1977. p. 287–301.

[93] Lampl L, Frey G. Hyperbaric oxygen in intracranial abscess. In: Kindwall E, Whelan H, editors. Hyperbaric medicine practice. Flagstaff (AZ): Best Publishing Company; 2004. p. 645–54.

[94] Kutlay M, et al. Stereotactic aspiration and antibiotic treatment combined with hyperbaric oxygen therapy in the management of bacterial brain abscesses. Neurosurgery 2005;57(6): 1140–6 [discussion: 1140–6].

[95] Kurschel S, et al. Hyperbaric oxygen therapy for the treatment of brain abscess in children. Childs Nerv Syst 2006;22(1):38–42.

[96] Davis JC, et al. Adjuvant hyperbaric oxygen in malignant external otitis. Arch Otolaryngol Head Neck Surg 1992;118(1):89–93.

[97] Narozny W, et al. Value of hyperbaric oxygen in bacterial and fungal malignant external otitis treatment. Eur Arch Otorhinolaryngol 2006;263(7):680–4.

[98] Eltorai IM, Hart GB, Strauss MB, et al. The role of hyperbaric oxygen in the management of Fournier's gangrene. Int Surg 1986;71:53.

[99] Gozal D, Ziser A, et al. Necrotizing fasciitis. Archives of Surgery 1986;121(2):233–5.

[100] Brown DR, Davis NL, et al. A multicenter review of the treatment of major truncal necrotizing infections with and without hyperbaric oxygen therapy. Am J Surg 1994;167:485–9.

[101] Shupak A, Shoshani O, et al. Necrotizing fasciitis: an indication for hyperbaric oxygen therapy? Surgery 1995;118(5):873–8.

[102] Korhonen K, Hirn M, Niinikoski J. Hyperbaric oxygen in the treatment of Fournier's gangrene. Eur J Surg 1998;164(4):251–5.

ELSEVIER
SAUNDERS

Emerg Med Clin N Am
26 (2008) 597–602

EMERGENCY
MEDICINE
CLINICS OF
NORTH AMERICA

Index

Note: Page numbers of article titles are in **boldface** type.

A

African sleeping sickness, 512–513

African tick bite fever, 504–505

AIDS, description of, 368

AIDS-defining illnesses, 368

Anthrax, 518–524
    clinical manifestations of, 520
    cutaneous, 520–521
    diagnosis of, 522
    gastrointestinal, 521
    inhalational, 521
    public health measures in, 523–524
    treatment of, 522–523

Antibiotic susceptibility, and
    community-associated
    methicillin-resistant *S. aureus*,
    434–435

Antibiotic therapy, delays in, in emergency
    department, 252–253
    for acute severe infections, timing
        of, **245–257**
    in bacterial meningitis, 249–250,
        261, 262–263
    in foodborne illnesses, 478, 488
    in meningitis, 303–305
    in pneumonia, 251–252, 390–392
    in septic shock, 251
    in urinary tract infection in elderly,
        333
    timing of, in pneumonia,
        253–254

Antimicrobial therapy, in pneumonia, 391,
    399–400

Antiviral therapy, and chemoprophylaxis,
    against influenza, 560–561
    in HIV infection, 380–381

Arachnoiditis. See *Meningitis.*

Avian flu, 273–275, 512

B

Bacillus anthracis, 518

Bacteremia, in elderly patients with
    infection, 321–324
        etiology of, 322, 323
        laboratory testing in, 323
        mortality associated with, 324
        sources of, 323–324
        symptoms of, 322

Bacterial meningitis, 259–263
    antibiotics in, 249–250

Bacteriuria, 425–426

Biological Weapons Convention, 517

Bioterrorism, category A agents of, 518
    infectious agents of, **517–547**

Bird flu, 273–275, 512

Blood, oxygen content of, determination of,
    573

Botulism, clinical manifestations of, 540
    diagnosis of, 541
    foodborne, 492–493
    treatment of, 541–542

Botulism toxin, epidemiology and
    transmission of, 539–540

C

Campylobacter jejuni, as cause of foodborne
    illness, 485–486

Cardiovascular complications, in HIV
    infection, 375

Central nervous system, anatomy of, 282
    rapidly fatal infections of, 259–266

Chest radiograph, automated, in
    pneumonia, 391, 399–400

Children, complications in, in HIV
    infection, 379–380